THE INDEX CASE

By Molly Macallen

Book One of
the MADDY SHANKS *Mystery Series*

THE INDEX CASE ©2022 by Alice Domurat Dreger

First edition published 2022.

Second printing, October 2022.

Designed by Cait Palmiter.

ISBN 978-1-387-84645-0 (Hardcover)

ISBN 978-1-387-84642-9 (Paperback)

Author's note: This is an original work of fiction and any resemblance to real-life events or real-life persons (dead or living) is entirely coincidental with the exception of quotations taken from actual historical works as identified in the text and below.

Quotations in this book are taken from the following works:

"We'll Be Together Again" (1945), composed by Carl T. Fischer, with lyrics by Frankie Laine, performed by Johnny Hartman on the album *Songs from the Heart* (1956).

Ambroise Paré, *On Monsters and Marvels*, translated with an introduction and notes by Janis L. Pallister (Chicago: University of Chicago Press, 1982).

Isidore Geoffroy Saint-Hilaire, *Histoire Générale et Particulière des Anomalies de l'Organisation Chez l'Homme et les Animaux, ou Traité de Tératologie* (Paris: J.B. Baillière, 1832-1837); original translation.

M.F.K. Fisher, *How to Cook a Wolf* (New York: North Point Press of Farrar, Straus and Giroux, 1954).

THE INDEX CASE

By Molly Macallen

-1-

Being passed again among the Catholics was not what Madeleine Shanks had had in mind. She had gone through just that, about a decade before, at fifteen years of age. And once was enough.

She let out a sigh – a sigh so long it came back around and almost startled her. She finished taking off the sweatpants, cotton socks, and flannel shirt that Detective Wolf had lent her, folding them up and putting them on the wooden chair in the corner, near the bathroom's door.

She pulled the stiff plastic shower curtain out of the tub and tucked it to one side, plugged the tub drain, and turned the water on a little to make sure it would come out of the tub faucet and not the showerhead. Getting the confirmation she wanted, she turned the hot water on high to start filling the basin. Opening the zippered canvas sack in which she had brought her toiletries, from the kit she pulled the three votive candles and book of matches she had packed back in Indiana just in case this Philadelphia house turned out to have a bathtub.

This bath wasn't anything like what she had dared to hope. She sighed again. Maddy had fantasized that John Wolf's home would sport a crisp white porcelain slipper tub set against a third-floor casement window, with a perfect view of the roofs and treetops of the old city of Philadelphia. Some kind of steeple view – that was what she'd had in mind. Facing obliquely west, to see the sky turn from the sunset to the dark.

This was a rather standard, old, rectangular cast-iron beast, rusted in spots where the enamel had worn off, set into a soulless wall of washed-out baby-blue tile. While this bathtub had probably felt like a great triumph for whomever had hauled it up and installed it in this second-floor bathroom of this little old Philly row house decades before, to Maddy it felt a disappointment. The bathroom had but one crappy old electric fixture – two bulbs of different wattage, behind frosted glass, mounted over the sink. All in all, it was about what she had back at her tiny flat in Bloomington. And here, the bathroom barely had a window – just a small one that faced the back alley. The light for an evening bath was just plain lousy.

But then, she reminded herself, this was exactly why she had brought the candles – in case there was a tub that needed help. At least it had an edge a couple of inches wide, good for holding her simple plain-glass votive holders. The sloping ceiling over the tub caused by its being partly stuck under the steep stairs that ran from this second floor to the third – well, that gave the bath a bit of character, didn't it?

And at least the place was clean – and clean in the way that suggested it was the owner's habit, not the result of one-time hasty preparation for this boarder.

At least she would have a quiet bedroom to herself?

But then she had finally reached a point in her life where having her own bedroom no longer felt like a luxury – just a basic necessity.

"Your pajamas have dried," she heard Detective Wolf say through the bathroom door as stiffly as if he were the door itself. "I'll leave them just outside right here."

"Many thanks," Maddy answered.

After hearing him descend the stairs back down to the first floor, she opened the door a sliver, reached out, and pulled in her cotton pj's. They were toasty from the drier. She held them for a moment against her naked chest, warming herself, and then put them on the bathmat next to where she had laid a towel.

She lit the candles and spaced them out around the tub. Then she felt the water and adjusted the temperature coming out of the tap. Unlike most of the rooms in this house, she noticed, the bathroom was free of crucifixes. Adding candles here didn't make it feel too much like being in church. This bath need not be a baptism, even if she *were* about to be circulated around the Catholics again like a blessed little statue.

While the water ran, as quietly as she could she opened the medicine cabinet and then the drawers of the small wooden chest next to the sink. No evidence of his wife – no prescriptions in her name, nothing in the way of shampoos or make-up a woman would have. Even if she weren't very feminine in habits, there would be *something* to indicate a woman if she were still here. So, wherever she was, she wasn't here. And she wasn't expected back.

"Where is your wife?" she had asked him over those excellent potatoes he had made for her, dotted with bits of torn fresh herbs from the plants on his kitchen windowsill. Rosemary and thyme. What was the third herb? Marjoram?

"You know I'm married?" he had replied, picking one piece of browned potato off her plate and eating it.

He nodded to himself, pleased with the flavor.

"Wedding ring," Maddy answered, "and the photos along the stairs."

"Got it," he said. "You eat a lot for a skinny girl – I mean, for a skinny *woman*."

Maddy remembered now in the bathroom how that need for correction – "girl" to "woman" – had made him get up suddenly from the table, as if in embarrassment. He went to check the moisture in the dirt of the herb pots, adding a little water to each from a small tin watering can just as the thunder picked up its drumroll again. The deep blue night started to break with silver flashes.

"So, where is she – your wife?"

"I'd rather not go into where my wife is."

His reply suggested she was at least alive and still his wife.

Maddy waited until the tub was full enough to seem reasonable – not so shallow that getting in it would feel pointless, not so full that her host would think her a mooch – and then turned off the water and the overhead light. She slipped herself into the tub and tried to relax.

Taking three deep breaths, she placed her hands on her thighs, under the water. She made a conscious effort to think about sex: *The thought of Giovanni waking her up in the middle of the night the one time he let her sleep over, him softly stroking the silky pubic hair just above her mons veneris with his thumb, as if petting a sleeping kitten. His whisper tickling her ear...*

But it was hard to think about anything other than the sense of having found herself in the wrong house.

She probably should have waited at 30th Street Station until it was clear that the storm had passed. Then she wouldn't have been caught in a downpour just after crossing the river bridge to get here. Then she wouldn't have arrived at his door in such a needy state. Just before she had reached Detective Wolf's worn stone stoop, the downpour did suddenly let up. But by then, the quieting of the sky made no difference. She was, by the time she arrived at his place, soaked to the skin, her hair as wet as if she had just washed it.

Back in Indiana, she had packed a travel umbrella in her suitcase. But there had been no way she could pull it out on the sidewalk in the pouring rain, no less manage the umbrella with her rolling suitcase and backpack as she dashed from the Amtrak station to here. Unlike New York City, Philadelphia seemed to have practically no awnings, no scaffolding, nothing for shelter from the rain. So, she had just run for it.

She had been to Philadelphia once before, but not for very long. Not long enough to learn her way around. Before she had left Indiana, she had worked on memorizing the map of these streets between the station and his house, and she had again studied the plasticized travel map on the long train ride to ensure she wouldn't have to stop and find someone safe to ask directions. But it hadn't been so easy in the night rain to feel confident she was going the right way. (Her heart had been pounding from more than the run.) The train was supposed to have arrived in the late afternoon when there was still plenty of light. Good old Amtrak, late as every time she had used it. But cheaper than a flight, still.

He had opened the door and asked, "Can I help you?"

"Mr. Wolf, yes?"

"Yes," he said, though he seemed confused as to why she was handing him her suitcase.

"It's a good thing I wrapped my computer up for the possibility of rain," she said, stepping past him into his living room.

He closed the door and latched it. She took off her backpack and put it on the floor, quickly pulling out the sealed plastic bag that held her laptop. She undid the wrap and breathed a sigh of relief that the machine had stayed dry. She set it on his coffee table.

She shook her hair out like a wet dog, pulled out her hairbrush, and transferred a hairband wrapped around the brush handle to her wrist.

"I'm sorry, who are you?" John Wolf asked.

Bent over and combing out her hair from the roots to the ends, she answered: "Maddy Shanks." She stood up, shifted her hairbrush to her left hand, and reached out her right. He shook it as if they had just made a deal. She apologized that her hand was so wet as she tried pointlessly to dry it off on her pants.

"*Maddy* Shanks? But – but I thought the person coming was named Matthew Shanks – *Matty* Shanks."

"Oh, that's funny," she laughed briefly, combing her hair one more time, pulling it quickly into a ponytail, and fastening it with the hairband. "You thought I was going to be a man! My first name is Madeleine. I generally go by Maddy."

"You can't stay here," he replied.

She had laid her suitcase on the floor, bent over and opened it, and started pulling out the damp clothes. She laid shirts, pants, a dress and a skirt out around his furniture on pieces that she figured wouldn't be damaged by being a little wet.

"I don't suppose you have anything dry I could borrow to wear just now?" she asked. "I don't want to sit down on your furniture as wet as I am."

"I can go and find you something," he answered. "But you can't stay here. I mean, tonight you can. But not for the months you're here in Philadelphia."

"Why not?" she asked.

"Because you're a young woman. It wouldn't be right."

She had just hit the suitcase layer with the ten pair of underwear, the plain cotton ones and the fancier numbers, and wasn't sure what to do. *Oh well*, she thought, and pulled the stack out, holding it between her hands.

He cleared his throat.

"Let me show you your room," he said. "Do you want me to carry your suitcase?"

"I've got it," she answered, zipping it up and following him up the stairs.

She liked that he didn't just assume he should carry it for her.

He led her to a bedroom on the second floor at the front of the house, a room with a queen-size bed draped in an old-fashioned quilt, with a three-drawer dresser and a desk in the corner near the curtained window overlooking the narrow street. A night table between the bed and the door held a lamp and a small clock-radio. On the far end, a wall of closet space had obviously been added; a house this age would not have had any closets. The louvered closet doors were of the sad 1970s variety.

The feel of the small, ivory-painted room – monastic, outdated, weakly rehabilitated for modern life, with the crucifix over the bed – immediately invoked the convent.

What have I done? she thought.

But then she realized it wouldn't matter. As she had done in the convent when she was fifteen, she would just work on her studies until it was time to move on. And in this case, she knew where she was going next – right back to Bloomington to finish her Ph.D. This was just a stop on the way to finishing.

And here – well, here, unlike in the convent, she couldn't be required to bunk with others, and she wouldn't be required to pray. And the stay would not be nearly so long. So, it would be *fine*. She could take the crucifix down, as he would surely leave her room alone. (He didn't want to see her underwear, apparently.) There was enough room here to do her morning hand-stand, her morning routine. Yes, she could do what she needed to do here, including if she woke up in the middle of the night in terms of pleasantly putting herself back to sleep with some deep breathing and some carefully collected thoughts of Giovanni....

But if it's the case that none of this Catholicism matters to my life as it is now, she wondered momentarily, *why am I bothering to think so much about it?*

She realized she was standing there staring at John Wolf with what must have been a stupid look, half-noticing the prominence of his collarbones under his t-shirt. He would make a good mounted skeleton. His bone structure was quite handsome, his head nicely proportioned with his frame. He would make a satisfying dissection.

"I'll go find you some dry clothes," he said.

She laid her suitcase on the floor near the foot of the bed and opened it back up. She took out the underwear, her socks, and bras, and laid them around the room to dry. He appeared at the door with a stack of loaner clothes for her. She met him at the door, looking him in the face as best she could, given that he was a good eight inches taller than her five-foot-three.

"You can't lodge here," he said again, looking over her shoulder and seeing her things laid about the room.

"What exactly is the problem?" she asked. "Are you an ax murderer?"

"No!" he cried out. "I'm a police officer!"

"Well, if you are really a cop," she said, "then you know perfectly well that being a cop and being an ax murderer are not mutually exclusive."

"Fair enough," he answered. "But I think it wouldn't be good for...for either of our reputations...to have you here."

She had by then put the clothes he had given her on the bed and gone back to the suitcase to unpack more. She came now to the brown-paper wrapped parcel Giovanni had given her. It had managed in the center of the suitcase to stay dry. She hesitated for just a second and then opened it, finding a pretty, light-wool dress with a matching jacket, both the color of café au lait. She emitted a squeal as she held the slightly wrinkled dress up before her.

John Wolf must have found it odd to know she had in her bag clothes she had not seen before. Not much caring, she laid the dress and jacket out on the bed and admired them. The stitching was quite fine, and it was all beautifully lined. He had done it again, found her something perfect. She opened the small white cardboard jewelry box that had been tucked in with the package. In that, she found a string of faux pearls with matching earrings – just right for the outfit, of course.

She put the little box back in the suitcase.

"Shit!" she suddenly yelled. "Oh. Sorry for cursing. I just realized I left my bag of food on the train. Damn it."

"I can make you something to eat!" John Wolf answered, seemingly in a happier tone. He made a move to go turn back downstairs. "How hungry are you?"

She quickly did the math of how to answer. She wasn't that hungry. But free food?

"I'm starving!" she cried out.

She followed him down to the kitchen, finding it at the back of the house, under the bathroom. The house could not be more than twenty feet wide and forty feet deep – a classic old Philadelphia row house sandwiched between two others, perhaps purchased by him before prices in this part of town had started to rise. Or maybe it wasn't worth that much? Even if the house had eighteenth-century bones, it was quite small and not in the nicest part of town. Along the street, some of the houses had been covered in vinyl siding, turned boxy and ugly. A few in the area had even been replaced by small, utilitarian apartment buildings.

But this house still showed its old pinkish brick, looking quite sensible about its age and its long life – extra sensible given the addition of painted cast iron grates on the first-floor windows. It had no dining room, just a living room and an eat-in kitchen on the first floor, largely divided from each other by the stairs. On the second floor, there was the bedroom for her in the front and the one bathroom in the back. The third floor must be just the master bedroom, she thought. There was a door at the top of the second-to-third-floor stairs.

Well, she could work at the kitchen table in the evenings and on the weekends if he didn't mind, when she needed to lay out all her papers and books to try to get some writing done on her dissertation. And otherwise, she could make do with the small desk in her room. It had a lamp – a lamp and a familiar book of devotions, one from the Marian Fathers, those hard-core fans of the Immaculate Conception.

(She could put that away with the crucifix.)

"I'm afraid I'm dripping on your floor," she said, interrupting him from pulling out two cast iron pans and a chopping board.

"Right," he said. "Go dry off and change – there are towels in the bathroom up on the second floor – while I make you something."

She went back upstairs and took the clothes he had given her into the bathroom. She peeled off all the wet layers – even her bra was soaked like a dish sponge – and hung the clothes up over the shower curtain rod. She dried herself off with a towel. Then she pulled on the sweatpants he had given her and cinched them up with the drawstring, rolling up the bottoms a few turns so that they would not drag on the floor. She pulled on the socks and put on his big flannel shirt, buttoning it up all the way except for the very top. She rolled up the sleeves and emerged from the bathroom to the smell of bacon and onions sautéing in a pan downstairs. The softness of his old shirt suddenly felt so soothing against her bare breasts and belly.

"You walked from the station?" he asked as she sat herself down in one of his kitchen chairs.

"Ran," she answered. "Given the rain."

She looked around noticing the red and white checkered curtains on the windows over the sink, the lack of photos or written reminders on the refrigerator, the absence of crumbs where the cabinets met the floor.

"That's not safe," he said. "The suitcase would give you away and slow you down, and it's dark. You should have taken a cab."

"Cabs cost money," she replied.

"Well, it's not really safe," he said again. "You could have called me. I would have come and gotten you."

"I didn't want to be a bother right off the bat. I guess I failed at that, huh?" she replied, tugging demonstrably at the shirt he had lent her.

He turned on the light of the hood above the pan to see better.

"You a beat cop?"

"Detective," he said. "Philadelphia P.D."

She watched him scrub a couple of potatoes, chop them roughly, and put them into a hard-boiling pot of water. Now he was cutting up a red pepper, expertly seeding and deveining it. It was clear he felt at ease cooking.

"You say I can't stay," she said, "but I'm thinking I've landed in the perfect place. A cop worried about my safety who also cooks. I can just focus on getting my work done while you take care of everything else! I mean, I'll clean up after myself and I promise not to eat your food in the future. I'll buy my own."

"No problem," he said.

The tea kettle started to whistle, and he turned it off and poured the hot water into a tea pot he had set up with two bags.

"But you can't stay," he added. "I'll make some calls tomorrow and figure out a place for you. The message I got said Matty Shanks. And I only said yes because Father Joe said you were desperate for a place to stay, that your planned housing had fallen through. He said he got a message from a priest in West Virginia that he knows who was told by a group of Dominican sisters there that a grad student from Indiana needed a place to crash for a couple of months while he did his grad school Ph.D. research here – *he*."

"You've got it all right except my gender," Maddy answered.

She wondered if he might offer her some milk and sugar with the tea. She didn't mind drinking it black, but her wet hair was leaving her feeling cold. Somehow sweetened milk tea seemed a more warming prospect.

"I had myself all set up for lodging with a woman historian who had an extra room here," Maddy told him. "She had said months ago that I could stay with her. But now she is pregnant, and her pregnancy is going badly, and her toddler is not sleeping through the night, and she bowed out of having me at the last minute. The sisters made some calls for me, as fast as they could. This is better anyway. Much closer to the anatomy museum. And you don't have any crying babies to keep me up at night. You don't have any crying babies, right?"

"You don't sound like you're from West Virginia, where the sisters are."

"I'm not – I'm from New York. Well, Long Island."

"You don't sound like you're from Long Island either," he answered, pouring out a cup of tea and putting it in front of her. Without her asking, he also put out on the table a sugar bowl, a half-gallon container of whole milk, and a spoon. "You don't sound like you're from anywhere."

"Yeah," she answered, stirring a teaspoon of sugar into her cup, "I get that a lot."

"So how do you know the sisters from West Virginia?"

"They put me up when I was fifteen." She topped off her cup with an inch of milk. "I didn't have family. My parents and my sister had all just been killed in a car crash. So, the parish priests had called around in haste, and I was passed off to the sisters. They took me in for a couple of years."

She expected that he would answer the usual kind of thing people did when they heard she was orphaned young – *I'm so sorry. How shocking. You poor thing.*

But he didn't. He said nothing. Maybe it was because he was a cop and tragedy was too often on his radar to cause him to blink?

"So, you're Catholic?" he asked, after a moment.

"My family was," she answered. "I'm an atheist."

She thought she heard him quietly harrumph but wasn't sure. She figured she might as well be honest with him. She would do a lot for free housing. But she would not have sex with someone she didn't like, and she would not pretend to believe in God.

"You okay with pepper?" he asked. "Black pepper?"

She said she was okay with everything.

He ignored the awkwardness of her last remark.

"How did you end up at Indiana?"

"From the convent, I went off to Georgetown University when I was seventeen. Talked my way into admission and a free ride. Finished in three years – I was worried about my scholarship running out, so I hurried to finish my undergrad degree. Since then, I've been at Indiana for my master's degree and my Ph.D. in history of medicine and science. They gave me a full ride. I'm on a dissertation fellowship at the moment. National Endowment for the Humanities. Before that, I had typical grad funding, teaching and stuff. No debt – I have to finish up soon, so I'll have no school debt, as I'm on my own."

"So, you're going to be a professor?"

"Yes," she said. "That's the plan."

"I would think that you would go for a more predictable profession – law, medicine, something like that. I mean, given that you have no family, no one to fall back on by the sound of it. You must be truly concerned about money if you avoid cabs even at night and feel bound to seek free housing here."

"You *are* a detective. Yeah, that would have made more sense, right? Law or medicine. You're right about me and money. My father did leave me a billboard, but it doesn't produce very much money. A billboard, of all things. Not that he expected to die and leave me that."

She stood up and walked over to the stove with her cup, to see what he was doing at the stove. The bacon was browning up nicely with the onions. Now he added the chopped peppers. He stuck a fork in the potatoes to test them.

"You know why I'm doing a Ph.D.?" she asked him rhetorically. "You get one life, and you never know when it's going to end. So, you might as well do what you like, right? As long as you have enough to eat. I like teaching, and I especially like doing history. You must get that. I mean, you must understand why I like doing history, since you like reading history."

"How did you know that?" he asked, looking her in the face quizzically.

She saw his eyes now for the first time. They were milk-chocolate brown, very similar to the color of his hair. She thought him good-looking but couldn't figure out why. Was it those prominent clavicles? Or the pectoralis major muscle attached to them ? The coloring of his face?

Smart eyes – that was it.

Mid-forties, she guessed, by his face and the photos.

"How did you know I like reading history?" he asked again.

"The books in the living room," she said. "Military history and political biographies. Not the stuff in my field – not history of science or medicine – but history, nevertheless. Makes sense. History is detective work. What you and I do isn't that different except *you* have to convince a jury and *I* just have to convince my readers. And for what I do – history of anatomy – there won't be too many readers. Mine might require a Ph.D., but my work is in some ways much easier than yours."

He tested the potatoes again and, satisfied they were done, he drained the pot in the sink by holding the lid on and leaving a small gap between the pot and the lid as he inverted the cookware. Then he took the lid off and shook the pot.

"Aren't you going to fry them?" she asked hopefully.

"Yes," he answered with a bemused smirk. "Don't worry, Miss Shanks. I'm just letting them steam off a little, so they don't get soggy in the frying pan."

He poured a little oil over the potatoes and ground a bit of salt on them.

"Working on your dissertation, then?"

"Yes," she said, "at the Burtonian Anatomy Museum. I have a lot to get done while I'm here in terms of research and writing to stay on track for graduation at the end of the academic year. They would probably fund me one more year, but I don't feel like I can risk delay. I'm studying nineteenth-century specimen acquisition – where bodies and body parts came from."

He let out a chuckle.

"You're right," he said, "our work is similar. But history of anatomy doesn't sound like a marketable skill."

"Shit!"

She was about to apologize again for cursing but realized that, as a cop, he must be used to foul mouths.

"I forgot I need to call my best friend to say I made it. Can I use your phone? I don't have one."

He nodded in the direction of the telephone on the wall, near the back door that led from the kitchen to the alley behind the house. She picked up the cordless receiver and dialed the number.

"Hey, Liz, it's me – made it fine. I mean, I got soaked in a downpour, but I made it fine."

"Shit!" answered Liz. "Is your computer okay? And your books?"

"Yes, I had packed my computer in a sealed-up plastic bag, all wrapped up, just in case, and it was dry. And I shipped my books to the museum, so they'll be fine."

"Give me the number again," Liz said, and Maddy read her the phone number off the tag on the telephone base mounted to the wall.

"I'm sorry I wasn't able to take you to the Amtrak station in Indy," Liz said.

"Fellowship deadline – I totally get it, Liz."

"Was it insanely awkward having Giovanni drive you?"

"Uh, no," answered Maddy smiling, watching the back of Wolf at the stove as he stirred the pan. "He and I did not find it, uh, awkward."

"Oh, you didn't," Liz said. "Tell me you didn't end up sucking face with him again."

"Don't make me lie," Maddy answered.

"You have to stop! He's twenty years older than you! And he's on your dissertation committee now!"

"He hasn't signed the paperwork yet," Maddy replied. "He told me that. So, it's okay right now. He was waiting to sign the papers until I left."

"Jesus, Mad. It's not okay. And his significant other might be moving to Bloomington to live with him. Seriously, you have to stop."

"I know, I know," Maddy replied.

"If you don't stop, people are going to say you got your degree by sleeping around. You're so much better than that."

"Right? But nobody except you knows. So, it's okay. Just shut up about it."

"What did he give you?"

"Perfect for first day at the museum!" Maddy said excitedly while trying to talk not too loudly. "Perfect for the first impression. A dress with a matching jacket, conservative, kind of a light brown. I mean, that sounds ugly but it's pretty. Great neckline – you know he knows the necklines. Just the right length hem. Lined. Perfect for conferences. And job interviews, too."

"With matching jewelry, I'm sure, because he doesn't want to trust your stash of shit baubles."

"You got it," said Maddy. "Necklace and earrings."

"And some kind of sexy stockings."

"He skipped that this time. Not sure why. Maybe he figures he's given me enough of those."

"You can't keep letting him dress you – and *undress* you – Mad Girl," said Liz. "I mean, I know it's hot. You know that I'm all in favor of hot. But seriously."

Then Liz said, "Geez, Pumpkin, why are you so chatty today!"

"Oh, let me hear him?" Maddy asked, and Liz momentarily put the phone down near her lap so Maddy could hear Liz's pet rat chattering. "Oh, I miss you already, little Pumpkin."

"I hear there are lots of rats in Philadelphia," Liz told Maddy with the phone back at her mouth, "but you probably don't want to snuggle with them. I think I'm getting this line just right – this generation is even sweeter than the last one, but they're still smart. Not as smart as the ones in our lab, but pretty clever."

"You don't want them too smart, or they might figure out it's you that keeps cutting off their nuts."

Wolf turned and looked at Maddy and she shrugged her shoulders at him.

He pulled a butter larder off the counter and placed it on the table.

"Okay, I gotta go," Maddy said. "Give Margie my love and tell her to run you on the wheel every day, so you don't get cranky."

"Going to the gym is gonna be no fun without you."

"Tell your *real* girlfriend to go with you! And don't call unless it's an emergency. I don't want to bother my host."

She watched Wolf crack two eggs into a hot second pan and move to put two slices of bread in the toaster.

"Wait, Maddy – are you going to have email?"

"Hey, John Wolf, do you have internet here?" Maddy asked.

Wolf shook his head.

"Not here," Maddy told Liz, "but I'm sure the museum will have an ethernet cable I can plug into. I'll email you from there."

16

"You really safe?" she asked.

"I'm safe," Maddy answered. "My host is not an ax murderer. I know because I asked him."

"And he's not a rapist?"

"Hey, Detective Wolf," said Maddy, "are you a rapist?"

"No," he replied. "Nor am I a petty thief, an extortionist, a racketeer, or an inciter of riots."

"Arsonist?"

"No."

"Scofflaw?"

"No."

"He sounds clean, Liz," Maddy told Liz. "Especially for a cop."

"A cop! I told you the rosary mafia would come through for you."

"I knew you were right. I just didn't want to go there again. But you were right. As usual. Give Pumpkin and Spice wet kisses for me."

. . .

Maddy would never have imagined that rye bread could taste so good with blackberry preserves. But she had had the sense, eating it with the rest of John Wolf's fine offerings, that this wasn't an accident. It wasn't that rye bread and blackberry preserves was all he had to offer her in the way of bread and jam. It was that he had discovered how remarkably and unexpectedly good these things tasted together.

Lying back in his bath, sad as this dim blue bathroom felt, she had no intention of getting passed to a different Catholic. Some might also put her up for free. Some might also keep house this nicely. A few might also be blessedly free of children. But most of them, she knew, would not cook this well. Most Catholics would never think to match blackberry to rye.

-2-

The big band music emanating softly from the clock-radio mostly drowned out the sound of the poker game downstairs. Still, from the desk in her room, even with her door closed, Maddy could hear now that someone was leaving.

She went to her door and cracked it open to listen. The rest of them were saying goodnight to Father Tad.

Maddy closed the door and went back to the desk. She poured herself the last of the Bordeaux into the tumbler she had brought upstairs for the purpose and tried again to translate from French the passage that had her stuck. Something about the patient having come from a farm and having fallen from – was that the French word for ox?

Back in Indiana, Maddy's dissertation director had suggested to her in one of the old man's moments of random but useful advice that translations to English seemed to go more smoothly if you drank a little wine from the region from which the text originated. As she had on hand Bordeaux, left over from dinner with Wolf and the two priests, she thought she might as well work on some French cases tonight.

So, was this death caused by a fall from an ox?

The detail didn't matter too much. This physician-anatomist, Jean-Marie

Marcotte, had been fascinated not by the cause of death in 1872, but by what he had found upon autopsy in the spring of that year: *situs inversus.* The dead man's major organs had formed in fetal development the opposite way of normal in terms of left-to-right – the liver and gallbladder had grown on the left, the stomach on the right – as if the body had been looking in a mirror of the sagittal plane.

There was no reason for the dead fellow to have known this. His organs worked fine; they had just been secretly reversed in a little joke of Nature's. Even to Marcotte, it had come as a complete surprise during the autopsy. A delightful surprise.

The trick had not been keeping the organs; that would be easy, as Marcotte considered the peasant family of the subject too ignorant to catch on if he returned the body stuffed with some meat other than its own. The trick for Marcotte was how to display this prize so that his colleagues would immediately appreciate that what he had in a jar of formaldehyde had been a case of situs inversus. He had decided to keep just enough of the bones to frame the trophy.

Maddy pulled out her French dictionary and looked up the word.

Ah, right, âne meant donkey, not ox. The man had fallen from a donkey, hit his head on a stone, and died. That's right – ox would be simply *boeuf.* She ought to know the word for ox from French menus. One fine side-effect of being an historian of anatomy was learning the words in many languages for animals and body parts. She had found it made ordering food while in Paris a little more certain.

She could hear now that the noise downstairs had changed in quality. The voices were a little louder, a little rougher, now that the priests were both gone. It reminded Maddy of how the girls in the convent dorm changed how they talked when the sisters had gone to bed.

She drank down the last of the wine and picked up the dark green bottle to look closely at it. The ivory label featured a sketched castle with a brook in the foreground. It tasted very good, much better than the simple table wine she'd bought for herself in Paris when she had been there for two weeks for a conference and a binge of research.

Father Joe had brought three bottles of this Bordeaux for dinner, apparently knowing Wolf would make some sort of red meat – a beef pot pie, as it turned out. But it was so much better than any beef pot pie Maddy had ever eaten. The crust flaked like the pages of a nineteenth-century newspaper. The gravy was laced with the flavor of mushrooms and *herbs de Provence.* He had used good cuts of meat.

She could smell the scent of woody mushrooms as soon as he cut into the pie.

"Is this why you were soaking those dried mushrooms since this morning?"

He had nodded.

"What kind?" she asked, thinking she needed to start organizing notes on what he did with food.

"I mixed porcini and chanterelles."

She thought, when Wolf dished her a plate of it, that she must have looked just like the rat Pumpkin did when Liz made chocolate chip cookies, standing on hind legs, nose and whiskers in the air, sniffing in delighted anticipation.

She thought back now to earlier in the day. Maddy had come back from the museum after cramming in a little more work that Saturday afternoon, at the end of her first week of work, and asked Wolf if he would mind if she changed and went for a run.

"I promise I'll shower and put on something decent before Father Joe shows up for dinner," she said.

He was just finishing making the dough for the crust, just having rolled it into a ball. He dusted it with flour, put it in a ceramic bowl, draped it with a dishtowel and put it in the refrigerator. He rinsed off his hands and shook them dry over the sink.

"Give me a second and I'll go with you," he said. "Show you where it is okay."

They had set out in what she knew was the direction of the art museum. At first, he seemed to be holding back, no doubt figuring their height difference meant she would be slower than him. But he soon figured out she was a fast runner and picked up the pace.

She wanted on the run to ask him for an extension of her lodging, to stop him from trying to push her to another place, but could not seem to bring herself to do it. The morning after she had arrived, when he got back from Sunday mass, he had still been talking about needing for her to go stay somewhere else, and she had managed then to convince him then to just lay off that relocation project for a week, to give her a chance to get her sea legs in Philly, get her mental bearings, get settled into her work without the stress of trying to find another place. And he had agreed then.

"Father Joe will be coming for dinner on Saturday," he had said, "and we'll ask him for his help then, finding you another place. But there's poker after dinner, you should know – just some guys I work with, and – and it may be loud."

"It's fine," she said. "I won't bother you all."

"But you should have dinner with us. I mean with me and Father Joe."

Was it that he wanted to make sure Father Joe knew the troublemaker he was dealing with, so that he did not relocate her into too religious a house?

Wolf seemed to her, running just in front of her, rather like a horse – like running came naturally as a form of movement, even if it was not easy to run on the sidewalks of these old streets, broken up into so many blocks, uneven from wear and bad upkeep. The September air held that marvelous combination of lingering summer heat and a hint of the cold to come. The leaves were just starting to fall into the gutters of the streets.

"How was your first week at it?" he asked, taking a corner rather rapidly. She turned on her heel to follow.

"Good," she said. "There's a lot of material, of course – I'm thinking a lot about how to organize it. By method," she breathed, "by anomaly," she breathed again, "or by characters."

He did not answer.

She wondered if she should ask him how his week had been – but what could a police detective say? Perhaps she should ask him what interesting thing he had seen that week. But then would that sound like she thought his work was generally uninteresting?

"What are you cooking?" she had asked instead. "Is the pie dough for a dessert?"

"No," Wolf replied, "I'll make us a chocolate mousse for dessert. With a raspberry sauce. That's Father Joe's favorite. Technically it's supposed to be served after it is chilled, but he likes it warm out of the pot. The dough is for dinner. It will be a beef pot pie."

"Oh!" she said, trying not to sound too excited. The pot pies of the convent had been terrible – thickened with gooey cornstarch, loaded with frozen vegetables. But she was sure his would be good. She had poked around his pantry and his cupboards, and it was clear he was serious about cooking. There were even cooking tools she did not recognize.

"You won't miss your nightly ramen?" he asked.

"No, indeed. How did you even know that's what I'm eating given that you've been working nights?"

"The trash," he answered, just as she thought to herself, *the trash, of course.*

He picked up the pace a little as they mounted a hill, coming into a section with more commercial development. She noticed he was starting to sweat a little under the arms and on the back of his neck.

"I don't suppose you have access to a gym?" she asked. "One with rings and such? Some mats?"

"You mean like for gymnastics?" he asked.

"Yes," she said.

"There's one I can get you into now and then," he said. "But it all depends on where you're staying in terms of convenience, since you have no car."

Maddy didn't respond.

She wished Wolf would stop this push to make her move. She had tried very hard to be no trouble – making sure to eat her own food unless specifically invited to eat his, to promptly wash and put away the dishes she used, to ask before taking up the bathroom for an hour with a soak, and to avoid making any calls, arranging to have them come to her when she knew he was likely to be out.

But then he had come home last night earlier than she expected him and had found her in the kitchen talking to Giovanni, wearing the most ridiculous combination – a bright red evening wrap-dress Giovanni had sent to her at the museum with the pink socks she usually wore with her pajamas, and she had just in time pulled the dress back together and hung up on Giovanni and slunk upstairs feeling caught by Wolf. Caught and stupid.

Wolf must have known what kind of phone call it was, though he said nothing.

"Can I contribute anything to dinner?" she asked now, looking at the soleus muscles of his calves.

"No need," he answered, pausing at a traffic light and pulling her back from the curb as a car drove by them too fast. "I've got the food and Father Joe will bring some wine. Father Joe will bring *plenty* of wine."

"Perhaps I could grab some flowers for the table on the way back?" she asked. "At the corner place? And put some fresh candles in the glass votives I brought with me, for the table?"

He replied that would be nice but added that she should not spend too much.

Now, up in her room, as the late-night poker game continued downstairs, she felt the petals of the white carnations between her fingers. Wolf had told her after dinner to take them upstairs with her, as he cleared the kitchen table for the game.

These blossoms were certainly cheap and simple. But with the green of the ferns and the dots of baby's breath, they had looked quite nice in the candlelight on the table. And Father Joe had specifically said, when he came in the back door off the alley and saw the table, that it was good to have a little wine and candlelight and flowers with good food and company to end the week.

He had blessed the food before they ate and noticed when Maddy did not make the sign of the cross or say "amen." The old priest didn't look especially pleased. He poured them each a generous amount of wine.

"John must have told you that I told him to expect a young *Catholic man* for a lodger, Madeleine," Father Joe said to her, tucking into the dinner with gusto, cutting up his steamed asparagus and dragging it through the gravy of the pie. "Matty, not Maddy."

He followed with a quick series of "t" sounds with his tongue. She noticed to herself that he did not bother to wear his clerical collar here.

"Well, of course *you know* that we confused *your sex*, Madeleine," he went on, "because Wolf says you must go because of your sex. I'm looking for a place for you. I mean, I will. Tell me how you know the sisters in West Virginia?"

"My parents and sister died in a car crash when I was fifteen," Maddy said, feeling strange that she was saying this twice in a week when she rarely told anyone. "I had no real family left, so, I was passed on to the Dominican sisters. For safe keeping."

"But you're not Catholic?" he asked.

"My family was," Maddy answered, looking at Wolf and sensing his discomfort. How might she change the subject? Ask Father Joe what was his own order?

"You were baptized and confirmed?"

"Yes, Father," she answered, hoping the honorific would satisfy him and he would leave her alone. It wasn't that his demeanor towards her was terribly critical. She just did not want to be stuck in this situation where she felt as if she were somehow embarrassing Wolf. As if she – or he – had failed somehow.

It was strange to be back in this kind of situation, where she felt as if her atheism was embarrassing those around her. Since starting grad school, she had grown so used to academia, where everyone simply assumed everyone else was a non-believer until proven otherwise. Although maybe, she thought now, she assumed too much in her desire to live a life in an ivory tower free of deities and repressed longings.

She looked at Father Joe's hands and noticed he had a mild tremor. He looked to be getting close to seventy.

A knock came on the back door as a friendly face looked into the kitchen through the small square window. Wolf sprung up and opened the door to another priest, this time closer to his own age, this time in a collar. Wolf threw his arms around this man, who returned the warm embrace. Maddy thought Wolf looked as if he had been rescued.

"I thought you weren't coming tonight!" said Wolf.

"Someone has to help you drink whatever Father Joe brought," the younger priest answered.

Wolf hastened to set a fourth place.

"Father Tad, this is Maddy Shanks."

"Pleased to meet you," Maddy said, shaking his hand. "Father Tad?"

"Yes, short for Tadeusz. Polish."

"Ah," answered Maddy.

That explained the Marian devotions in her room. She knew them to be a Polish order.

"And you are?" asked Father Tad.

"No longer of the faith," answered Father Joe for her, rather matter-of-factly, pouring wine for his colleague and suggesting Wolf open the second bottle and the third, too, to let it breathe. "Madeleine was just telling us that her family were all killed in a car accident when she was seventeen – "

"Fifteen," said Maddy and Wolf simultaneously.

"Fifteen," repeated Father Joe. "And that's how she ended up with the Dominican sisters in West Virginia. They took her in, you see."

"Mercy," said Father Tad in a way that Maddy thought was rather clever – a religiously appropriate response that sounded reasonably, too, like a sympathetic swear.

His hair was thinning, but he had a liveliness about him that she rather liked.

"We will arrange a novena for your family," Father Joe told Maddy. "John, you will get us their names."

"So, the sisters didn't manage to keep you for their own ranks, eh?" said Father Tad, trying to lighten the mood.

Maddy shook her head. She was looking at the pie. She was glad Wolf had made such a large one. With four eaters, there seemed little hope of leftovers that he might tell her tomorrow to go ahead and eat. But there was at least hope of real seconds tonight. The carrots and peas somehow tasted like he had gotten them out of a farm field five minutes before cooking. Was that because of the earthiness of the mushrooms?

"Apparently the sisters did not secure the faith in her!" observed Father Joe, taking the second bottle from Wolf and refilling his own glass.

"Right," Maddy said, thinking that if she didn't acknowledge it, they would never move on. "I'm not a proselytizing atheist looking to destroy the Catholic Church or anything. Just a simple non-believer." She drank back her wine. "I guess that's why Wolf has to get rid of me."

"I don't *want* to get rid of you!" Wolf exclaimed. "You shouldn't take it personally."

He cut another piece of the pot pie and served it to her plate even though she had most of the first piece left. He did not do the same for the others. She looked up at him and caught his eye for a second.

"Thank you," she said. "It's excellent. I mean it's truly excellent. Not just not-convent-food good."

"I thought you would like some real meat after a week of your carrot-and-hummus lunches," he answered.

"John is one heck of a cook!" exclaimed Father Tad, taking a long drink from his water glass. "I may have rushed some of those last confessions a bit. But I am always glad to get an invitation for dinner here."

"I can understand why," Maddy replied. She got up, placing her napkin on the table, and took Father Tad's and her own water glass back to the sink to top them off. She returned and sat back down, carefully straightening out the skirt of her dress, the way Sister Mary Grace had made her practice.

She had picked out this patterned cotton frock after her post-run shower figuring it was about right – not so fancy as to appear over-dressed but nice enough to seem respectful of being invited to share this dinner. The fake pearls from Giovanni gussied it up just right. When she'd come down to the kitchen, Wolf looked at her and gave a small nod of approval. It felt to her the way she thought Pumpkin must have felt when Liz planted a firm kiss on his little head. Reassuring even if performed across the species barrier.

"Did you lose your faith when God took your family, child?" Father Joe asked.

Maddy did the math and realized he was already on his third glass of wine.

"I never had faith, Father," she answered in a voice she was trying to modulate between too quiet and too firm.

"Did you pray for it?"

"Why would I pray for something I didn't want?"

She now remembered praying as a child for a treasure chest full of money and nothing happening. She remembered praying to wake up one day in a different family, perhaps the Goldsteins down the street – they seemed so happy – and nothing happening. If God would give you only what *he* wanted, this prayer thing, she had realized, seemed at best a total waste of time and energy, at worst a pathetic dependency. Like her mother's on her father.

"You didn't blame God?" Wolf asked. "For their deaths?"

"No," Maddy answered. "No, Wolf. I blamed somebody else." When no one answered, she added, "I hope I am not being offensive."

"You are speaking the truth of yourself," Father Tad said, holding the edge of the table momentarily in his hands and looking her in the face. "How could that be offensive?"

"Do you need me to usher this Sunday, Father Tad?" Wolf asked, obviously trying to change the subject.

"That would be fine, John. Always happy to have your help."

"I was thinking, Father," Wolf went on, "that you might ask Mrs. Swinton about whether she might have a spare room for Maddy."

Maddy let out a sigh, realizing too late that it would be audible.

"In a way, John," said the younger priest, "I would think Maddy would present more of a problem to you were she still a practicing Catholic."

He smiled an impish smile and Wolf cleared his throat.

Maddy figured out what Father Tad meant – that Wolf would not find an atheist very attractive. She was not much of a temptation. She felt the corollary must also be true – the more Catholic he proved himself to be, the less his company would interest her.

She wished, though, that she did not have the sense she was embarrassing him with her worldview. And she wished she could pull Father Tad aside and ask him where Wolf's wife was. Perhaps there would be a chance later.

"What time are the boys coming for the game?" Father Joe asked. "Will we be seeing Wes, of the blue eyes?"

Wolf nodded and said nine o'clock.

"I'll stay to watch the game, but we'll put you in a taxi back to the rectory after you've said hello to the boys," added Father Tad.

Wolf appeared to Maddy as if now he were embarrassed.

She smiled at him, trying to give him a good imitation of the nod he had given her earlier.

To her surprise, he smiled back, looking a little grateful.

"Tell us what you're working on here in Philadelphia, Maddy!" suggested Father Tad in an overly enthusiastic voice.

She proceeded to explain the basics of her dissertation and of her research at the Burtonian Museum – that she was trying to understand how medical men acquired bodies and body parts in the nineteenth century, particularly for anatomical collections. She told them that the museum was helpful not only for its own collection but for its library, which held a great store of texts related to anatomical acquisition.

"Sometimes," she explained, "a body was procured by an anatomy collector long after it was buried because it was dug back up and something interesting was found."

"Well, that's desecration of a grave," said Father Joe, his rosacea now blooming from the Bordeaux.

Father Tad simply ignored his remark. "Like when?" he asked Maddy, quite interested.

"It happened with the body they call 'The Soap Lady,'" Maddy answered. "When she was supposed to be decomposing, because of the soil she was in, her flesh instead turned to something like soap. She's kind of like a giant bar of soap!"

The three men said nothing but stopped eating for a moment. Maddy just went on eating, using her knife to push onto her fork another piece of asparagus and pie. (It was best eaten together.) She chewed, moaned a little at the flavor, swallowed, and took a drink of water.

"Well," said Father Tad after the quiet pause, "well, one cannot comment on the state of this lady's soul. But at the resurrection, her body will surely be quite clean!"

The four of them burst out laughing.

-3-

Maddy finished off the translation of one more nineteenth-century journal article – this one in German capturing the story of how a physician came to obtain the amputated leg of a soldier along with a cannonball. The cannonball had led to a crush injury, which had led to gangrene, which had led to the amputation. Which had led to the prize pairing of the injury (the taxidermed remains of the leg) and the etiology (the eight-pound munition, only a bit scarred).

She kept thinking about the little dish of chocolate mousse in the refrigerator, the one Wolf said she could have later if she wanted. It sounded as if the game downstairs had hit a momentary lull. There was a scraping of chairs, the sound of beer bottles clinking as they were moved, and she could hear someone coming upstairs to use the bathroom. She decided she might as well now go get the leftover dessert even if she looked a little silly still wearing this dress and the pearls from dinner.

She came into the kitchen holding the empty wine bottle and glass just as Wolf turned from the sink.

"Oh!" he said, surprised to see her. She handed him the bottle and glass.

"I just came down for that cup of mousse," she said. "I hope that is okay."

"Of course, Maddy. Maddy, this is Manny, Crappy, and Wes."

She shook each man's hand. She could tell which one was Wes. Father Joe wasn't wrong about those remarkable blue eyes. They were, she thought, the color of bluebells in the spring. Almost a little violet.

"And here's Neller," Wolf said, gesturing to the man who had just come back from the bathroom.

"Charmed," said Neller, bowing a little to her. "Are we cutting you in for a hand?"

"I was just coming down for something to eat," Maddy explained, accepting from Wolf the dish and a spoon.

She walked back up the stairs and soon found she was being followed by the guy Wolf had called Manny. She wondered if it was his real name or a nickname.

"Can I help you?" she asked as she hit the second-floor landing and felt him close behind her.

"Just gonna use the John," he said, gesturing to the bathroom. "You using John?" he asked, winking at her.

He had the look of a guy who had smoked too many cigarettes. In fact, he looked, she thought, a little like a thug. She wondered if they sent him out undercover to play one.

"Excuse me?" she asked, genuinely confused for a minute what he had asked.

"Joke," he said. "Joke about you and Wolf. Eh, never mind. There's a reason we call him 'Mr. Clean.'"

She walked back into her room, closing the door behind her, and sat down at her desk to keep working. She could hear Manny go into the bathroom and loudly bang up the lid and the seat of the toilet.

She wished the telephones in this house weren't limited to the one in the kitchen and the one in Wolf's bedroom, the one she sometimes heard him on above her late at night when the station seemed to be calling. She wanted to talk with Liz the way they did at home late at night, at her place or at Maddy's. Maddy should have asked Wolf if she could take the cordless one from the kitchen upstairs, if the signal reached. She couldn't very well go back down again now.

But Maddy was craving the normality of a near-midnight conversation with Liz, about work, about life, about the politics of academic disciplines. She wanted to hear what was going on at Liz's lab and to tell Liz about what had been going on with her own work. The museum's collections and library were a goldmine – just as everything she researched in advance had indicated they would be – and the work here felt almost too easy. Maddy was starting to wonder if her whole dissertation topic was too simple, if editors and job committees would find her work not very scholarly because it was rather straightforward. These days, everyone preferred novel theorizing to descriptive history. And it wasn't like Maddy wasn't capable of theory....

She could imagine having this conversation with Liz and Liz saying, "You know what? Men never worry when the data comes easily to them. They think they've *earned* it. We think it means we're *stupid*. You're not stupid, Mad Girl. The data's coming fast and easy because you did everything right."

Suddenly, Maddy heard her door open. She turned quickly in her chair to see Manny standing in the opening.

"Oh, sorry," he said, looking around her room and then looking at her. "Wrong door, I guess."

He exited, leaving her door ajar.

She got up, closed the door, and locked it. Now she changed out of the dress into jeans and a sweatshirt and sat back down to work. She figured she had better not tell Wolf about Manny coming in her room. He would think it one more reason she ought to be in some other house.

. . .

The noise of the house dropped so suddenly, Maddy wondered if Wolf had gone out with the rest of the men. She unlocked and opened her bedroom door and made her way down to the kitchen. Wolf was very quietly cleaning up.

"You don't need to worry about waking me up," she said. "I'm still up. I'll give you a hand."

"You don't need to," he said, but he took from her the empty beer bottles as she handed them to him.

"Can I ask you something?" she asked. "Do you ever play the records you have in the living room?"

"Yes. I just haven't been while you are here because I don't want to bother you."

"Music rarely bothers me," said Maddy. "And it's your house."

Wolf went into the living room. She could hear him trying to find a particular place on an album to leave the needle. He came back a moment later to the sound of Johnny Hartman singing jazz in his low voice, a piano behind him.

No tears, no fears. Remember there's always tomorrow.

She wondered if he put this song on for her? But then it moved on to the main line – *We'll be together again* – that song about two people in love being separated.

"I hope we didn't keep you up," Wolf said to Maddy, pausing from listening, as if he had just remembered she was there.

"It's *your* house, Wolf!" she answered. "And I got a lot of work done."

Handing her a damp washcloth to clean the table, he said he was glad. As she washed down the table, for a moment she could hear Wolf quietly singing along to the recording. His soft song sounded like he felt relief to have this music back. She wished she had asked him about the records sooner.

She wiped the table harder in the sticky spots, scooping the crumbs into her hand, bringing them to the sink. She rinsed her hands and the cloth and took it back to the table to wipe down the chairs.

"They taught you how to clean in the convent," said Wolf.

"They *made* me clean the in convent," Maddy laughed, and he laughed back. "The food here is way better. I'm happy to clean for it."

He looked pleased with himself, and she realized, from the way his mouth seemed quick to smile, that he must be a little inebriated. She had not seen him this way before.

"So, do you do gymnastics?" he asked her, making a twirling motion with his finger. "You asked me about a gym for that?"

"A little," she said.

She tucked the chairs under the table and said, "Watch this."

She took a second to get herself in the right position and did a perfect flip backward, her knees tucked at the apex.

"Damn!" he said, clapping his hands three times.

She thought it a bit childlike – out of character for him.

"I'm somewhat surprised I can do that comfortably with that pot pie and mousse in me."

"Yes, yes," he said, as if she had raised something he had meant to bring up. "I am sorry that Father Joe gave you a hard time over dinner."

"Shit, Wolf, that wasn't what concerned me. I was concerned I was putting you in a bad spot."

"How so?"

"Making you look bad for putting up an atheist."

"I should turn a young woman out? Onto the streets? This would make me more Christian?"

She realized in that moment that what she'd been thinking was true must in fact be true: he was one of those rare birds who thought about his actions in a way consistent with his professed faith. Common among the sisters. But something Maddy had found less common in men.

"Where would all you Catholics be if you didn't have me as a subject of your charity?" she asked rhetorically. "I should sin more so you can get more points for saving me. You get to heaven, and no skin off my nose."

She meant it as a joke, but she could see he wasn't sure how to take it. She asked him for a broom and dustpan. Wolf opened the door tucked under the stairs and pulled from the basement landing the tools she wanted.

"Oh, that's the way to the basement?" she asked. "Is that where your washer and drier are? Can I use them tomorrow? I'm running out of clean clothes. Cities are tough on a living body."

"Of course," he said, waving her over. "Come here, I'll show you."

He flipped two switches to light the stairwell and the basement. She began to follow him down and then, about five steps from the bottom, saw between her and the washer his exercise bench with the weights.

She froze mid-step. Seeing the exercise bench and the weights, it felt as if all of her organs had flipped to the other side, all at once. Of course, that was impossible – quite impossible, she told herself.

There's no such thing as acute-onset situs inversus, Maddy, she said to herself

"Never mind," she said to Wolf.

"Never mind?" he asked, turning to see her startled and stuck. "Never mind?" he said again. "I don't understand. I know there are few spiders. Is that it?"

"Goodnight," she said, and backed her way up the stairs, sliding her hands along the rails behind her. "Goodnight."

"Wait, Maddy," he said, rushing up the stairs after her.

He ended up on the landing at the same time as her, standing too close, facing her. He looked into her eyes and tried to figure out what had disturbed her.

"How about I show you an easy dessert to make, one that will keep your belly full through the night?"

She nodded. She did not feel that she could simply disappear upstairs. He must be wondering what was wrong with her. She felt apologetic even as that practiced voice in her head told her there was nothing to apologize for about this.

"Come over here to watch," he said, pulling her gently by the elbow to the stove.

He took out a medium-sized pot with a handle, ran enough water into it to fill it about a third of the way, and put it on the front right burner to boil. Then he plopped a rounded-bottom double boiler into the water, lined up its handle with that of the pot below, and cracked two small eggs into the well of the boiler. He quickly added a tablespoon of confectionary sugar and a dollop of vanilla extract. Finally, he added a bit of Amaretto and water and, firmly holding the handles together in his left hand and the whisk in his right, started rapidly whisking the mix.

"What is it?" she asked, looking into the pot. Smelling the rich vanilla and amaretto, her physiology was starting to feel less like her body had been suddenly slammed against a wall.

"It will be kind of a creamy vanilla-egg custard. I'll shave on some chocolate at the end, if you like."

She watched him keep whipping the egg mixture as the water started to heat up. The mix began to foam. She was taking deep breaths in a studied fashion, and she sensed he could tell.

"Here," he said, handing her the handles of the double-boiler and the whisk. "Take over for a minute."

She did the best she could to keep whipping the foaming egg in circles without banging the whisk too hard against the metal of the double boiler. He pulled out of the cupboard a small serving bowl to have ready, and also poured a small glass of port. Then he took back over the whisking of the mixture. The record playing in the living room ended and the needle started to make the lisping sound of being caught near the label.

"Go pick something else," Wolf said to Maddy, tilting his head toward the next room.

She went to the living room, pulled out another album at random, and put it on. It was a collection of old railroad blues. As the music started, Wolf came into the living room and gestured for her to sit on the couch. He presented her with a spoon, the bowl of chocolate-laced yellow egg custard, and the glass of port. He settled himself down in the armchair nearest her.

"See," he said, "you can make this when you need something warm and sweet. Easy."

"Easy," she said, "if I happen to have a double-boiler, a good whisk, and Amaretto."

She tried a little bit of the soft, warm custard with the spoon and nodded at him appreciatively. Any remaining stress hormones seemed to be chased off by this lovely egg cream. She had another spoonful. It had ever so slightly a boozy flavor – it tasted a little like a rum babka. She noticed that the curls of chocolate Wolf had shaved on top were accentuated by the vanilla extract and the almond flavor.

She paused to take a sip of port and then realized she kept looking at the front door. She glanced at him to see him looking at her and then glanced away quickly.

Wolf looked from her to the front door and back and let out a sigh.

"Listen, Maddy," he said. "Okay. I'll tell you where my wife is. I don't mean to scare you by withholding that information. She's in the hospital."

She wasn't sure why he was telling her this now. But she also didn't want to stop him from explaining.

"She's been there about two years. Happened just after 9/11. They call it a persistent vegetative state. It's a kind of coma. Well, you study the history of medicine, so you probably know what I'm talking about. Random accident. She was in a car that got hit by a falling construction crane. Random. She's never woken up."

"I'm sorry," said Maddy, putting down the bowl on the coffee table. "It was here, in Philly?"

"Yes. And you don't have to stop eating. Don't stop eating. It's no good when it's cold."

She took the bowl back up.

"So, look. That's why her clothes are in those plastic bins in the basement. In case she wakes up and comes home. That's why you saw that."

Maddy realized he thought that those bins were what had caused her to back out of the basement. The plastic bins of women's clothing on the shelves. She had barely registered those in her quick retreat.

"I keep her clothes," he went on, "because if she *does* wake up and come home, I don't want her to think I gave up on her."

"You think she will? Wake up?"

"If that's what God wants," he said.

She wanted to ask Wolf if *he* wanted his wife to come home, but she thought she'd better not. She held the bowl in her left hand, leaning it on her thigh, and used her right to take another sip of port.

"Wolf, did you want some of this, or can I eat it all?"

"I made it for you, not me."

While he watched her, she finished off the custard, dragging the side of her index finger around the bowl and licking her finger clean to make sure she had gotten it all. She drank away the remainder of the port and put the dishes on the coffee table.

The man on the stereo was singing about the firebox of a steam engine and a woman he had lost. Maddy wasn't sure how to ask Wolf what she really wanted to know now.

"How often do you see her?"

"About three or four times a week these days," he answered. "Well, more like two or three, I guess. I'll go see her tomorrow after mass. She doesn't recognize me. She doesn't recognize anybody."

"But her eyes – they are open?"

"Her eyes are open sometimes, and she seems to maybe look around. And if you put your finger in her hand, she will grasp it. But the doctors explained to me that is just an instinct. I don't see any change. They tell me there's little-to-no hope of – of any real change."

"So, she has a feeding tube?" asked Maddy.

He nodded.

"And you don't think to..."

He wrinkled up his lips at her.

"If someone lets an animal starve to death, we arrest them for cruelty. That's cruelty."

"Okay," she said. "I'm not going to argue the point with you." She didn't like how that came out. "You can tell *I* would not want to starve to death."

He snorted at her a little.

"I think you might wake up from a coma simply from hunger, young lady."

"Hospital food would hardly give one a reason to get out of bed. But the prospect of *real* food, well. So, Wolf... so, that's it? You're stuck married, without another relationship – " she wondered to herself why she was being so uncharacteristically delicate – "you're stuck *without sex*, maybe forever?"

He nodded.

"Well, *that* sucks."

He nodded.

"Why don't you – I mean, don't you think God would forgive you for having another...relationship?"

"I took a vow. I am still married to my wife. Even if she does not know me."

"But I mean, denying yourself that – for *years* – "

She realized she had her hands out in front of her in the gesture one makes when a person is being unreasonable.

She put her hands in her lap.

"I like sex," she said.

He leaned back in his chair and looked up at the ceiling as if to avoid her gaze.

"I like sex, too," he said. "But I believe in having it within the context of marriage."

"I like sex a lot more than that," she said.

"Yes," he said, standing up and taking her bowl and glass to the kitchen. "You are happy to be...dressed up."

She said nothing in response. She was wondering if he meant what she had worn for dinner. No, that wasn't what he meant, she was pretty sure.

He returned from the kitchen and sat back down in the chair.

"So, do you like that red dress he sent?"

"How did you know it was sent to me?' she asked.

"It wasn't in your suitcase when you arrived – I didn't see anything that color – and then you were wearing it. So, I figured it had to have arrived while you were here. I figured you probably didn't buy it, based on your frugality. It looks expensive. It looks nice. Nicely made. And I figured that guy sent it to you, based on what you told your friend Liz on the phone the night you arrived. I guess he hasn't signed the paperwork yet?"

"Geez, living with a detective is something," she answered, pulling her feet up onto the couch and tucking them under her. "No secrets for me, I guess."

She started to think maybe she should find another place.

He gave her an awkward look and then looked down. She felt badly for it.

"Well," she added, "I don't know what you think, but I don't think the red one suits me as well as the brown. The brown is more conservative, anyway."

"More conservative?"

"Less...bold."

"You know what?" he said, as if she had not just made the last observation. He looked weirdly bright now. "I just thought of something. You know what doesn't fit you? Your *name*. I have never thought 'Maddy' suited you. Maybe it's because I expected you to be a Matty. But it just doesn't feel right. You don't seem like a Madeleine."

"Do I seem like a chocolate éclair?"

"Ah, a French pastry pun," he answered. "Very good. No, no. I've got it. I think between your nibbling of carrots and your fast sprinting and your ability to jump high in the air *and* your attitude toward – your interest in – "

She was trying to figure out what he was getting at.

"Well, I think with all that, with who you are, I should rightly call you 'Rabbit.' You seem much more a Rabbit than a Maddy."

"A rabbit who lives with a wolf?" she asked, delighted now at his concise description of her person. "Well, that will give you more cause to kick me out. A wolf can't have a *rabbit* around without making a dinner of it. Although I'm sure you'd make a very tasty dinner of me."

"Now, now," he replied, smiling, "you will recall the lion and lamb can get along. Was that in Genesis?"

She threw her head back and rolled her eyes.

"You have it all wrong! Not a lion and a lamb, and not in Genesis. Which one of us is religious? The *wolf* and the *lamb* shall feed together, and the *lion* shall eat *straw* like the bullock," she corrected him, wagging her finger. "And it's in Isaiah, not Genesis."

"Well, hell, who wants to eat *straw*? And I may be a lion or a wolf, but – no offense – you're no *lamb*. Definitely a rabbit."

He yawned, his jaw off to one side.

"So," he asked, "what does *your* religion – your philosophy – really hold, O Rabbit? Where does atheism get you?"

He wasn't asking in a hostile voice. She could see he was pleased by something. Perhaps it was the nickname. Perhaps it was getting her to talk, to stop looking at the front door.

"I believe," she started, "that we are all responsible for ourselves. In my life, a God gets no credit, and a God gets no blame. I hold *people* accountable. That's what my atheism gets me. You must believe in holding people accountable, too, given your job? If everything is up to God, why be a cop? Especially a detective. Why try to effect justice on earth?"

"One has to do *something* while on earth," he answered, "and it seems like it's not a bad job for someone who wants to be good."

"And being a cop in a real city might get you to heaven faster."

He leaned forward with his elbows on his knees.

"Are you just an earthly St. Peter, then? Giving the score *after* the fact, after it's all well over? Don't you want your work to be about more than what happened in *the past?*"

She looked at him and wondered how he could figure out so much about her but not have understood that her reaction in the basement was not about the bins.

"Don't you want your life to be about more than the *past*, Rabbit?" he asked again.

"This from a man who denies himself the pleasure of sex," she replied, "maybe forever more because of a vow made years earlier in completely different circumstances. Don't *you* want more than the past?"

"This from a woman who saves her pennies, who denies herself the pleasure of a great weekday lunch, because she knows she has to save money and work hard all day to take care of her long-term future. Hummus and carrots and work. Hard work, all the time."

She nodded, smiling. "True enough. You have me."

"Yup. You think about your long game just as much as I do," he said. "You know if you didn't, you'd blow it all on something good to eat. Yup, you'd stop work for a few hours and go have a real, hot Philly cheesesteak with a fine, cold brew."

"Great!" she answered, throwing a small square pillow from the couch at him. "Great! Now *every day* this week, come lunch time, I'm going to be looking hopelessly at my little sack lunch thinking I could just go out for a cheesesteak and a pint. That's going to make it hard to work."

He yawned again in the same off-center way.

"Go to bed, Rabbit," he said, standing up and reaching a hand out to her.

She took it and stood up. There she was, again, eye-level with his clavicles.

"So, you're not going to mass with me tomorrow?" he asked, much more seriously.

She shook her head and gave him a look like he must be a little bit crazy.

"Just thought I should ask. Father Joe is going to ask me if I asked you. Do you have to work every day? No Sabbath?"

She stretched up her arms and yawned.

"You know, Wolf," she said, letting her arms flop to her sides, "the terrible and wonderful thing about an academic career is that the work is never done."

"That's too bad. Because I thought tomorrow I could take you for a cheesesteak when I get back from the hospital. So, you know the right place to go if you want one for lunch."

"Get behind me, Satan," she replied. "I have a degree to finish."

She was glad to hear him laugh at her.

-4-

"Well, can't you just *lie* about what you're working on while you're here?" asked Shirley Anseed, the Burtonian Museum's chief curator. "Then I can just act all shocked after your dissertation comes out and it turns out it is about where all our darlings came from? I just need plausible deniability about your work, sweetie."

Shirley took another one of Maddy's French fries, dunked it in the dollop of ketchup on Maddy's plate, and ate it slowly. Maddy remained quiet, trying to figure out what to do about Shirley's awkward request.

Maddy understood why Shirley was asking this of her. When Maddy had written to Shirley from Bloomington to tell her she wanted to come to the museum for a few months and do research for her dissertation, Shirley had warmly welcomed her.

But Maddy hadn't fully explained then what she was working on – that her focus was specifically on specimen *acquisition*. And so, before Maddy had arrived, Shirley had not thought about the possibility that the prominent gentlemen-physicians whose medical society owned the Burtonian Museum might worry that Maddy's work would lead to serious questioning about how some of the artifacts had come to be there. It hadn't occurred to Shirley that Maddy might be seen as a dangerous mole in their midst. It certainly hadn't occurred to Maddy.

Shirley signaled to the pub waiter that she'd like a refill of her water glass and then poured into her beer glass the rest of her bottle of stout. She reached over and did the same for Maddy with her beer.

"Drink up, Maddy," said Shirley, "and listen, don't panic or anything. This is not that big a deal. It's not like anyone is going to read your dissertation! Only your dissertation committee is going to read it, if they even do. It's just that repatriation has become a big thing with the Indians – I mean, the Native Americans – and, well, the old guys don't want the place opening up and emptying out like we're having some kind of anatomical garage sale. We're, uh, kind of *fond* of the collection. Particularly given that it's taken a hundred and sixty years to assemble and it's one of the best in the world."

Shirley drank down the last of her beer and then added, "We also happen to think science matters more than sentimentality about the dead."

"I know," said Maddy. "I don't disagree."

The waiter came over with a pitcher and refilled the two water glasses. As Maddy watched him wipe up the bit that spilled onto the table from tumbling over the ice cubes, she wondered to herself why she hadn't considered the possible political implications of her dissertation topic.

But of course she *had*, at least to some extent. She had been interested in the topic not just because of the stories, not just because of the historical detective work involved in figuring out how each item came to be in the possession of this or that nineteenth-century physician or surgeon or anatomist or museum, but because she was interested in the issue of power. She was fascinated by the question of who controlled what body or body part, which relic, which lock of hair. So, of course her work was political. How naïve could she have been about how the keepers of anatomical collections would see her?

She remembered now back to her first day at the museum, the week before, when she'd arrived in the dress-jacket combo from Giovanni and Shirley had provided her a tour of the collections not on public display – the drawers and cabinets and jumble of remains in jars on dusty shelves down in the basement, where the staff had their offices. Within two minutes of the tour's start, Maddy realized what Shirley was doing. This was her professional-welcome schtick – a standardized tour she'd give to people she considered insiders in medicine and science, meant to look impromptu but in fact well-rehearsed.

Shirley pulled out one pungent drawer of desiccated fingers saying, "Phew, we've got to change the box of baking soda in there." She asked Maddy what she thought a large phallic-shaped bone might be, waiting for Maddy to say, "I don't know," so that Shirley could respond, "Too bad, because we don't know either. The tag fell off."

Even knowing it was a well-practiced comic routine, Maddy found it impossible not to immediately like Shirley. She name-dropped in a way that felt not like she was trying to put Maddy down or hold herself up, but rather, it seemed, that she was subtly assuring Maddy she'd hook her up with powerful people – and that she was looking forward to the day she could name-drop Maddy, too. She was, like Maddy, so comfortable with human artifacts, able to have a sense of humor about abnormality, pathology, death. She was tall, too, in a pleasant sort of way – so tall compared to Maddy, she seemed a little like one of those clowns at the circus with the stilts hidden under billowy pants – and she fussed over Maddy like a dear old aunt, showing her where to stash her lunch, telling her who to avoid on the staff, and asking Bill, the maintenance guy, to run an extra ethernet cable to the desk Shirley had arranged so that Maddy wouldn't have to bother anyone when she wanted to connect her laptop to check her mail or look something up on the internet.

"And get Ms. Shanks a decent lightbulb, Bill, while you're at it! One that Thomas Edison didn't personally manufacture."

Granted, the desk Shirley had given Maddy sat in a very dark part of the basement, under a bunch of old cobweb-prone pipes running along the ceiling. It was located in a room that had only a tiny bit of natural light even on the brightest days, from a window-well facing the street. (Maddy knew it was getting to be closing time when she could feel the quickening of the shadows of the people hurrying past at evening rush.) But it was a dedicated desk, just for her, in a prestigious institution with little space to spare.

Shirley had been good to her.

"I have an idea, Maddy!" said Shirley now, with her toothy conspiratorial grin framed by her dark-brunette bob. "Here's what we'll do. We'll have you give a guest lecture for the old boys, and you'll suck up to them and entertain them and make them feel all appreciated and understood, and then they won't worry about you. Plus, some of them might take an interest in you, and it never hurts to have wealthy doctors as your patrons. You just have to play History Geisha for an evening."

Maddy took another bite of her hamburger and thought about this. It wasn't a bad idea. It would mean another invited lecture to put on her c.v., and it would give her some practice in a fairly low-visibility setting. If she screwed up the delivery of this talk, it wasn't going to be like if she screwed up at a conference for her own discipline. These were M.D.'s who were never going to sit on a search committee for a job she needed. And no one from a future search committee was going to be there to see her suck up to these guys.

"Okay," said Maddy. "I could give a talk about some discoveries that saved some lives. Let them know I believe medical science is an incredible public good."

"That's the idea!" exclaimed Shirley.

"There *are* a bunch of useful findings that came from autopsies and specimens in the period I'm looking at, of course. I could pick something in your museum's collection as the focal point of the lecture."

Maddy took another bite of her hamburger, chewed, and swallowed.

"I know," she said. "I could focus on that specimen of the cancerous testis from the unnamed society lady found on autopsy by Dr. Wilmore Booth. I can talk about that specimen you have and the general discovery that undescended testicles, including in patients who had been assumed to be normal females, are at special risk of becoming cancerous."

"Perfect!" yelled Shirley, a bit loudly for Maddy's taste. "That has everything. Sex, cancer, death, upper-class hermaphrodites, heroic medicine – they'll love it. We'll do a wine and cheese thing beforehand. Get the old fellas feeling warm and generous. Maybe serve some nuts, ha! You can wear that number you wore on your first day, with the pearls, and put your hair up in a bun, and they will be powerless before you. The ones with big egos will fantasize you will write about them, and the ones with small egos will fantasize you will write about their mentors."

"And the ones with the middling egos?"

"They're the useful ones. You definitely want them there."

"You sound a little cynical, Shirley."

"I am a practical woman, Madeleine Shanks," answered Shirley, faux-gravely. "Strangulated hernias must be treated emergently! Toxic megacolon must be avoided if at all possible! And doctors must be understood as believing that all historians are there to cherish their particular professional lineages. You can't fight nature, sugar. Before you give the talk, I'll give you the important docs' bios and headshots, so you can act like you've heard of them. I'll call Dr. Wilhelm's number two, Dr. Goncharov, and ask him if I can set it up with Dr. Wilhelm as the official host. That will bring a crowd."

"Dr. Wilhelm – he's the big-deal bone-and-growth specialist – dwarfism mostly, yes?"

Shirley nodded without speaking, because she had just taken a forkful of her salad into her mouth.

"I don't know a lot about contemporary physicians like Dr. Wilhelm," Maddy added, "so I could use your help with that before I have to deal with them. As you know, I do *dead* people."

"Well, I like to think of the living as the future-dead," Shirley answered, wiping her mouth with her napkin. "And Dr. Wilhelm is a *very* big deal. His obit will make the New York Times. Short-listed for the Nobel in physiology, they all say. Decades of NIH funding, uninterrupted, marking him as the envy of everybody in the med research biz. He *has* pulled off just about forty years of remarkable work on growth mechanisms. And you know, he's beloved by *the little people*."

Maddy knew that "little people" was the generally accepted term for people with dwarfism, but the way Shirley said it made it sound rather humorous. She made it sound like a title, with perfect annunciation and equal emphasis on each word: *The Little People*.

Shirley could tell her delivery had pushed Maddy to amusement. So, she continued.

"My dear Madeleine, did you know that in England dwarfs are called 'persons of restricted growth'? Doesn't that make them sound like someone went and bonsaied them?"

Maddy was just taking a sip of water and spit it back out into the glass, breaking into a hard laugh and then a cough.

"Nobody trimmed *my* roots, as you can see," said Shirley, sweeping her hands down around her long torso in a gesture of proud display. "You – well, you look like you didn't quite get enough fertilizer, Ms. Shanks. Or maybe they didn't repot you when it was that time."

Maddy kept coughing and laughing.

"Stop!" Maddy begged. "I'm going to die of respiratory failure."

"Well, don't do that – I haven't gotten you to sign a form yet, promising me your body for the collection."

"I don't think I've got anything interesting anatomically," answered Maddy.

"You never know till you're on the autopsy table," said Shirley. "You know that better than most people. You might just have a big ol' cancerous testicle in there, a downright handsome specimen, for all you know."

"My regular menses would suggest otherwise. And the gynecologist probably would have noticed a lack of uterus when she inserted my I.U.D. So I'm pretty sure I'm a standard female."

"You never know," said Shirley. She waved at the waiter for the checks.

"Let me get your lunch," said Maddy. "You've done so much to help me out."

"I won't fight you today, but don't make a habit of it. I know what grad students get paid, even if they have a fellowship."

The truth was Maddy was buying Shirley lunch in case she needed soon to ask her help finding cheap housing. Living with Wolf was perfect from Maddy's point of view. It was easy, quiet, and safe. The way her room evoked the guest rooms at the convent had turned out to make her feel weirdly comforted, as if she had graduated from the girls' dorm there to the grown-up space in that feminine fortress. And Wolf was even kind in that non-demanding way Liz had about her; when Wolf had realized Maddy couldn't bring herself to go down to the basement to the washer and dryer and also couldn't bring herself to even explain why, without comment or question he had rotated her laundry through the machines for her, bringing her the basket of warm clothes so she could take it all to her room to fold and hang.

But it was clear that Wolf still wanted her to move out soon. And she couldn't trust that the next Catholic home she was passed to would be as bearable. She might have to give up on the rosary mafia's help soon. Shirley's web of connections might just have to be tapped. Buying Shirley this lunch counted as a good investment.

...

Maddy came back to her desk to find competing email messages from Giovanni and Liz.

No, no, no, wrote Liz. *I understand that this thing with Giovanni arose in completely different circumstances where he was just on a two-semester sabbatical visit from Pitt, and of course back then it never occurred to you he'd end up applying for a job in your department, or that he'd get it, or that he'd take it – or that he would land on your dissertation committee, for fuck's sake.*

But now there you are and there he is and you just can't anymore – even for fuck's sake. There are other fish in the sea, Mad Girl. Granted, there are few other fish who are going to make you look so good. But this is just going to leave you or him or both of you in a terrible situation. Move along, chica.

On another topic completely, my P.I. is driving me insane. He doesn't seem to understand why I'm doing the current assay the way I'm doing it even though I've explained it and think it is very clever. When I become a Principal Investigator, I will be thrilled to have a grad student as smart as me.

Also, I miss you. And I'm sure Pumpkin misses you. (Spice is not bright enough to know you are gone. He's disappointing me a little in the intelligence department.) Call me when you can and I'll call you right back so Wolf doesn't have to pay the charges.

And from Giovanni:

The Penn program is taking me out for dinner after my lecture there next week, so I can't take you out for a meal when I'm there, but you can come meet me at my hotel when I'm back from the dinner. The wrap dress – bella, wrap up my favorite present, and I'll unwrap it.

I haven't signed the paperwork yet, and soon I'm going to have to. If I put it off much longer, they're going to think I have no faith in you as a student.

Say yes.

Maddy closed her computer and sighed.

Say yes. Was there a sexier imperative a man could utter? It packed in everything – desire, power, deference. She was lost in the thought of him undoing the tie of the dress, feeling his thigh up against hers.

She turned her squeaky 1950s-era swivel chair toward the wall and leaned back to face the tiny window near the ceiling. Through the filthy glass, she could see along the sidewalk a baby carriage move from left to right with a slow, grandmotherly gait pushing it. Then came a yellow dog on a leash followed by a pair of quick, androgynous black pants.

She was trying to figure out what to do. She wanted to meet Giovanni at his hotel. He was good at dressing her, but he was so much better at undressing her, undoing her, while he kissed her on the neck and muttered things half in English and half in Italian. With her limited knowledge of French, she could half-figure it out. All of which led to a delightful confusion, like she was lost in the sexiest parts of a translation dictionary.

And in his hands, she felt a bit like an artwork in creation, the way he paused to look her over and signal appreciation with his eyes before engaging further the tools of his fingers, his lips, his – hamstrings. Oh, that lovely place where his thighs met his torso.

How good that place did smell.

A skinny squirrel stuck its face in the window and looked at her, then jumped back and ran away. The city squirrels of Philadelphia looked remarkably like rats....

Ugh. It was never supposed to be like this with Giovanni. When he had come for his sabbatical from Pittsburgh, he was just supposed to be there for one academic year. He'd just gotten tenure at Pitt, so of *course* he would be going back to Pitt after the sabbatical year. No one changes institutions right after getting tenure, and no one gets hired by another university at that point in his career. The job they had advertised in her own department in Bloomington – the one they ended up hiring him for – wasn't even supposed to be for someone in his area of research. They had advertised for someone in the history of modern physical sciences. It was just because they all liked him so much that he ended up with the job offer.

This thing between him and Maddy – it had started a few weeks into his arrival when they had exchanged a particular glance in the mailroom as they were both arriving to pick up their mail. He had opened an envelope that matched one she was opening. They had received the same invitation to a reception given by the dean for those in the college who had current National Endowments for the Humanities funding. The head of the NEH was coming to town, and the dean wanted to show off the college's chops. Giovanni had NEH funding for his sabbatical; Maddy had it for her dissertation research.

"You going?" asked Giovanni, holding up his copy of the invitation and waving it at her.

She answered that she felt she had to go but didn't have anything that seemed right to wear.

He motioned to her to sit down with him on the mailroom couch. He took a sketchbook out of his messenger bag. She could see, as he turned the pages to find a blank one, that in it he had sketched scenes from his research trips all over Europe – an anatomical theater in London, wax obstetrical models in Florence, the façade of an old bookshop on some narrow street. Finally, he opened to a clean page and sketched a dress he said would look good on her.

She had turned pink at what he drew; he must have imagined her taller and more graceful than she was? But no matter. He was right that, with her hair up, she would look particularly good in that neckline, one that started high around the carotids and came down to the sternum in a sharp-v. He had penned it with a skirt that flared out slightly and a wide belt tied around the waist.

"But where would I find such a thing?" she wondered aloud to him, just as another grad student had walked into the mailroom and looked at the two of them huddled over his sketchpad. "There aren't so many eighteenth-century wax obstetrical models in the U.S.," she added, hoping it would sound to the other student like that's what they had been talking about.

Four days later, he had called her into the office he was using, signaling her silently in the hallway with a twitch of his finger, to give her a big white box with a dress just like the one he had drawn, to wear to the event. It was made from a marvelous fabric – in an eggplant purple – and draped so perfectly. He would not say where he had found it and brushed off her suggestion that she pay him back for it.

"A gift," he said. "Be gracious and accept it. But don't tell anyone."

And just after the dean's reception, when they went back to his place, he was twitching his finger in an even more delightful way, and she was discovering the deliciousness of his sweat. He made such a break from work, from the slow provincial life of academia in Indiana, and from guys her own age, who always felt too young to her. And the conversation before and after was smart. Plus, he supplied good wine. With good olives.

When the department had signed Giovanni Mastromonaco up for the job, her dissertation director Professor Carlyle had said to Giovanni in front of Maddy, "You'll join Maddy's dissertation committee!" as if there was no question. It was only logical; Giovanni's work on early-modern epidemics was close enough, in the scheme of disciplinary spheres, that it would make little sense if he were in her department and *not* on her committee. She needed a fourth member, too.

But this was just so damned awkward. What they had been engaged in was supposed to have been a silly dalliance, an erotic escape, not a professional complication for either one of them. He had told Maddy that he and his partner back in Pittsburgh had a semi-open relationship, an agreement that it was fine to have fun when in different states – "don't ask, don't tell."

But now his partner would likely be coming to take a job in Bloomington, too, or at least coming to visit regularly, and that was just going to make it all the weirder. Just meeting her was going to be incredibly awkward.

But one more time with him? Maddy was pretty sure he had managed to get this talk invitation at Penn specifically to come see her while she would be here. It didn't seem to be a coincidence.

A good hotel room in a real city, that red dress – she could buy a new bra, front-closing to go with the theme of a dress that opens in the front – and what the hell, maybe try garters if they were not too expensive. Or would it look like she was trying too hard?

Maybe she'd figure out a way to ask him what he would like to find between her and the dress.

How, though, was she going to manage this with Wolf? He said he wouldn't be working nights next week, which meant he would be home and would see her leaving in that red dress...and she would have to tell him she might not be back that night, so he would not worry.

Maybe she could claim she was visiting a woman friend in New York for the night and take the dress in an overnight bag? But then what? Change in the lobby restroom of the hotel before going up? The front desk staff would think her a sex worker. Change in his room? That took all the heat out of it.

Besides, Wolf would surely see what was going on. He didn't go into her room – she knew that for sure, because he had said to her yesterday out of the blue, "You know you can take that crucifix over your bed down, if it bothers you," not realizing she had already taken it down days earlier. But even though he didn't go into her room, he seemed very good at seeing right through her. Why else had he so deftly taken, washed, and returned her laundry, without remark?

Not that she should care what Wolf thought of her and Giovanni. It was none of his business. Nevertheless, fooling around with Giovanni in a way that Wolf would figure out felt a bit like bringing a ham-and-cheese sandwich to a Jewish home.

And what was she supposed to think of Giovanni's delay at signing on to her committee for the purposes of fucking her a little more? She hadn't asked him to put it off. The delay seemed to be for his own sake. Which did not exactly speak to him putting her career ahead of his pleasure.

Which did not exactly speak to him being a decent guy.

Plus, now, whether he praised her work or criticized it, his reading of her work was always going to be mentally framed for her in the four-poster bed of the Bloomington house he had rented that year.

Liz was right. This was a mess.

The only way out of this would be some elaborate excuse delivered to Giovanni, out of the hearing-range of Wolf.

But whatever that excuse for not showing up at his hotel room, it would not eliminate her longing to have Giovanni's touch again. She wanted to feel just once more, him slowly sliding his hand down her ass, down toward the hem of whatever he had put her in. The dresses he bought her were always so finely lined, and it had been a true revelation to her – the phyllo created by the layers of his warm hand, the outer fabric of the dress, the cool satin of the lining, the enervated surface of her skin, her pulsing blood vessels underneath.

"Maddy!"

Maddy jumped in her chair and turned quickly around.

"Oh, sorry to startle you, kid," said Shirley, leaning in the doorway. "You've got a phone call."

Maddy followed Shirley into her messy office and picked up the receiver. "Hello?"

"Rabbit, I'm sorry to bother you at work."

"No problem, Wolf," she said. "What's up?"

"I have to work later than I had expected so I need you to go to D'Alio's before they close at six and pick up the lambchops I ordered. I don't want Bernardo ticked off at me. I'll call and let him know you're coming for them."

"Okay," she answered, wondering if he meant that he was having someone else over and if that meant she should pick up and drop off the lambchops and bug out of the house for the evening.

"Wolf, do you need me to do anything with them – or to set up the table for – I mean, if you're having guests – "

There was a pause.

"Sorry, Rabbit," he said, "I thought you'd be home for dinner tonight."

"Oh, you meant for me?"

"Yes," he said. "I don't have to work tonight. I was just going to make me and you lambchops tonight. Do you not like lamb?"

"I love lamb," she answered.

"I know some people think they don't like lamb. But that's because they haven't had good lamb, made correctly."

"I *love* lamb," she said again. "Much better than straw."

"I guess I should have checked to see if you were free for dinner – I just assumed – "

"It's fine," she answered. "I just don't want to assume. I mean, it's fine *you* assumed. Yes, I can do that. I can go get them."

"Thanks. Gotta go," he said, and hung up.

Maddy hung up Shirley's phone and thanked her.

"You eat straw sometimes?" Shirley asked. "*Definitely* leave us your body,

Ms. Shanks. This sounds more interesting than you let on at lunch. A ruminant stomach? How atavistic!"

Shirley pulled out a cadaver donation form from the top drawer of her desk and handed it to Maddy along with a pen.

"Okay, sure," said Maddy without hesitation. She truly didn't care what would happen to her body once she was gone.

Maddy scribbled her signature on the paper, added a date, and handed it back to Shirley. Shirley signed on the line for a witness.

"I called Dr. Wilhelm and he is coming over to meet you," said Shirley, popping a piece of gum in her mouth and handing Maddy a piece. "So, get rid of your beer breath and comb your hair while I print off his bio for you to memorize. If you need to distract him from your real dissertation topic, just talk about your intellectual fathers and their fathers' fathers and their fathers' fathers' fathers. Eventually you two will discover you're academic cousins. Then he'll have to treat you as kin."

-5-

That Maddy had let out not only a scream but literally jumped out of her chair had delighted Shirley and the visitor, both of whom were nearly doubled over with raucous laughter behind Shirley's desk.

Shirley kept trying to stand up and make the introduction properly – "Dr. DesJardins, this is..." – but looking at Maddy's post-alarm disheveled appearance, she just kept bursting into more laughs, her eyes watering. She grabbed a tissue to wipe her tears and handed another down to the visitor, who also seemed to need one.

"Jesus Christ, Shirley," Maddy murmured, trying to settle herself back in the chair. "Honestly."

"Everything okay?" asked Bill, the maintenance man, sticking his head in the door. He had heard the commotion from down the hall. "Oh, hey, Dr. DesJardins! I didn't know you were in town."

Bill came over to the visitor, reached down, and shook his hand.

"Great to see you, Bill," said Nicholas DesJardins, now composing himself. "Shirley and I were just testing the future Dr. Shanks to see if she's afraid of monsters."

"Sounds like the answer is yes," said Bill, smiling and heading back out the door.

Maddy wondered if she should get up again to go shake Dr. DesJardins' hand and introduce herself. But she was sitting there trying to figure out how to undo having made something of an ass of herself.

Shirley had completely set her up. Just as Maddy had been starting her morning cup of coffee in her own office-hole, preparing her note-taking materials to head up to the museum library upstairs, Shirley had stopped by Maddy's door to call her into Shirley's own office. Shirley had told Maddy there was an out-of-town visitor she wanted to introduce to Maddy.

Maddy had followed Shirley into her office. Shirley took her seat behind her desk and Maddy sat in the chair across the desk from Shirley.

Maddy asked Shirley, "So, where is the visitor you wanted me to meet?"

And just then, Dr. DesJardins popped up from behind the desk, yelling "Hello!" and jumping up a little so that his small face cleared the edge of the desk.

Maddy couldn't figure whether it was simply that she didn't know there was another person back there or if it was that he was a dwarf adult that had startled her so, making her jump up and scream and duck as if she'd seen a bat flying at her. It wasn't like she'd never met a person with dwarfism. But you don't expect a grown man a little over three feet tall to suddenly appear from behind a desk and yell a hyper-friendly "hello" at you.

A grown man, she thought to herself. Funny expression, that. Like: *when I was little.*

The man now came around the desk with his right hand outstretched.

"Nicholas DesJardins," he said. "My friends call me Saint Nick."

"Madeleine – Maddy Shanks," said Maddy, reaching out her own hand and standing up instinctively, as one does when one meets someone else who is standing. She immediately felt like a fool for towering over Nick. She should have stayed seated.

"Hey, are you trying to intimidate me?" he said, looking up at her with a mock-scowl while shaking her hand, causing Shirley to keep laughing.

Turning to Shirley, he added, "You didn't warn me that Ms. Shanks is a giant, Shirl."

Maddy sat back down, wondering how red her face was at this point.

"I'm sorry," she said to which Nick replied, "Never apologize for your height around me. You don't need to be ashamed of it. You didn't choose it."

Shirley pushed her own chair around to the front of the desk and Nick climbed onto it with Shirley pulling in another chair from the side of the room and sitting herself down, so that the three of them could sit as a group.

"So, if you are St. Nick," asked Maddy, "how big are your elves?"

"Ooooo!" said Nick to Shirley. "I like this one! How long are you in town, Maddy?"

"A couple of months total," Maddy answered. "I'm working on my dissertation in the history of science and medicine. The collection is important for my dissertation subject."

"Teratology or pathology?" he asked.

"Both," answered Maddy. "I'm interested in it all."

"Nice," he responded. "You don't discriminate between inborn and acquired. None of that *born this way* shit."

"Can you imagine if the little people community made that distinction?" Shirley asked.

"Oh, but they do, Shirl," answered Nick. "I've seen it at the conferences, where there's a disdain among the inborns for the people who come with acquired short stature. Not very pleasant but it's there."

"Yeah," answered Shirley. "You're right."

Maddy thought about it and realized what he meant; there were indeed ways to end up short enough to count as having dwarfism not because of genetic destiny but because of something that happened to you that halted normal growth – a childhood disease or sometimes treatment for a childhood disease, like some cancer treatments, or even psychological trauma. Maddy had always had to wonder if she herself would have been taller than her five-foot-three if The Jerk had not severely restricted her calories the way gymnastics coaches sometimes did with girls. Her parents and her sister had been a few inches taller than she had ended up.

"So, let's test your medical knowledge, Ms. Shanks!" said Nick, interrupting her thoughts. "Why am I interesting?"

"You mean besides your dwarfism?" Maddy asked.

Nicholas DesJardins nodded.

"You were born with cleft lip, too."

He let out a whistle and Shirley bumped him gently on the shoulder with her fist, saying, "I told you she was sharp."

"Good eye, Dr. Shanks! Good eye! And you're getting a Ph.D. and not an M.D.? Maybe a waste of that good eye. Or maybe I should go back and complain to the surgeon who did my primary lip repair. Maybe it's not as good-looking a job as I think!"

"No," Maddy replied. "It's good. Most people wouldn't see it."

"It's generally not what their attention is drawn to," said Nick, chuckling again.

Maddy took another look at Nick's face, feeling like she had license now to stare a little closer at what she had noticed – the trace of a surgical scar above his upper lip. The old name for cleft lip, "hare lip," was just right, as it did look rather like the shape of a rabbit's upper lip when a child was born with it.

She thought about the six-month fetal specimen of a baby with cleft lip upstairs in a jar, donated in 1895 to the museum by the physician who acquired the body after it was stillborn. As Maddy had stared into that jar and tried to sketch it in her notebook, she had had to wonder if the mother had had any idea how her child's body ended up, developmentally or geographically.

"Cleft lip indeed, coincident with dwarfism, which makes me a rare and valuable bird," Nick said, blowing on his fingernails and polishing them on his shirt in a dramatic gesture. "And I have not just a cleft lip but what we think is an honest-to-God midline defect."

"Signs?" asked Maddy, realizing a moment later this could come across as a rude question considering that the developmental problems that show up with the midline defects can include not only the face, brain, heart, and spine, but the genitals, too – anything that fell on the vertical center line of the body.

"Just lip and heart, so far as we know," Nick answered, pulling his left foot toward him to tie his shoe. Maddy noticed that his shirt had French cuffs with cufflinks made of silver, matching his tie clip. "No signs of schizophrenia. And I've just cleared forty, so. We think my brain formed according to the normal developmental playbook."

"Nick is a clinical psychologist," Shirley explained. "Ph.D. from Columbia. He lives in Ohio now. He's in Philly to see Dr. Wilhelm. Maddy met Dr. Wilhelm a few days ago."

"I'm trying to start a bidding war," said Nick.

Shirley shifted in her seat uncomfortably and asked him what he meant.

"Oh, I didn't tell you – I've got another doc interested in me. Younger fellow, Dr. Coman, out of Cleveland Clinic. I figure I can start a bidding war between him and Dr. Wilhelm – see who will give me a better deal for access to my celebrity bod."

Shirley made a sour face and Nick laughed at it.

"Shirley doesn't like the idea I might see *other doctors*," said Nick, in a loud whisper to Maddy. "She's the exclusive recruiter for Dr. Wilhelm's team."

"I'm happy to have anyone do good science and good medicine," answered Shirley. "But it's hard for me to believe you're going to find some-body more qualified than Dr. Wilhelm and his team."

Looking to change the subject, Maddy asked Nick how he got into clinical psychology. He replied that as an undergrad at Yale he had taken a couple of classes in the field and become fascinated with it, so with the encouragement of a mentor, he decided to pursue a Ph.D. in clinical psychology at Columbia.

"And why did you end up in Ohio?" she asked.

"My wife's family is from there," he answered. "I lost my wife to lymphoma a year ago."

"I'm sorry to hear that," Maddy said. "But you're staying put in Ohio?"

"Yes, for now anyway. We put down roots there and my neighbors all know me and I know them, which makes my life easier, and I've got an active clinical practice with people who have come to depend on me. So, I'm not interested in moving right now. Were your born with anything special? Any hidden charms, Ms. Shanks?"

"No," said Maddy, "nothing of interest physically."

"Psychologically, then?" asked Nick, smiling at her.

"Totally monstrous – totally acquired," answered Maddy and, seeing him cock his head, she laughed to make clear she was joking. "I'm kidding," she added. "Joke about being raised Catholic."

But now he was only looking at her with more interest.

"What's your dissertation on?"

Maddy looked at Shirley and understood from the glance back that she ought to be careful how she described her focus given Shirley's political concerns. She thought about how to explain her work in a way that would be both honest and vague.

"I'm interested in the history of power dynamics between people who had – well, interesting bodies – I don't think of them as 'monstrous' any more than you really do – I'm interested in the history of the power dynamics between them and the medical and scientific men who studied and treated them. Nineteenth century is my main area. Mostly American plus some European."

"Very good," said Nick, nodding. "Very good topic."

Maddy was looking at his face, to look for his age. He said he had cleared forty and that looked just about right – he looked to be in his early forties, with the telltale dermatological topography around the eyes. (Maddy had always wondered how the morticians removed those from her mother's face and made her look so young.)

"And you've found...?" Nick asked.

"Forgive me if what I'm going to say is terribly obvious to you with all your education in the history of anomalies," answered Maddy, "but the common assumption is that doctors and scientists back then had all the power. Because they have so much power now, people think that must have been even more true back in the days of things like the brutal enslavement of Africans and the legal subjugation of women. But in earlier times, when medicine and science were relatively less mature, some people with unusual anatomies managed to maintain the upper hand – while they were alive, anyway – particularly if they were white and came from money. But even sometimes if they weren't. An interesting body could sometimes give you power to overcome points against you for race and class and gender."

"Ah, race and class and gender. Those things certainly do matter as birth-rights," said Nick. "Look at me – I didn't get to Yale and Columbia just by my good looks and book smarts."

"Shut up," said Shirley jokingly, looking more at ease since the conversation was going well. "You know you're a brilliant and attractive guy."

"Aw, stop buttering me up, girl," Nick said to Shirley. Turning to Maddy, he added, "Shirley just wants to get in my pants. She wants to know how far my midline goes."

They all laughed for a moment.

"So, nineteenth century – that means you probably don't remember Ambroise Paré's thirteen causes of monstrosities?"

Maddy scrunched up her face trying to remember them.

"I know you're talking about Paré's *Monstres et Prodiges*," she said. "From 1573. I can probably name a few. Let me try. I know that God and the Devil are two of the causes he named for birth anomalies?"

"The first is the glory of God, and the second, His wrath!" answered Nick, standing up on the chair and pointing to the ceiling for added drama. Then he pointed to the floor. "The thirteenth is Demons and Devils!"

He sat back down.

"So, you're just missing all the ones in between, Maddy. That's better than most people do. But you're lucky they didn't ask you this question on your Ph.D. qualifying exams."

"Wait – the mother's imagination!" said Maddy, naming another she could recall. "And something about semen – I mean, 'seed'?"

"Better than most, indeed," Shirley said to Nick. "You have to give her credit."

Nick then stood up on the chair again and launched into the full list from Paré's text, one of the earliest dedicated to the question of what could cause children to be born with unexpected body types. He delivered it as if it were an important monologue from Shakespeare.

The first cause is the glory of God.

The second, His wrath.

The third, too great a quantity of seed.

The fourth, too little a quantity.

The fifth, the imagination.

The sixth, the narrowness or smallness of the womb.

The seventh, the indecent posture of the mother, as when, being pregnant, she has sat too long with her legs crossed, or pressed against her womb.

The eighth, through a fall, or blows struck against the womb of the mother, being with child.

The ninth, through hereditary or accidental illness.

The tenth, through rotten or corrupt seed.

The eleventh, through the mixture or mingling of seed.

The twelfth, through the artifice of wicked spital beggars.

The thirteenth, through Demons and Devils.

"Goodness," said Maddy when Nick had finished his recitation and sat back down. "I never considered how many of them have to do with semen. All that talk of seed."

"Oh, yes," said Nick, interlocking his fingers and laying his clasped hands in his lap. "We talk nowadays about always blaming the mother, but Paré's list invoked mostly *male* power, don't you think, Maddy? God, the Devil, and the father's bad seed."

"My personal favorite is the mingling or mixing of seed," giggled Shirley. "I guess Paré did not approve of threesomes."

"Or women who cheat," said Maddy. "I assume that's what that one is about. A woman who sleeps with one man and another soon after. Unto her shall *not* be born the King of Bethlehem."

Nick looked delighted at Maddy's responses.

"You ever been to the annual, Maddy?" he asked, leaning forward slightly.

"The annual what?"

"Conference," he answered. "National Association of Little People. I ask because it's in D.C. this year, in a little less than a month – easy trip down on the train from here."

"No," answered Maddy, "but I'm sure it would be interesting."

She was saying this to be polite. This was not the kind of conference that would have a lot of discussion of the kind she was interested in – history of medicine and science.

"I think you might find the modern power dynamics interesting," Nick told her, and Shirley nodded. "But I also ask because I help put the program together and I'm wondering if we should have you give a talk about the history. I've always felt it's something the community should know more about. It helps us understand how stigma is culturally specific, something I'm always trying to emphasize to people there and back home in my clinical practice. Everybody's dealing with stigma, but they don't get it's culturally specific and always has been. Always will be. We could change that culture."

Maddy's eyebrows went up in curiosity. He continued.

"The point you made, about race and social class and gender mattering, well, it might help the community start to talk about those things and how they matter within the community. We've got elephants all over the room stepping on us sometimes! Bringing somebody in from the outside can help us talk about the elephants."

"You might want a different metaphor if you talk about it there, Mad," said Shirley, putting the tip of her index finger on her chin. "Avoid the circus imagery?"

"Ha!" responded Nick. "Elephants and dwarves and landmines, oh my! That's what we've got in the room. But that's what makes the annual a blast – that, and a lot of good company. And some assholes. Seriously, it's an interesting gathering and I'd be happy to set you up if you like."

"That would be an honor, Dr. DesJardins," said Maddy genuinely, realizing he was right that it would probably be fascinating and would also help Maddy think about how to present her work in a way that interested people who lived with the conditions she was researching. "I would love to have that opportunity and that experience."

As if he could read where her mind went next, he went on:

"We've got no money left in the budget this late in the game. Can you get yourself there – pay your own way and all?"

"For sure," answered Maddy. "I have research travel money I can put to it."

She was especially glad right now that Wolf was saving her so much money.

"Great. I'll see what I can set up. Write down your name and email address for me and I'll copy you on the email about it to the program committee. That way they will have to say yes."

Shirley reached behind her to grab a pad of paper and a pen from the stacks on her desk. She handed them to Maddy and gave her gave her a look that equated to a thumbs-up. Maddy had managed to impress Dr. Wilhelm a couple days earlier and Dr. DesJardins today. Two for two; not bad.

-6-

It seemed quite impossible that Margaret Lovisa could be speaking from inside the sealed jar of preservative fluid.

First of all, how could one speak in a jar of liquid without inhaling the fluid and drowning?

Second, how could Lovisa be speaking so calmly to a perfect stranger as if all were normal when Lovisa was stark naked?

And third – not least – she was dead.

But there Margaret Lovisa was, telling Maddy that Maddy could interview her if she liked – ask her what she pleased.

And Maddy was politely telling her back, while trying to make sure to look at her face and not her gnarled hands or her exposed genitals, that there was no need. Lovisa was so recently dead (just two or three years gone?) that her history, like her small body, had presumably been preserved quite well by Dr. Wilhelm. There wasn't anything Maddy felt she needed to ask.

"I don't do oral histories," Maddy told her, awkwardly. "I'm not that kind of historian. I do *dead* people."

"But I *am* dead!" protested Lovisa, lifting a cup of tea from a matching, finely painted saucer and bringing it to her lips. The pattern looked to Maddy to be Royal Albert, Old Country Roses. They had had a partial set of that china at the convent, pieces that someone had donated from an estate.

"I *am* dead!" protested Lovisa again.

"But your eyes – " said Maddy.

Lovisa was just a little over three feet tall – about the height of Dr. DesJardins – but being in the jar on top of the table meant Maddy could look her straight in the eyes. In fact, Maddy had to look up to her a little.

"Your eyes – " Maddy said again.

"Windows to the soul!" answered Lovisa.

Maddy looked to the left to see the aquarium that held Wolf and his wife, frozen, looking at the camera, smiling. But they did not seem to be smiling exactly? And their clothes did not hang on them quite right. Their garments should have been ever so slightly lifted, inflated by the preserving fluid. Instead, they looked as if they were out in the plain air. They were both so still. Completely still. Not like Lovisa, so mobile.

Just then, Maddy became aware of Dr. Wilhelm and his colleagues being behind her. She turned to see them there. The residents and attending physicians were filling up seats in the rows of an anatomical theater. Wilhelm stood between Maddy and them. She looked over their ranks: the tall and sad-faced Russian, the ruddy-cheeked Greek, the dull-affect fellow with the dull name of Jones.…Not a woman among the lot of them. Not all white, but not a woman.

"Will you not take off the dress, Miss Shanks, and let us examine you?" Dr. Wilhelm asked with his clipped Austrian accent in his stiff manner, looking over his reading glasses, standing before his colleagues and trainees, sounding a little impatient.

She knew what they would see under her dress. Maybe they knew, too. That horrid growth protruding out from her belly, made of a tangle of metal, like a hairbrush.

No; barbed wire.

No; steel wool.

She could feel its shape, its harsh edges, through the fabric of her dress. Even without feeling it, she knew it was there. It had been there for so long. And they would see, if they saw it, that it was inoperable. Inoperable and fascinating to everyone but her.

She realized with a start that she had signed a cadaver donation form, the one Shirley had handed her. She could not get that signed form back.

Her eyes started to water, and Dr. Wilhelm was asking her, "What? Are you a child?"

This only made her fall toward a full-on fit of crying. For it was of course what The Jerk used to say to her to try to stop her from crying – "What? Are you still a child?"

She felt so deeply foolish for breaking down in front of these men. All these men expecting her to perform, and she could not. But maybe like The Jerk they would be content if she would just lie there and let them do what they wanted. She tried to think of the whale.

She could hear Margaret Lovisa now behind her, saying, "Don't be foolish, you know perfectly well that when you're dead, none of it matters. It doesn't matter then whether you do this or that, whether they do this or that to you. You know it doesn't matter once you're dead. That's why you signed the form!"

Maddy felt Lovisa's small hand touch her shoulder from behind and let out a whelp. Then she could feel the hose tangled around her legs, and she could see the fluid coming from the hose starting to rise, as one of Dr. Wilhelm's residents in a modern white coat was holding the end of the hose, filling up the glass tank in which she was now standing, filling it with the preservative – and another was lifting her dress to see the growth –

And now she could hear someone banging on the side of the tank yelling, trying to get her attention as she was crying, struck with panic –

"Let me in!"

It sounded like Wolf? But was he not locked with his wife in the aquarium?

"Unlock the door, Rabbit! *Maddy, unlock your door! Now!*"

She untangled her feet from the bedding, sat up, stumbled to the door and unlocked it. Wolf forced the door quickly open and pushed past her, looking rapidly around the room, going to the window to see it was closed, looking under the bed and in the closet. He was in the sweatpants and t-shirt in which he slept, his hair disheveled.

"Are you okay?" he asked, coming near her.

She had trouble answering.

"Nightmare?" he asked.

She nodded, standing there shaking and cringing a little. She wiped the tears off her face with the back of her hand.

"When you fell at the gym this evening, did you hit your head?"

She shook her head "no."

"Should not have fed you that linguine," he said, rubbing the back of his neck hard with his hand. "The sauce was too heavy. It was terrible."

She did not answer.

"Should not have told you about the rapes," he said a little quieter.

She shook her head left to right twice. She realized then that he would think she meant she agreed – that he should not have told her about the rapes – but what she meant was that that was not it. It was not the rapes.

He did not say – as she thought he should or that she should – that they should not have had that argument. He did not say, as she wished, that he forgave her for the stupid things she had said after too much wine, about how crazy he was to keep his wife on life support and leave her suspended between life and death and leave himself in the same state of suspension –

In the same suspension. That is why she had had this dream, of he and his wife suspended in that aquarium, Margaret Lovisa in her own suspension, the fluid.

Well, that and what she had seen at Dr. Wilhelm's office that day. That and the conversation with Nick DesJardins a few days before....

"Can I call Liz?" she asked in a small voice, feeling like she was back in the convent asking one of the sisters in the middle of the night if she could please have some aspirin. It was one of the things for which she could ask that sometimes helped. She could not ask to call anyone; there was no one to call. She dared not ask for diaries in which to write her thoughts; someone might then see them. She used the notebooks they gave her only for her studies.

"Of course, you can call Liz. You can call anybody you want."

He turned on the light in the stairwell for her and led the way down, handing her the phone receiver while he poured a glass of milk and then warmed it up using the microwave.

"Liz?" she asked, trying to sit down calmly but in fact collapsing into one of the kitchen chairs. "Oh Margie, I am sorry. Can you please put Liz on? It's Maddy. Liz? I am sorry to call you in the middle of night."

Wolf could hear Liz assure Maddy it was okay. Maddy's tear ducts started to weep like wet washcloths being rung out over the sink. He could hear Liz ask Maddy what was wrong.

He stirred the glass of milk with a spoon, put the glass down in front of her, put the spoon in the sink, and went back upstairs.

-7-

"But Mad," said Liz, after listening for a few minutes, "you know this was just an exceptionally weird nightmare. Just a terrible dream."

Liz was talking in a normal voice, no longer in a whisper, since she'd moved to her living room so that Margie could go back to sleep.

"It's holding on to me. Like a cobweb I can't brush off, Liz," said Maddy.

She was on Wolf's living room couch now, under a blanket with one small lamp turned on behind her. Wolf had gone back up to bed on the third floor, and Maddy was speaking as quietly as she could.

"It just feels like this dream is clinging to me."

"It's because it is the middle of the night, Mad. Your sleep hormones have a hold on your brain, and they are holding you just outside of rationality. It's hard this time of night to walk back into rational thought."

Maddy did not reply.

"Talk to me about where all the parts of this came from, and then you will see it was just your brain mixing up all the files in the cabinet of your mind. That's what happens in sleep."

"But I think – I think it was seeing something – something significant – "

Liz stopped her and told her to take a deep breath and just answer her this: Why were all those doctors in the rows, watching her, with Dr.

Wilhelm in the lead?

Maddy explained that Dr. Wilhelm had been setting up a talk for her to give to the doctors of the medical society, about the history of anatomy. With Shirley, Dr. Wilhelm was setting up the details of the event and making invitations for it. So of course, in the dream, they were all sitting in the rows of an anatomical theater, because she was going to soon have to give a talk to them all in reality about the history of anatomy – about anatomy and power.

"But you've noted that they were all men in the dream. And Dr. Wilhelm was asking you in the dream to take off your dress?"

Maddy explained that was because Shirley had joked to Maddy that Maddy would have to be a "history geisha" to them for an afternoon, that she would have to charm and distract them from the fact that she was working on specimen acquisition.

"Admit why else," Liz nudged. "Admit why else they were all men and you were expected to take your clothes off."

"I know you're right, Liz."

"Say it."

"Because on Thursday – wait, that's today now, isn't it? It's like three in the morning now, isn't it. So, right, later on today, you know, I'm supposed to see Giovanni. I get that. I get that that part of the dream wasn't just about Dr. Wilhelm and the talk I have to give. It's because I feel like I'm in a mode where I know I'm supposed to be presenting myself professionally, I'm *wanting* to present myself professionally, and I'm being asked to take off my clothes. And it feels wrong. I know, Liz. I get it."

"Okay. I know that seems kind of obvious. But I want to point out you *know* it is making you feel gross. It's not just me saying it's a problem. You know it's a problem."

Liz waited to see if Maddy would answer, but she did not.

"Wait, Mad, why were Wolf and his wife there, and why in an aquarium tank?"

Maddy explained that in the dream she could see them exactly, life-size, reproduced from a photo Wolf had in a frame hanging in the stairwell that went from the first floor to the second. That was why their clothes were not behaving like they would in fluid. The dream simply had them life-size instead of contained in five by seven inches.

"I have looked at that photo, when he is not home, again and again, trying to understand why he holds on to her, why he keeps her alive with food and with antibiotics to fight infections. I said stupid things to him to-night at dinner about his situation. About her suspending him. God, I was so stupid and insensitive."

"You?!" said Liz sarcastically.

"Shut up," answered Maddy with no humor in her voice.

She went on to explain that Wolf had told her over dinner just before they argued that he looked into the eyes of his wife to try to see if her soul was still there or if she had left, if it was time to let her body go, too. And Maddy had answered that he had let his wife suspend *him*, that his wife had put him in a kind of persistent vegetative state by virtue of her own.

He had gotten so angry at Maddy that he had told her to fuck off.

"And he never talks to me like that," said Maddy to Liz. "He literally would not speak to me after that."

"Talk about biting the hand that feeds you, you idiot," said Liz. "Did it occur to you that you were beating up on him because you don't feel so great about the relationship choices you're making?"

Maddy didn't answer, and then asked how Pumpkin was doing.

"You're not changing the subject on me," responded Liz. "You don't get to call me in the middle of the night and wake up my girlfriend and then ask me about a rat. You know I'm here for you, but come on. So, tell me why this other person – what was her name – in the jar?"

"Margaret Lovisa," said Maddy. "She was a dwarf. Dr. Wilhelm studies growth and he had her in a jar of preservative in his back office, at his research office."

"You mean in the dream."

"No, Liz," said Maddy, "for real. He had me over to his research office yesterday. I guess he invited me there to impress me. He knows I'm interested in anatomical collections and so he was showing me his. He had a bunch of fingers and a mounted skeleton of a dwarf. And she was there, Margaret Lovisa. He told me her name and some of her history. And in the preservation – well – her eyes were sort of open."

Liz didn't respond. She wasn't sure what to say.

"I don't know if those were her real eyes or glass replacements. She looked kind of sleepy but, well, like she was looking back at me. And I was struck, Liz – I mean, I know it is stupid to say it – but it felt, looking in her eyes, like she was looking back at me and her soul was still there."

"That sounds like what Wolf said to you. That doesn't sound like something you would say."

"Well, I'm saying it now. I don't mean it *literally*," Maddy replied, rubbing her forehead with her free hand. "I don't mean I suddenly believe in souls. I just mean – well, it's one thing when there is a preservation from the nineteenth century, when there is a naked person in a jar and it all happened in the nineteenth century. I'm *used* to that. But I was a little startled to see a twenty-first century preservation of a person who had been a patient of his like this, in that style of the nineteenth century. It felt – "

Liz did not fill in the pause.

"It felt, Liz, a little like you go to someone's house, some white person's house, and you discover they have a black person as a slave, serving them. Like it's the fucking early-nineteenth century?"

"What else did he have?"

"Multiple bodies. And tissue preservation – slides, and cell cultures. You know, now it's a lot of cellular metabolism studies and genetics. He only needs bodies because he also studies the bone and ligament growth and you need cadavers to get at that. He told me that. That there's nothing like a complete specimen. There was that mounted skeleton of another former patient. I forget that man's name now. It just – I guess it bothered me. It seems strange because I'm so used to seeing people preserved and mounted and all. Maybe it's because I met a person with dwarfism the other day? A clinical psychologist....Anyway, usually it doesn't affect me, human anatomical preserves. But Dr. Wilhelm's collection – it really unsettled me."

"Yeah, *well*," answered Liz.

"I don't know, maybe it was his manner? But maybe it was what Shirley said."

Maddy explained that Shirley, the curator, had given her some advice: that when Maddy was talking and writing about people with anomalies, she should always imagine the person before her had a child of their own with that very anomaly. To avoid saying anything insensitive. Maddy figured Shirley gave her the short lecture because she was afraid Maddy might think everyone at the little people conference would be as comfortable with dark humor as she and Dr. DesJardins. Whatever the reason for the talking-to, Shirley warned her to remember there are limits to how much you can joke. That these are real people, some just different from the social norm, some with real pain and suffering.

"I think that's why Margaret Lovisa was alive in the dream? – what Shirley said about remembering these are real people? Or maybe it was just seeing her. Like that."

"Does her family know she is there?"

"I don't know," said Maddy, "but I would guess so. She gave her permission – Dr. Wilhelm told me that she wanted him to have her body. That she was very grateful to him for his clinical care and especially his research. That she had been clear she wanted to help his research, have something come of her suffering."

Liz didn't say anything.

"She had had pain from back problems, from hip problems. He said her suffering ended with a quick death."

"But did she want him to have her body, well, *like that*?"

Maddy answered that she had no idea. The forms in all likelihood, she said, had been general cadaver donation forms. (She didn't tell Liz she had signed one herself on museum letterhead with Shirley as a witness. Nor did she tell Liz that, when Maddy had later asked Shirley if she had signed the same form, Shirley had said, "No way! I have to work with these people. I'm being cremated." It was an answer that made no sense to Maddy.)

"Want to talk about why you had those metal growths show up again?"

"Do we need to?" asked Maddy.

"No," Liz said.

They were a recurrent theme in Maddy's nightmares – tumors of barbed wire, of twisted metal, of steel wool, always ulcerated from her uterus. Broken through the skin, visible, painful, freakish.

"You think *every bad dream* is about The Jerk," said Maddy. "Maybe not every bad dream is about him and what happened to me."

"Or maybe every bad dream no matter how it starts welcomes him to show up. The way a light attracts insects. Only he's attracted by the dark – the dark parts in your brain. He shows up when you think you can't do it – that you can't finish your degree and go on with your life. You're always afraid he's going to pop back up and ruin it all, right?"

Maddy did not reply. She realized the blanket wasn't enough to keep her warm. Maybe it was just because she needed to pee.

"Is something going on that might be making your memory tap there – tap The Jerk?"

Maddy didn't answer. She had not thought about it until Liz asked this but she realized now that Liz was probably right: the sexually coercive position she felt herself in with Giovanni was probably scratching at those memories of The Jerk's sexual coercion that had started when she was twelve. And it couldn't help to have had Shirley joking about Maddy having to make herself something of a sexual object to men in power, suggesting Maddy lie about the scene, lie about what she was there to do –

Lying about lying about.

The phrase popped into her head, like a rhetorical joke from a treasonous part of her grey matter. She could not believe she was spending so much time thinking about The Jerk since she'd gotten the Philadelphia. Was it just being on the East Coast again? Was it that he just showed up in her subconscious as the embodiment of her anxieties about never finishing her degree, about failing?

Maddy told Liz to hang on while she went and used the bathroom. She soon picked back up the phone. She wanted to change the subject, but Liz was right about her off-kilter mental status. It felt like she had one foot still in the dream and one in reality, as if she were walking along a street with one foot up on the curb and the other in the gutter. Like a balance beam she couldn't seem to mount.

"Wolf got me time at a gym this evening after work, before dinner, some time on the mats, some time on the rings. I had asked him to help me find a gym for that."

"Oh, well, no wonder you'd have allusions to The Jerk in that nightmare! No wonder the metal tumors showed up again. No matter how much you feel like you have yourself back, Mad, being so close to New York and doing gymnastics is surely going to bring back thoughts of The Jerk, given that he was your coach there – out east. I'm not saying you shouldn't go to the gym and do those things – do gymnastics – I think you *should*. You absolutely should. I think you're right you have to own yourself with that physical work. But it has to stir up some things."

"I know," said Maddy. "I got stuck at the gym this evening when I was working on an aerial. And I kind of fell. I think because The Jerk was there for a second, in my head. There's something about the blue of the mats that evokes a certain memory...."

After a moment's pause, she added, "Oh, yeah, that's right – in the dream, the dress I was wearing was exactly that blue. The blue of the mats."

"Did you tell Wolf?"

"Tell him what?"

"About The Jerk?"

"No," Maddy answered. "Of course not. Why would I tell him that? But his basement – his basement is just like The Jerk's. I mean, not *just* like it, but it has weights with a bench and I couldn't bring myself to go down there to do my laundry. I'm working on it. I think by next week, I'll be able to go down there and do laundry."

Maddy paused to remember Wolf silently handing her the basket of her clean clothes.

"You know, Liz, Wolf is kind of the opposite of The Jerk."

She realized immediately that that sounded wrong – like she was comparing a sexual relationship to her relationship with Wolf.

"What I mean is I'm not at all in a position today like I was back then," Maddy added quickly. "I'm perfectly okay. I keep reminding myself that The Jerk has been out of my life for a decade and I don't have to have him in my head."

Maddy could hear that Liz was getting herself a glass of water.

"So, Mad, you understand this dream was just a bunch of layers of anxieties, a bunch of anxious references – a kind of club sandwich of anxiety – and it doesn't mean anything?"

"I don't see how you can say it doesn't mean anything," answered Maddy, standing up to take the empty milk glass back to the kitchen. "Obviously I feel guilty about what I said to Wolf. Obviously, I feel conflicted about seeing Giovanni later. Obviously, I feel gross about presenting to these doctors – "

"Fine. But you knew all these things."

"I don't think I knew how disturbed I was by Dr. Wilhelm's collection. That feels like the one cobweb I can't brush off. Or maybe it's the rapes."

Liz asked Maddy what she was talking about.

"Wolf told me there's a serial rapist they're trying to catch. Attacking women in their homes. At first, when he started talking about it over dinner this evening, it just sounded like the shit you hear on the news – you know, basically a morbid curiosity of a story – but then, well, he got upset telling me some about the latest one, telling me what will probably make it to the news, and what won't make it into the news – some of it was so disturbing. I think that's why he flipped out when he heard me screaming and crying in my room. Why he almost broke down my door."

"Jesus," answered Liz. "And you wonder why you had a nightmare after he told you about a serial rapist? Are you safe there?"

"I live with a cop," said Maddy. "A cop who brings a gun home every day and puts it on the kitchen counter with his keys and his wallet before he takes it upstairs. A cop who won't fuck anybody because he loves his wife just that much and because he's just that Catholic. A cop with grates on the first-floor windows and three locks on each door. Hard to believe I could be safer."

"So why did you lock the door to your bedroom? You said Wolf had to bang on the door to get you to let him in?"

Maddy didn't answer. She didn't tell Liz that, for reasons she could not quite articulate, she had started locking her bedroom door after Manny the creep had come in her room, that night of the poker game.

"And what about when Wolf is not home? Are you safe then?"

"Come on, Liz," said Maddy. "Statistically, I'm about as safe as any woman can be. Meaning – well, you know as well as I do: the odds of being sexually assaulted by a familiar are a lot higher than by a stranger. We both know that."

At that, the two of them went quiet.

"How's Margie?" Maddy finally asked.

"Tired of me working so much. I think she thought all that time you and I spent together was going to turn into time she and I would spend together, once you went to Philly."

"So, she didn't get we were just both working most of that time together?"

"I tried to tell her that!" answered Liz. "But I guess she thought you and I were goofing off all the time we spent hanging out working in the same spaces."

Maddy thought to herself that if Margie had heard the conversations they did have, she would have realized they were almost all about work – figuring out how to handle a research problem, struggling to write a paper or a grant, working out some professional challenge involving collaborators or rivals or the people with the power to dole out resources.

"Well," said Maddy, "that's what you get for dating someone who isn't an academic. They don't get us. But that's the upside, too."

"Yeah," agreed Liz. "That's what makes being with her a *relief*. She isn't an academic."

"That and the sex," said Maddy, and she gave out a small laugh.

"That and the sex," said Liz. "She's wonderful in bed. God, her body, her hair, her smile. And her paintings are genuinely magical. And you know me – I'm not an art person. You gonna see Giovanni later today?"

"I don't know," Maddy sighed. "I know I shouldn't. I also know that knowing I shouldn't is part of why it's so hot. And, fuck, I love the heat."

Liz muttered something that Maddy couldn't quite make out, but the tone suggested she did understand.

"My plan is this: I'm going to his lecture at Penn this afternoon and I'll have my backpack plus the dress and heels and all that in a separate tote bag, so the dress doesn't get crushed. I can't wear it to the talk or I'll be totally overdressed and look ridiculous. When he goes off to dinner with the faculty, I'll take myself out somewhere for dinner, read a book, and then use the restaurant bathroom to change before I meet him at his hotel."

Liz said the plan made sense, but she said it without enthusiasm.

"I just don't want you to feel crappy about this afterwards, Mad," said Liz.

"You don't want me calling you in the middle of the night to tell you I did something stupid that gave me a bad dream?"

"We are a stupid, stupid species, but smart enough to invent the telephone," Liz answered by way of not really answering. "Listen, you're not going to be able to sleep now, Mad Girl. The dream won't leave you alone if you go back to bed. You'll lie there and stew and make it worse. So just get up and work."

"On what?" Maddy asked.

"What do you want to work on?"

"I want to look up Wilhelm's work. I want to see what he might have said about Margaret Lovisa. I want to see if he's written anything in his published medical reports about this clinical psychologist I met – Nicholas DesJardins. And the other people he's treated, especially the people who became his full-body specimens after death. It's bothering me."

"So why don't you do that?"

"No internet here," Maddy explained. "Plus a lot of the papers will probably require me pulling copies of journals at a medical library. Not sure the museum library would have them."

"So, for now, do something else. Translations. Do one or two of those."

"Okay. You go back to sleep, Lizard," answered Maddy. "And thank you."

She hung up the phone back in the kitchen, went to her room, closed her door behind her, and switched on the lamp on the desk. As she bent over to pull her laptop out of her backpack, she noticed her bed had been made and turned down. The tangle of her sheets had been made calm. She noticed Wolf had also added an extra blanket, folded neatly at the end of the bed.

She opened her door again, just a few inches, and looked up the stairs at his. For the first time she could recall, he had left his bedroom door open.

She closed her door again, turned the lock, and looked back at the bed. What was it about the way the sheet and blanket were turned down so neatly that evoked the shoulders of the human form?

Then Maddy remembered suddenly a snippet of a different dream – when had she even had it? It was a dream of burrowing her nose just south of a masculine clavicle, that tight spot near the shoulder with a trampoline's give, just above the armpit. Naked, flesh against flesh, feeling so nicely fucked, hearing herself let out a moan of happy abandon. Nothing wrong.

The dream seemed in her mind for a moment as large as the night sky of the West Virginia convent's mountaintop, then suddenly as small as a single star of light. So disorienting was this oneiric shadow sweeping over her. But who even was it in that dream? Giovanni?

The sensation gone, she sighed and set herself up to translate another text. This one, from 1881, was about a set of conjoined twins – omphalopagus, stuck together at the umbilicus.

(Would she be stuck together at the umbilicus with Giovanni later that day?)

"Omphalopagus," thought Maddy, focusing her concentration as she had first learned to do for floor routines. "Omphalopagus. As named in the taxonomy and nomenclature of Isidore Geoffroy Saint-Hilaire, coiner of the term *teratology*, based on the root *teratos*."

Teratos, meaning "monster" or "marvel," and yet, in the 1830s, the French anatomist Geoffroy Saint-Hilaire had moved well beyond the medieval visions of Paré of monsters and marvels to create an anatomical philosophy, a means of understanding all forms of human flesh, no matter how startling. There was a profound rationality to all body types for him; all were connected together in the natural logic of development. He did not know of genes, yet his understanding presaged the genetic code – with his belief that all possibilities are contained within the natural world. No need for appeal to the supernatural. *Nature is one whole*, Isidore Geoffroy Saint-Hilaire insisted. No human flesh was monstrous, really. Nothing was beyond explanation.

There are no organic forms which are not subject to laws; and the word 'disorder,' taken literally, cannot be applied to natural productions.

However goofily Romantic in his grand visions the early-nineteenth-century Geoffroy Saint-Hilaire might be, Maddy did so prefer his textual company to that of Paré, the sixteenth-century invoker of wizardly beggars and rotten seed, of the Almighty and the Devil. For Geoffroy Saint-Hilaire, every body was created subject to a rational law of biological development. Every body came and went simply natural. Nothing was truly abnormal because everything made sense, once you understood the developmental causes. You just had to dig deeper, catalogue more, think across it all. (Think, not pray.)

<h1 style="text-align:center">-8-</h1>

Funny, the medical reference librarian thought to himself. Funny how a person could be earning a Ph.D. in history and not have heard of the Freedom of Information Act. But then historians tended to be so specific in what it was they wanted to know about, just like neurologists, and surgeons, and oncologists, and everybody in the specialties. How far might the human race advance (and how quickly!) if researchers were interested in what the other fields wanted to know?

He was pleased to have had the opportunity to educate the grad student about the Act and some other useful tools for subjects more modern than what she said was her usual period of focus. As he'd told her, too many medical researchers saw the Freedom of Information Act as a tool only of journalists rather than a useful option for anyone interested in obtaining un-published reports and budgets and communications from the last fifty years or so in medical education, public health, medical research, and the like. It was perfect for historians working on contemporary issues. Because much of modern medical research and public health was funded or regulated by the government, much was potentially available through a FOIA request. Whatever was in the government's possession, one could at least ask to see.

She had looked to him a little young for a grad student. But maybe he was just getting old?

Her outfit conformed to the standard of her discipline: khaki slacks; simple short boots with enough of a heel to make them a little dressy; a neat, white, button-down shirt; a short string of pearls; finished with a light-brown jacket from what must have been a suit. All she was missing were the elbow patches. But those were usually confined to the male of the species.

Following his explanation of the Freedom of Information Act, the grad student had told him she wasn't sure she would want to bother with it. But then, after she appeared to think about it for just a moment, she reeled off a number of questions that he thought good ones: What wording would speed up or slow down a response to a FOIA request made to the National Institutes of Health? What might increase or reduce the odds of being charged a fee by the NIH for the FOIA response? And would the researcher whose grant reports were the subject of her FOIA request be notified of her interest?

When asking the last question, she had mentioned knowing the confidentiality code of librarians – that librarians do not tell other people what a patron wants to see or to know. She had asked him if the same privacy rule would be followed by the clerks who would answer a Freedom of Information Act request from her at the NIH. She said it would not be that big a deal if the researcher whose work she was interested in knew that she was looking. But he might find it a *little* funny that she wanted to look at his unpublished material.

The librarian explained to her that FOIA clerks were not professional librarians but that, in his experience and based on what he had learned at conferences, FOIA clerks also did not tend to be people who were looking to complicate their jobs by notifying subjects of relatively ordinary requests. So, as long as what she was looking for was easy for the FOIA clerks to pull, photocopy, and send on to her, odds were good that they would not bother to mention her formal request to anyone. Legally, there would have to be a record of her request, and anyone could see a copy of her request if they wanted to. But the researcher whose materials were being requested would be unlikely to be notified in the normal course of business.

It was interesting to him that she didn't want the researcher, whoever it was, to know she was looking at his grant reports. She did not even seem to want to tell the librarian in whose work she was interested or even hint at what she was trying to find out. She must have been seeing or seeking something out of the ordinary? Something politically dicey? Something about which she didn't want to be scooped by another researcher? Perhaps she fancied herself having stumbled on a cure to cancer or something else important that a researcher hadn't noticed in his own work, and she wanted to keep it to herself until she put all the parts together and secured credit.

Or maybe she had just been tasked, as a grad student might be, with writing a laudatory biography of some living person for a surprise celebration of his long-life's work.

But her face had seemed more troubled than if she had been focused on some relatively dull task like biographical research for a fête. As she talked to him, she kept taking her hair out of her ponytail, pulling it back from her face, and fastening the hair back into the loop. Like a nervous tic.

He walked over to the bank of photocopiers to look at the bound journals she had pulled, the ones from which she had been photocopying articles: *The Journal of Growth and Metabolism; The American Journal of Clinical Endocrinology and Metabolism; Nature.* Mostly periodicals on bones, human development, and cellular metabolism, ranging from the 1960s through the present day. If the reference librarian bothered to go through each, he could probably figure out which researcher's work formed the common thread here. But there was no good reason to spend hours doing that.

Whatever the issue was, it had certainly occupied *her* for a good three hours. The stack of photocopies had become large enough that she had a bit of trouble fitting it into her backpack when it was time for her to go. He could tell, watching from his desk, what she had been doing – going backwards through citations: pulling work cited in an article, looking at those, tracing the references there back to earlier articles, pulling the earlier ones. He could tell because of the way she was flipping from the bodies of the texts to the references at the end, holding the index finger of her left hand on the body, the index finger of her right hand on the references, making fast notes, then going to get more journals to photocopy more articles.

It was the technique of someone who knew she didn't have a lot of time at a given library, who had to efficiently maximize collection of sources, who would look more closely at the content later. It was the technique of somebody who was good at library research.

He noticed she had been glancing at her watch more frequently as the time neared 4 p.m. She had asked him how long it would take to get to Logan Hall, and right at 3:55, she had packed up and waved to thank him and started to dash off, taking her backpack and zippered tote bag. He had had to run after her to tell her she'd left her suit jacket, and she'd grabbed it from him and thanked him and kept moving fast.

She seemed to him much faster, in gait and in research skills, than the typical historian. But then not so many historians came into this library. Perhaps his sample size was too small to judge.

-9-

Maddy was sitting up high in the rear of the lecture room near the windows. The late afternoon sun licked at her back as if it were the long, hot tongue of a giant cat as she tried to remember the little brain biochemistry she knew. Was there a specific hormone that produced that mental feeling in one's chest, the feeling of a sinkhole of emotion into which everything around it was falling?

Liz would know if there were such a hormone. Maddy just knew the feeling. Were this sinkhole on the edge of a southern Indiana highway, she thought, there would be the pavement of the shoulder crumbling in, and then perhaps the white line that marked the division between the driving lane and the shoulder also giving way into the crevice, and then the weeds growing next to the pavement tumbling in – the dandelions and the thistle and the crab-grass – as the hole deepened and widened.

But here, here it was her human thoracic cavity becoming the sinkhole, bringing down into it the edges of the lungs, the tube of the trachea, perhaps next the front ribs, all collapsing inward.

"You are over-reacting," she thought to herself. "Buck up."

The host was standing at the front of the small lecture hall giving Giovanni Mastromonaco a gushing introduction, speaking of his two books, his peer-reviewed articles, how fortunate Indiana was to have drawn him away from Pittsburg. The audience was smiling along and nodding, the faculty and the graduate students eagerly anticipating his talk, which would no doubt be very good, for, as the host noted, Professor Mastromonaco included in the slides for his lectures not only photographs of the early modern medical instruments and the texts about which he was to lecture but also his own sketches of various devices and scenes.

Giovanni was smiling modestly at his host's introduction, looking around the room, and for an accidental moment caught Maddy's eye.

She looked down quickly, taking her pen to her notebook. She began a doodle of nothing in particular: a tree, a charismatically tall tree, with rough bark and limbs that sloped down like the way Shirley's long arms sloped at her sides when she was trying to find her keys in the piles of her office.

As she doodled, she was remembering that time Giovanni had picked her up for a drive, on a beautiful Wednesday afternoon. He had given her beforehand just two things to wear – a spring-green gingham sundress and a pretty straw hat with a bright white ribbon. She had taken the hint and worn nothing else but a pair of white canvas flats. They drove out to Cedar Bluffs, and parked. He carried an over-the-shoulder bag into which he had packed a picnic blanket, an ice-cold bottle of prosecco, two hard-plastic cups, and a pint of perfect raspberries.

They had walked up to the bluff, off the trail, and when it was clear after a half-hour of walking that they were not going to run into anyone else, he had taken off her hat and put it atop his bag on the ground, leaned her up against a tree like this, just like the one she had drawn, and confirmed with an approving grunt that she had nothing else on under that dress.

How lovely had been the feeling of his one hand positioned between the tree and the back of her head, cushioning her head as he kissed her lips and kissed down her neck and pulled down her neckline with his other hand. How lovely the feeling as he gently ran his lips over the curve of her left breast. How wet he found her when he turned her toward the tree and put her hands up against the bark and lifted the back of the dress and came into her from behind, muttering a string of possessives and nouns in Italian in her ear, reaching his hands around her, one on her breast and one between her legs. And afterwards they'd lain about on the blanket in the sun and he gave her a cup of the wine, and fed raspberries into her mouth, one by one, so as not to stain her dress, he said.

She'd thought to herself at that moment on the blanket in the dappled sun that it didn't matter what happened with the two of them later, because this moment was perfect. As he observed aloud to her something that he had just figured out about the European plague, she thought to herself this: *Isaac Newton might have used The Calculus to figure out the entire area under the curve, but sometimes the best thing to do is to just live in one section under the curve, one perfect section of the area under the curve, for just a few hours.*

She had almost said this to him aloud but she was afraid that, if she did, he would ask her why she was thinking about the history of early-modern physics when he was talking about the history of the early-modern plague. And it would sound like she hadn't been listening.

Someone came up near to Maddy to close the shade just to the left of her, to make the room darker so that the slides of the lecture would show up better. Now Giovanni was well into his talk on the intersection of art and medicine in the eighteenth century. He was speaking of the culture of the Grand Tour, the bachelor sons of the wealthiest aristocrats and merchants making their way through Europe from famous ruin to famous city, and the concomitant role of the physicians in managing these young men's acquired syphilis infections.

Giovanni was deploying double entendres at which the audience was laughing, first as giggles and then with a bit of a tumbling roar, and Maddy realized the person who had come to close the shade was now looking at her curiously because Maddy was not laughing along. She quickly pretended to be as amused as everyone else.

She wanted more than anything in this moment just one thing: to pull out of her backpack the stack of photocopies she had just collected at the medical library and go to work on that.

But this narrow lecture room seat with its little fold-up desk would be maddening for such work, work that would require a real table. So she just kept doodling and pretending to listen.

She decided to situate this tree in a neighborhood now. So here was, on her paper, a neighborhood with a three-story rowhouse to the left side of the tree and an identical and attached rowhouse to the right, both with stoops, and *oh*, she thought, *what I wouldn't give right now to be in this drawing, in that little row house, working on this stack of photocopies, trying to figure out why Margaret Lovisa is still stuck to my arms.*

But would she find Lovisa in Dr. Wilhelm's published record? Would she find Lovisa in the articles she had just photocopied at the library?

People in nineteenth-century jars were often easy for Maddy to find in the pages of medical history. In fact, as a general rule, the farther back you went, the easier it became to know something about the person who had become the anatomical artifact. Whichever doctor or surgeon or researcher had scored the specimen would have published a report on it and quite often in that report would be what was known about the person whose body or body part it was. That was part of the game – the scholarly standard – the trophy display. The record would tell you at least the person's initials, if not his or her full name, place of birth, residency, occupation, family history, and more. By the late-nineteenth century, there was sometimes even a full photograph of the person as she or he appeared in life; before that, there were often sketches of the person – full-on sketches of their face, their posture, their person.

But medicine had changed in the last hundred years, pulling to the front the doctor or researcher, receding to the back the specimen's source. (Was her knowing this why, in the dream last night, Lovisa had ended up behind Maddy, Wilhelm in front of her?) The ostensible reason was respect for the patient's confidentiality. But as much as anything, Maddy knew, it was about putting the research in the foreground. In most cases nowadays, the specimen was not even discussed as if it had *ever* come from a real body. It was just tissues or cells or genes – devoid of any personal history.

But the old-fashioned way that Dr. Wilhelm had kept Margaret Lovisa in the back of his research lab in that large glass container – perhaps she was preserved in his pages somewhere, the way she was in his research office? Perhaps Maddy could find her and see her again, this time in words, and try to understand what was so troubling to Maddy. Maybe it was that her body remained and yet her history felt lost. When there was a whole body like that, there ought to be a written history. And there were several whole bodies in his lab....

Maddy had asked Shirley that morning as brightly as she could what Shirley knew about Lovisa. (She did not want to show Shirley that something was bothering her; it seemed, well, *unprofessional*.) Shirley had replied that Lovisa had been in her early fifties when she died, that she had been divorced, with no children, that she had a good sense of humor. (Maddy figured that meant Lovisa had laughed at Shirley's jokes.) Shirley said Lovisa had been a valued copyeditor for a small book publisher. She went by Maggie, generally.

"And how did Maggie Lovisa die?"

Well, said Shirley, it was *such* a funny story – "not so much funny as in *ha-ha* but funny as in an odd coincidence."

Maggie had come to Philly to see Dr. Wilhelm, and Maggie had come to see Shirley upon her arrival to town, as she always did. But Maggie had ended up collapsing and dying the day *before* seeing Dr. Wilhelm at the clinic. So she never made it to the clinic that time, which was terrible because perhaps Dr. Wilhelm would have detected something was wrong and saved her life?

"Anyway, of course Maggie had promised Dr. Wilhelm her body, so there *it* was, and there *he* was, and so he of course did the autopsy and then he used her body for research, as had been Maggie's stated wish. So, some good came of it!"

For some reason, knowing Margaret Lovisa also went by Maggie felt disconcerting to Maddy. Was it that knowing Lovisa had had a nickname made her just that much more human to Maddy? (Was she not fully human to Maddy before?) Or was it the similarity of "Maggie" to "Maddy"?

Maddy was starting to feel annoyed with herself for feeling this *off* about it all. She wondered if she would feel this way were it not for having met Dr. DesJardins.

"Why were you late coming in this morning?" Shirley had asked her, perhaps just to fill the silence that had ensued after Shirley told Maddy how Lovisa had died.

"I had an issue with my housing that I had to deal with," Maddy answered. "I may have to deal with it again this afternoon."

Maddy was not going to explain to Shirley that she had had to meet Father Tad that morning at Rittenhouse Square to talk about Wolf and about Wolf's wife and about the nature of confession. (Her own damned fault for the things she had said to Wolf last night over the heavy linguine.) Nor did she think it made sense to tell Shirley that she was thinking she ought to spend the afternoon at Penn's medical library looking up Dr. Wilhelm's work, to try to find Maggie Lovisa. So she had lied about her morning and her plans for the afternoon....

As Giovanni went on with his lecture, slide by slide, Maddy had to admit to herself that the longing to work now was not just urgently wanting to get started on seeing what had been happening with specimen acquisition in Dr. Wilhelm's research lab. It was primarily to belie what Giovanni had done to her at the informal reception just before his lecture. Work would require her to forget about her humiliation for a while. Work might stop the sinkhole.

Maddy had rushed over from the medical library to show up in time for the pre-lecture punch-and-cookie affair held in the hallway outside the classroom and had confidently walked up to Giovanni expecting him to greet her warmly. Instead, he had looked at her like – well, he had looked, she realized now, like a man caught – and he had said to her, "Maddy, I was not expecting you."

He seemed to glance about.

And when she thought he was joking and she laughed, he added, shaking her hand and pulling her in to speak close, that, because he had not heard from her in the last couple of days, he had made *other plans.*

He added that it appeared the jacket from the dress-jacket combo fit her well, but he thought it would go better with the dress itself. Was there something wrong with the dress, he asked? As if he thought she was purposely snubbing him.

At that point, she did not have time to explain that the red dress was in the tote bag, to explain obliquely why she was wearing now what she was wearing, to see if he still wanted to try to meet up – because the host had come up to them and Giovanni had introduced Maddy as a grad student from the Indiana program who happened to be in Philadelphia working on her dissertation research. And when the host said that the program should have Maddy give a talk while she was here in Philadelphia, Giovanni had said Maddy wasn't ready, and the host should ask her again after her dissertation was done.

Which had stunned Maddy into uncharacteristic silence.

Because – as Liz would surely exclaim angrily when Maddy told her about this – no one who is anything like a mentor or a friend turns down a talk for a graduate student, certainly not a talk offered to a student who will have to be on the job market shortly. And you *certainly* don't turn down a talk invitation to your grad student from a prestigious department in your own damned field. To do so indicates a lack of confidence in the student, marking her down in the eyes of the person who suggested it while also destroying the opportunity for an important line on her c.v. and a chance to network-build.

Liz would surely add in righteous indignation that Maddy was widely considered to be one of the top students – if not *the* top student – in the whole fucking department – a department considered one of the best in the world in its field – so when exactly did Giovanni think she would be "ready" to give a talk? Particularly considering she had already given a number of invited lectures in her own department and papers at conferences.

The host had looked embarrassed for Giovanni and Maddy both and said to Maddy that she should at least leave him her email address so that the host could connect her with the grad students in their program, so she could come to their parties while she was in Philly.

Yes, she could go to *grad student parties*. Giovanni would think her "ready" for that.

Before the host left and another faculty member came up to greet Giovanni, he had had just enough time to say to Maddy that she should rest assured he had signed the paperwork.

Now, when she pictured his pen pressing against the page that indicated that he would be on her dissertation committee – the page that specified who would certify that she had fulfilled the disciplinary and university expectations for her Ph.D. – she imagined that it was that pressure of the pen's tip on the paper that started that thoracic sinkhole.

How stupid could she have been. What an idiot.

-10-

Wolf had not been expecting the Rabbit home for dinner, but as he tasted the soup again, he found himself pleased that she was. She had seemed quite out of sorts when she had come in the door, dumping her backpack and her tote bag in the kitchen and heading quickly upstairs to change to go running. He knew from his own experience that when you are out of sorts, there are few things as satisfying as a good tomato soup with a grilled cheese sandwich. Which happened to be exactly what he was making.

He calculated that he had enough food to stretch it to feed them both, even with her substantial appetite. The soup was sweeter than he had expected it to turn out, but then these were late-season tomatoes and sweet onions. He would adjust the cheeses to make the flavor of the sandwiches a little more sour and a little more bitter, to complement the soup. The sandwiches would be mostly Gruyere with a little bit of blue cheese, and he'd use the pumpernickel loaf he had been thinking he would serve the next day with the corned beef.

The soup still needed a little thickening. Cream would be the obvious choice, but John Wolf pulled instead from his refrigerator a potato. Adding dairy to the soup could just taste redundant to the cheese of the sandwich.

Potato thickening would not compete.

Wolf wrapped the potato in a paper towel, ran it under the sink, and put it on a plate in the microwave to cook on high for seven minutes. He would then peel it and mash it into the soup and use the immersion blender to get the consistency to even out.

He recalled to himself that Father Tad had called at seven-thirty that morning to say he needed to talk with Maddy about the housing issue. Wolf had told him she was still asleep – that she had had a bad nightmare and had been up for a long time in the middle of the night and was now sleeping later than usual – but Wolf could leave her a message from Father Tad before he left for work. Wolf also told Father Tad that he and Maddy had had an unpleasant argument – that, the night before, Maddy had said to him over linguine some obnoxious things about his decision to keep treating his wife.

"To be honest, I would rather go in to work before she's up so we don't have to continue the argument," said Wolf. "I can leave her a note to meet you. I'm sure she will be up soon. She never sleeps very late."

Father Tad responded that he would talk to Maddy about the argument in the hopes she would not continue it but explained to Wolf that he needed primarily to see Maddy to tell her that Father Joe had found her another house and to offer that option to her.

"Although I think it is the wrong house for her, John, and I need to explain that to her, even though I need to offer it to her, as that's what Father Joe wants."

"Does it not have a bathtub, Father?"

Wolf had told Father Tad about Maddy's evening habit in the hopes the next house they found her would allow her that nightly respite. But he had soon realized it sounded funny. His friend had cleared his throat and replied that the bath that wasn't the issue. Firstly, the house was very far from the museum. But much more importantly, it was a household of five young women considering the religious life. And the way Father Tad saw it, sending Maddy into such a setting was about as high-risk to these women as sending in a young Valentino, given her religious views.

Wolf understood the point.

So, Wolf had left Maddy a note on the bathroom mirror saying that Father Tad wanted to meet her at 9:30 at the southwest corner of Rittenhouse Square. Wolf told Maddy in the note what to bring for Father Tad: a large coffee with two sugars and cream. He didn't include in the note that he had asked Father Tad to please try to get Maddy a piece of lemon poppyseed cake from the Polish bakery so that Maddy could try it. It was the best lemon poppyseed cake in the city, the almond so perfectly balanced with the other flavors.

When Father Tad had called him back hours later, ringing Wolf at work that afternoon, he told Wolf that he had talked to Maddy and that she was very sorry about what she had said to Wolf the night before. She was upset enough that she had asked somewhat sullenly if Father Tad was going to give her two Our Fathers and three Hail Marys and absolve her of what she had done.

When he had asked her if that was what she wanted, she had explained to him that no, that was *not* what she wanted. Because, she had said, the Catholic Church's system of confession meant you go and say you are sorry to someone other than the person you hurt. You tell some random priest and he absolves you and tells you not to do it again. And then you go and do it again. And then some priest absolves you again. And you never actually apologize and learn your lesson.

She had told Father Tad (as Father Tad had then told Wolf) that Maddy thought this system of confession and absolution lacked a basic understanding of how self-discipline works for humans, and that what she needed to do was to go and apologize to Wolf himself. She trusted, she had told Father Tad, that Wolf would *not* be infinitely forgiving with her as Father Tad saw his God to be and that knowing Wolf would *not* be infinitely forgiving would stop her from being stupid and insensitive again.

She had told Father Tad she hoped Wolf would forgive her *this time* but that she also hoped he would be clear that he would *not* forgive her again and again. She had also told Father Tad rather matter-of-factly that she didn't need a man – and certainly not a priest – to moderate her relationships with other human beings.

"She said all this politely enough, John," Father Tad had added, after a moment of silence. "Madeleine Shanks is blunt, and she can even be rough, but she is strangely polite about it. Perhaps that is the influence of the sisters. Or living in the Midwest for her graduate work. In any case, it means she doesn't come across as merely rude. She also did not hog the poppyseed cake, which I appreciated. And she brought me a coffee, which you must have told her to do."

When Wolf had not immediately answered (because he had been mulling what Maddy had told Father Tad about apology and confession and self-discipline), the priest had continued:

"Anyway, she asked me to call you at work and tell you she will apologize properly when she sees you next. She also asked me to remind you of the line in the Lord's Prayer – *forgive us our trespasses* – because she says that's exactly what she is. A trespasser to your home."

Rabbits aren't born to respect fences, Wolf had thought to himself.

Father Tad then had asked Wolf if he understood that Maddy was quite good at getting information out of people. Wolf had answered, trying not to sound pleased about this, that yes, he understood her to be that way.

"Then John," said the priest, "you will understand how it is that she got out of me what happened with your wife, with the accident. What you found out."

Perhaps, Wolf thought, it was just as well that Maddy heard from Father Tad, and not one of his workmates or someone else, that when the construction crane had fallen and hit the car in which his wife was riding, she was not the only one in the car. The crane had also hit and killed his best friend, a fellow officer, a man who had no good reason to be in that part of town, at that time of day, with Wolf's wife. Maddy would now understand that Wolf had lost in that moment not only his best friend and probably his wife but also his understanding of his closest friendship and of his marriage. Perhaps now she would lay off the subject of his marriage and his wife.

The priest told his friend that Maddy had also gotten out of him the information that before the accident Wolf didn't cook much, and that the reason he had taken up cooking was that Father Tad had counseled him that there were many bodily pleasures that one could enjoy on earth in moderation without sin, and that Wolf had hit upon cooking.

"What did she say to that?" asked Wolf.

"She thanked me for being your spiritual advisor and then she told me she thought I should seriously consider giving Sunday's sermon specifically on the redemptive power of the Maryland crab. Figuring you might listen. I am taking her suggestion under advisement, keeping in mind that you would need me to bless that dish, however you cook them. Because, John" – the priest cleared his throat – "you never know about crabs."

"Duly noted," answered Wolf.

Father Tad said then that Maddy had also asked him to tell Wolf that she would not be home until very late – that she had a friend from Indiana who had come to town – and would Wolf please not latch the door from the inside, so she could get back in without ringing if she was very late?

"Yes," said Wolf, and he thought to himself he'd better stay up, to make sure she got home.

Wolf had been on the phone with his car mechanic, stirring the soup, when Maddy had come in the back door hours earlier than he had figured she would. Looking sour, she had just dumped her bags and told him quickly, since he was on the phone, that she was going to change and go running and that she wasn't going out tonight after all. She had looked at the table and seen he had set himself a place, with a soup bowl and a small plate. She had gone upstairs and soon come back down, her face scrubbed clean of all make-up, her hair secured with a tight headband, her running clothes and shoes on. He had been just off the phone and adding a matching place-setting for her.

She had looked at the table and then looked at him with some degree of what appeared to be exasperation. At first, he had thought she was exasperated with him. Was she annoyed that he presumed she would want to have what he was cooking for dinner?

Soon it had become clear from her gestures and sighs that her issue was somehow with herself. She had positioned herself right in front of him, moving uncomfortably, as if this positioning were a physically challenging thing to do, and she had looked him in the eye. He had thought it looked a little like she wanted to punch him, like a child annoyed at another.

"Thank you for letting me have dinner with you again," she had begun. "Now I have to apologize."

She had repositioned herself and sighed again.

"Listen, Wolf. Listen."

"I am," he had said.

"Listen, Wolf. I don't ever want to be a religious person. I could never *imagine* myself being one. But that doesn't mean there haven't been times in my life when I have felt something like envy for people like you – people who are able to believe that there is a purpose in everything, who are able to believe there is a God taking care of things. It seems like a very good coping strategy and I sometimes wish I had a coping strategy that good."

She had seemed almost to wince from the thought of it.

"Similarly, I realized today that it's damned clear I have never felt anything even remotely similar to the love you obviously have felt for your wife. But that doesn't mean it isn't real – that you haven't experienced it – just because I have not. I have enough sense in me to be a little envious of that, too, even though I realize that having that kind of love means having your heart broken is vastly more crushing than any romantic insult I have ever received."

He had wondered if she meant to use the word "crushing" or if the allusion to the crane was simply a Freudian slip.

"My lacking religious and romantic experiences similar to yours," she had continued, "well, that may mean I am incapable of true empathy as far as your situation goes. But that does not mean it is okay for me to be an insensitive asshole. What you decide about your wife is your business, not mine, and I am very sorry – I mean that I am *very* sorry, John Wolf – that I somehow suggested that what you are doing is irrational, or unloving, or illogical, or unjust. The way I behaved last night over that linguine was stupid and insensitive and arrogant. And the longer you let me live here, the more you will discover that that is my very nature – to be stupid and insensitive and arrogant, even when someone has the decency to be feeding me. The only thing that keeps me from being a complete and utter asshole is that I have enough insight to know I can be an asshole. You should throw me out."

He had been about to speak when she had held up her hand.

"You can't throw me out yet. The house Father Joe has found for me is full of young Catholic virgins planning to be nuns and, were I to move in with them, they would be put at great risk from my corrupting atheistic rationality. I might even teach them some history of science. Gasp. So, you have to put up with me a little longer for the sake of five or six virgins. I know that will be motivating enough for you to keep me temporarily. If you can take me to that gym one more time, I think I will be able to do my own laundry in your basement and not bother you with that."

He had wondered what going to the gym would have to do with doing laundry. But he didn't ask.

She had moved toward the kitchen door to leave for her run, out the back alley. When she had gone to pull the door closed behind her, Wolf had grabbed the edge of it and yelled at her.

"Listen, Rabbit! I forgive you. But don't do it again! Or else!"

She had turned and looked at him, mumbled "thank you," and ran off. He thought she might have smiled as she turned.

He had gone back in the house to continue cooking but paused just inside the door.

Normally, Wolf had thought to himself, Maddy did not carry a second bag to work as she had that day. Normally, he would not look in her bag. But she had seemed so out of sorts, something had to have happened to change her evening plans. She was gone on her run and would not know.

Unzipping it just a couple of inches, he had seen right away the red of the dress. He had zipped it back up.

Now, as Wolf blended in the potato, he thought about how much he admired the way historians used verb tenses. It was one of the things he had noticed from reading histories – how historians would be very careful about use of the tenses that the English language had to offer. He had learned some tricks from it, useful to him sometimes when questioning a suspect, when he wanted to make it sound like he knew more than he did without actually lying.

The tense the Rabbit had used in referring to his love for his wife had been just such a clever use. She had referred not to "the love *you felt* for your wife" (past tense) nor to "the love *you feel* for your wife" (present tense) but to "the love *you have felt* for your wife." He couldn't remember what that tense was called, but he knew that, while it allowed for past love and future love, it assumed little as to constancy.

...

Looking at the clock and seeing it to be almost eleven-thirty, Wolf handed Maddy the bowl of egg custard, dotted this time with lightly crushed, small round berries over which (she could smell and see) he had shaved a little bit of nutmeg and a little bit of vanilla bean.

The berries emitted the shocking color of – of life? Exactly the color of the blood of a papercut, she thought. A brilliant, happy red.

"Fresh currants," he said, anticipating her question. "I have a source."

He added that he hated to interrupt her from such intense work but he thought she needed something more in the way of food if she was going to work past midnight, because it had been a long time since the soup and sandwich.

She said in return that she was sorry to be taking up the kitchen table quite so long.

"Does anyone else need the table?" he asked rhetorically. "It's late. Eat."

She put down her pen and took up the spoon.

"I don't get a glass of port with it this time?" she asked.

He poured and brought her a glass of brandy and sat down across from her. She was holding a little bit of the dessert on her tongue, letting each flavor find the right taste bud – a do-si-do pairing of this and that in her mouth.

"Can I make an observation to you, Rabbit?"

She nodded and took a sip of the drink. It warmed up her cheeks immediately.

"There are many lousy emotions in life," he said. "But I do think that the very worst – the one that feels the very worst – is being let down by someone you were counting on."

At first, she thought he was referring to him having been let down by her. Or by his wife? (He must have known that Father Tad had told her that morning about Wolf's discovery of his wife's affair.) But then Maddy understood from something in the way he said it, something in the way he was looking at her, that he was referring to her *own* disappointment. He couldn't know about Giovanni but Wolf must have put together the pieces and figured out enough about her day.

She took another spoon of the custard and held it for a moment in her mouth before swallowing. She sipped a little more brandy and understood now from her tastebuds why this version of the egg custard – with the nutmeg – had called Wolf to the bottle of brandy and not to the port.

"Being let down by someone you were counting on," he continued, "well, it has a way of attracting every other lousy feeling. Loneliness. Sadness. Jealousy. I know that feeling. And I know that work – working hard – that is a good way to step out of it. I just wanted to say I am happy for you that you know that about work, too."

"Thank you," she replied.

"Also, I promise to make Maryland crab soon," he added. "But we will have to invite Father Tad for that. So he can bless it."

She smiled a little at him.

"Can I tell you a joke I almost told Father Tad today?" she asked, and he nodded. She told him this one:

A young man goes to confession and he confesses to the priest that he has had relations with a young woman.

The priest expresses disapproval. He asks, "Was it Mary O'Hannigan, lad?"

"No, Father," says the young man.

The priest asks, "Was it Sally Mulhaney, then?"

"No, Father," says the young man again.

"Well, was it Molly Finnigan, my boy?"

The young man says no again.

The young man comes out of the confessional booth. His friend asks him how it went.

"Pretty good!" the young man answers. "I got five Our Fathers, ten Hail Marys, and three good leads!"

Wolf just chuckled at first. But then he started laughing, and then he laughed as hard as Maddy had ever seen him. She delighted in having brought this on, as she ate the rest of the custard and drank the rest of the brandy. His laughter finished right about the time she finished the treats. She handed back the bowl, the glass, and the spoon.

As he took them to the sink to wash them, he asked her why she was working on late-twentieth century medical texts – modern medicine – when she usually worked only on publications before 1900.

"I need to find someone I met at a research lab," Maddy answered. "A woman who died. She came back in that nightmare last night. I want to see if I can find her in the records."

"I don't understand," said Wolf.

"I don't yet either," said Maddy.

How interesting it was that that joke from years ago would suddenly come back to her this morning, right after the nightmare. A joke about accidentally obtaining good leads....

About two years earlier, Maddy had confessed to a professor who was now on her dissertation committee that she thought she was bad at staying focused on a topic. Other students seemed very good at following the narrowest and most direct path to the end of a paper. But Maddy could not seem to stop herself from chasing down an interesting lead even if it appeared only tangentially related to what she was supposed to be researching.

The mentor's answer had surprised her. She had told Maddy that Maddy had an unusually good nose for subjects – that she had noticed how Maddy could see in a text a line of inquiry that other students would never see. She knew where to look for interesting things.

"Don't cover your nose," she had said to Maddy. "It may take you a little longer, it may be a harder, or less – well, less popular a method – the way you do history in our field, the way you sniff things out and connect things other people don't connect. But Maddy, your nose makes your work genuinely original. Follow those scholarly instincts. They're unusually good."

Now, fresh off the deeply satisfying smell of shaved vanilla and nutmeg, fresh off sniffing through dozens of papers by Wilhelm, Maddy just could not drop the feeling that there was something about Wilhelm's approach – the anachronistic nature of it? – that made it worth her understanding even more, at least perhaps in comparison to what had been done a hundred years earlier. There was something so interesting – so strange – about a nine-teenth-century approach to collecting in a twenty-first century research lab.

She had found what appeared to be at least two clear references to Lovisa – references to postmortem tissue specimens obtained by a 53-year-old woman with diastrophic dysplasia. There were also three earlier references when Lovisa was alive to a patient who seemed to match her age and diagnosis. These references each came with more citations Maddy would have to pull next. But regardless of whether she found more about Lovisa specifically, what she wanted to understand more was why he kept the collection at all, the way he did.

She had also found what appeared to be four references to Dr. DesJardins – a man his age with pituitary dwarfism (that was what he had, yes?) and a midline defect....

Was it just Dr. Wilhelm's interest in the history of anatomical collections that led to what – or rather *who* – was now a specimen in his lab? Or did Dr. Wilhelm have an understanding that the collection of whole-body specimens, the preparation of a whole skeleton, still could matter to science, when everybody else had long since turned away from whole bodies to small bits of tissue?

Why did he seem to veer in his published work from almost bragging in his papers about his own postmortem collection years ago to lately not writing much about it? He had not hesitated to show Maddy his assemblage in his lab. But was that because he knew she was used to such things from her own work, and he figured it wouldn't trouble her?

And if she was so used to it, as she liked to think, why *had* his corpus of corpses troubled her? There was something here she needed to grasp even if put her working in the wrong century.

"Wolf – about my nightmare – I just want to be clear, it wasn't anything you said, about the rapist, or anything else you said, really. It was about work, more. More than anything else, it was about work. Do you think sometimes the subconscious can give us useful leads for work?"

"Absolutely," he said, sitting down across from her again. "More than once, I've figured out something in the corner of my brain and I've just had to wait for it to come to the center. And then of course verify it."

To verify it. So, obviously, he did not go on faith on everything. Not for his work as an officer of the law. She wondered if part of the reason he prayed was to take his mind off something that needed his subconscious-ness, something that needed freedom from his consciousness. She remembered doing this in the convent. When she felt overwhelmed with the thought that she was now without family, without any real form of security save her intelligence and the high-cost charity of the church (and perhaps, as a distant back-up, the disorganized, dangerous care of the state), she would pray along with the sisters – not to access God but to stop her mind from obsessing on the problem she could not yet control. The repetitive words would carry her into a calm where her mind could untangle the knots at a more effective pace. The words of prayer were like a train bound for a destination under the conducting of someone else.

"Do you have nightmares a lot?" Wolf blurted out, as if he had been holding the question for hours and minutes, as if had just seen something change in her face that made it possible for him finally to ask.

"Not too often," she said. "I hope – I don't think I will bother you too often with them."

Then she felt suddenly – for just a moment – what she figured her ancestors would have experienced as the presence of a ghost or a vision, for the recollection of a different dream suddenly appeared back into her view. Maddy had had this dream after she finally went back to bed that morning, back to the bed neatly remade by Wolf just after her nightmare.

It was winter but not cold, and she was skating on the frozen Schuylkill River. She was skating because Wolf had reached out his hand to her from the other shore and she had taken it. It was right near 30th Street Station, where she had gotten off the Amtrak train, the part of the river she had crossed by bridge to hurry to his house that first night in the pouring rain. But now, in this dream, it was winter, and night, and she was down on the river, skating the river frozen and silent – no one else seemed to be in the city, although through the windows of the buildings she could see warm light. She could hear the Philadelphia Symphony playing in the distance, the Blue Danube Waltz, and there she was with Wolf, skating a duet that they both seemed to know. Neither of them spoke. There was only the movement.

"Don't you think it's strange, Rabbit," he said, interrupting her recollection of this lullaby dream and chasing it away unknowingly, "that we both lost people in car accidents? I mean, accidents involving cars."

She pulled her mind back to the table.

"Car accidents are one of the most common causes of disability and death," she answered quietly, as if reading from an actuarial table. She was trying to rapidly record what she could remember of the dream in her conscious memory so she could bring it back again later, to think on it, perhaps even to feel it.

"I have certainly met others like us, Wolf – people who lost people in cars."

(The distant sound of the violins. The feeling of him skating next to her, going in the same direction. The ice, perfectly smooth, as if the Zamboni had just come by. The darkness, the river, perfectly quiet.)

"Did your parents and your sister die in the car?"

She looked at the wrinkle in his brow, wondering what he was hoping for.

"My father and my sister did. My mother made it alive out of the car, and they got her to the hospital, but she died soon thereafter," she answered. "I know because I asked the mortician's son and he told me the truth. Everyone else told me to stop asking and just pray for their souls. But I kind of felt like I had to know how they died. It was kind of like a necessary part of believing."

"Believing what?" he asked.

He expected her to answer *believing they were dead*. But with the Rabbit, he was never truly sure what to expect in reply.

"Believing I would no longer ask my parents for anything, ever again?"

He noticed she intoned it as a question.

"I see," he said.

She remembered now the last time her parents had let her and her sister go into New York City on their own, on the Long Island Rail Road to Penn Station, up the C subway to the Museum of Natural History, not too long before the accident. The dozens of times they had gone to the museum with or without their parents, her sister had always wanted to go be in the gem room to stare into the glass cases of jade, amethyst, and azurite, to admire the quartz samples that came in so many colors. But Maddy preferred the Hall of Ocean Life, and without the parents going with the two girls on the most recent trips, Maddy had taken the chance to lay down a long time under the giant blue whale just as she had when she was very little. She had long ago learned that if she laid there long enough, the great beast suspended twenty feet above would start to move, ever so slightly. The whale would start to swim. On the last trip, just before the accident, she imagined that, if she laid there long enough, the resin of the magnificent model might magically turn to mammalian flesh. The strong, dense flesh over her would be this whale, this beautiful, majestic whale, and not –

She looked now at Wolf's honest face, his smart eyes, the bone of his jawline, and settled her gaze for a moment on the bow of his clavicles. She turned her eyes back up to his, and they stared into each other's eyes for what felt to her like the time it takes to watch the sun set: always a little longer than you think it will take; always a little longer than you think you should look.

He blinked.

"So, what did you learn from your work tonight?" he asked, blinking again.

"A librarian suggested to me today that I could use – well, I could use a kind of a special request system to obtain some materials from the National Institutes of Health," she replied. "I've never used it but I think I will try that route tomorrow. It should let me see a little deeper. I'm trying to understand the acquisition of a series in what amounts to a private collection. Do you mind if I ask the NIH to send me the results here? It would probably be a biggish envelope."

"Not at all," he said, "but if neither of us is here, the postman might leave one of those package notes and you'll have to go down to the post office to get it. Why don't you just send it to the museum?"

She wasn't sure what to say. She didn't want to tell him that a package for her sent to the museum would be delivered by way of Shirley and she didn't want Shirley asking her what she had requested from the Freedom of Information Act Office of the NIH. Shirley would not like Maddy looking into Dr. Wilhelm's grants to try to see what he had said about his collection.

"Liz said she has sent me something here, too," Maddy told Wolf now. "A photo of the two of us she wanted me to have. She said it would be here soon. Oh, and my billboard lawyer emailed and he's probably going to be sending me a new contract here in the next few weeks. I'm sorry," she added, looking at the kitchen table covered with her papers, "I've set up shop here, haven't I? And when I move on to another place, you'll have to track me down for mail sent to the wrong place? Ugh."

"It's fine, Rabbit," he said, standing up and pushing his chair in.

"But –"

"It's fine. Hey, tomorrow is Friday. Can you stop by the fish market for me on the way home? I got passed along what looks like a good recipe for a Thai curry fish dish, from a sergeant who's Thai. I'll give you a list of fish that would work for it. Or you can just pick any white-fleshed fish that smells fresh – whatever doesn't smell fishy. Cod or haddock or whatever. A little over a pound."

"Of course," she answered.

"I'm going to bed. Sleep well. Sleep better than last night."

"I hope at least I let you sleep better," she said.

What a funny idiom that is, she thought: *smell fishy*. The smell of something recently dead and out of place. Dead humans would presumably smell that way if humans ever let each other just rot.

-11-

Thanks to Giovanni's brush-off a couple of days earlier, Maddy was spending the night with every guy she had ever slept with. What was it about being rudely dumped that always called the whole cast to one's late-night bed?

Here was Colin, who would presumably still be available for the occasional fuck when she got back home to Indiana. Colin liked to mention his crazy research travel schedule and his associated National Science Foundation grant deadlines as the reasons he had to avoid a committed relationship. (He studied the lifecycle of monarch butterflies, which meant flying all over North America all year round to follow his subjects.) When Colin had dropped why he couldn't commit for about the third time, Maddy thought about telling him she wasn't looking for a relationship. But then it occurred to her that maybe he kept mentioning that his butterflies came first because he liked talking about his professional success. Or maybe he just liked feeling in control of his and Maddy's sexual relations that way. Whatever his motivation, the effect of his work schedule was what she wanted. So, she left it alone and just learned to say "got it" when he mentioned it again. He was always mentioning it here, in bed, again.

She and Colin had met because a frat boy doing delivering for Phoenix Dumpling reversed their orders. It was the first time in Maddy's life she had ever ordered delivery and she had only done so because she was out of groceries and totally buried in work with deadlines approaching and it was swampy as hell outside. She did the math and decided the cost of cranking up the air conditioner when she got back drenched from the walk would be about the same as paying for delivery. And having someone else bring her the food would save her time.

Figuring if she was going to pay for delivery she might as well make it worth it, she had ordered five dishes. As soon as she realized she had been delivered the wrong order, she called Colin's number from the receipt and told him she thought he probably had her food since she had his. She pointed out that she had ordered way more than he ordered so he needed to either pay up or switch orders.

"But I have already eaten your crispy wontons," he answered. "Because I meant to order those. It seemed justified."

"Damn it," she answered. "Well, then I'm going to have to eat your egg-roll. But you'd better not eat my pork-veg noodles because those are supposed to last me three meals this week."

"Three meals from one order of noodles? What are you, like ninety pounds?" he asked.

"I'm a starving graduate student," she laughed at him.

"Of course you're starving," he replied. "Try eating a whole meal. I could come over. Do you want me to pick you up some pizzas on the way or something? I'm faculty. I can afford it."

They had ended up talking and eating together for an hour – he was insanely amusing in an unknowing way when talking about this butterfly larvae – then making out. After that, until his next trip, they made a regular thing of take-out, beer, and sex. Professor Butterfly (as Liz called him) had a pleasant efficiency about him that Maddy appreciated, particularly when she had a lot of papers to grade. And she liked that he was a good decade and a half older than her.

"We good?" he would always ask Maddy at the end. The one time she answered, "No, I didn't get enough," he obliged her implied request without complaint, without mention of work that needed doing. That was nice.

He seemed to call her promptly whenever he got back into town.

"Phoenix Dumpling?" he would ask without saying hello. The first time he did this, she thought he had gotten the wrong number and she had almost answered, "No, this is not Phoenix Dumpling."

She just wished he'd floss between the meal and the fuck. His teeth were kind of close together and sometimes she found a bit of scallion cooked in soy sauce in there.

Before Colin, there had been Sundeep, an engineering post-doc that she met by sharing a table one crowded afternoon at the Runcible Spoon. As usual, no one at the Spoon seemed to be waiting tables – the staff had a habit of all going out back for smokes together – so he'd asked her if she would watch his things while he went to try to get another cup of tea. He asked her if she wanted anything and she gave him a five and asked for a coffee with a little cream and a muffin.

"Get me anything except the vegan zucchini-orange," she said. She added that vegan zucchini-orange muffins were probably illegal in the state of Indiana and if they weren't, they should be. He just looked confused at this joke.

When he came back with their drinks and food (blueberry-walnut-cinnamon) and he started back up on his work, she could see he was going over c.v.'s. He just kept sighing.

"You on a search committee with no good job candidates?" she finally asked, feeling like she ought to express some sympathy for his pain.

"These are resumes of potential wives," he explained. "My parents sent me these and I am to sort through them and indicate which ladies I wish to meet when I go back home."

"Seriously?" she asked.

He nodded, extended a hand, and said his name was Sunny. He had a lovely way of smiling with his ears that she could not figure out. They wound up at Nick's for calzones and after a couple of gin and tonics she suggested they go back to her place so she could try acting out the various resumes to make it easier for him to pick. This had led to a fair degree of amusement particularly as she kept trying to do an Indian accent and to wrap herself in scarves and he kept telling her with a grin that she was being extremely culturally offensive. When she finally went down on him, playing a woman named Nalini, he told her Nalini was definitely going to get an interview.

The pleasure of his company, which featured a string of clever maneuvers with her scarf collection, had lasted a few months, all the way up until he confessed to Maddy he was falling in love with her and so had to stop, given his situation. He could not disappoint his parents.

She objected: "Children are born to disappoint their parents. You're supposed to disappoint them. I disappointed mine. That is why I am never going to have any children. Why create novel beings who will by their very nature be utter disappointments to you?"

He had no reply. She wondered if he was just telling her he loved her as a way to dump her politely. But Liz sensibly told her that she might as well believe Sunny and take the compliment on the way out the door.

For a while, Maddy assumed she and Sunny would still run into each other on campus or around town but somehow, they never did.

And, back in college, there had been Michael – *climb on in, Michael, join the party* – simple Michael, whom she had dated while she was at Georgetown, starting in her second year and ending when she had to head off to Indiana for grad school at the end of her third year. He'd been a virgin and she told him only that she had had some prior experience with someone but that it had been no good. She never told him that the reason she wasn't a virgin was what The Jerk had done to her.

Her therapist at Georgetown, a woman named Paula, had come up with the notion of Maddy making her first sexual relationship after The Jerk with someone who was a virgin, someone who would bring little expectation of how Maddy should feel and act, so that she could be relatively free of requirements.

Maddy vividly remembered what her father thought of therapists because of the one time when Maddy's mother had told her father that a family friend was seeing a psychologist. Her father had answered in contempt, "She doesn't need a therapist, she needs a priest!"

By the time when Sisters Thomas Aquinas and Mary Patrick drove Maddy and her brown cardboard boxes of second-hand clothes and books through the gates of Georgetown and helped Maddy find her first dorm room at the university, Maddy had read all she could find about the university's counseling services and she was determined to make use. Having had a chilly father who said things like "You don't need a therapy, you need a priest!" struck her as something that suggested you could probably use a therapist, particularly if you were a seventeen-year-old abusively deflowered atheist orphan being dropped off by a pair of Dominican nuns at a Jesuit school.

Maddy had taken advantage of the counseling services at Georgetown almost as soon as she had arrived. The financial aid package the school had given her – Maddy referred to it as "The Catholic Orphan Special" – included free counseling up to once a week while school was in session. She'd first been assigned as a therapist a man who felt all wrong to her but he at least had the good sense to conclude after two visits, "I think you need Paula Slocum as a therapist, not me."

In her initial intake, Paula had ascertained that Maddy wanted a therapist's help because she wanted to figure out what to do with the detritus of her existence. To Maddy, this need seemed obvious – isn't that always why one sought a counselor? – but it took a smart woman like Paula to get it quickly. As Maddy had done with the first therapist, Maddy told Paula rather plainly about it all, speaking like she had rehearsed it before she arrived: She was raised by crazy Catholics on abortion picket lines but never had the faith. Her coach started a relationship with her when she was twelve and had started fucking her outright when she was thirteen. Then her family was killed when she was fifteen and though she never did get faith, she figured she'd be safest with the nuns and took the offer to go live under their care. Now she was here because she had talked the admissions office into taking her and giving her a full ride.

"The Catholic Orphan Special."

Paula had thought about this all silently for about two minutes and then asked Maddy two blunt questions:

Did Maddy have any interest in trying to be Catholic?

No. None.

Did Maddy want to learn how to enjoy sex?

Yes. Please.

And with this, Paula dove right in, explaining to Maddy that ordinarily she had to try to fix students who wanted to stay within the cultural framework of the Catholic Church. If that was what they needed to be well overall in their lives, she had to help them with that; that was her professional duty as she saw it.

But, Paula told her, if Maddy was essentially out of the Church and wanted out of the whole damned Catholic worldview, then if Maddy would promise not to tell anyone, Paula would help her understand how to move past the Church, enjoy sex, and be free.

Paula started by giving Maddy a copy of *Our Bodies, Ourselves* and a hand mirror, and Maddy read well beyond what Paula assigned for the first week, understanding for the first time the components of her vulva – her labia majora, her labia minora, her clitoris, the introitus to her vagina. She used her hands to understand the bones of her pelvis, feeling them through her skin and muscle while looking at drawings of skeletons. It was as if she had been given a map to a treasure island. Only the island was her.

Paula encouraged her to masturbate and to do so using just her fingers – to avoid things like dildos and vibrators until she learned her own feel, her own smell, her own response – to not to worry right now about her vagina, where The Jerk had been, but to explore her clitoris, her labia, her breasts, where he had never intentionally bothered to go.

He had only ever fucked her missionary style and he had never bothered to do anything but get off in her, and then get off of her, all as fast as he could. But Paula said that was in a way a good thing – there was so much left where he never had been.

"Go to the places where he never really went," Paula told her. "There are plenty of them. Go slowly. Don't judge yourself for whatever you find or feel or remember or think. Just do what feels good and if something feels bad, pause, breathe, and try to go back to good. If that doesn't work, pause and go exercise – go feel the rest of your body at the gym. Then try again later. Not too much later."

And Maddy did this as much as having a roommate allowed and came back each week to talk more to Paula, to tell her what part of her anatomy she had explored, to tell her what had felt good and bad in her thoughts and her body, to tell her little bits of the story of her mother and her father and The Jerk.

By the second year of their work together, Paula told Maddy she thought Maddy was ready to try vaginal intercourse anew and she helped Maddy figure out who she might tap. First, she sent Maddy to Planned Parenthood, to get an I.U.D. and a proper screening, to make sure The Jerk hadn't given her anything she should know about.

When Maddy's tests all came back clean, she stopped on the way back from the clinic at the local florist and bought herself a small palm tree for her dorm room, something that felt necessary for reasons she could not ascertain. It came in a vibrant cobalt blue ceramic pot, and was now, six or so years later, big and healthy. Maddy always left it with Liz when she went away for more than a week, so it wouldn't die. Liz said the rats liked digging in the pot's dirt and she figured their pee was good for it. It always seemed happy when Maddy got back home and took it back from Liz.

As for potential sex partners, Paula liked the idea of Michael, a virgin Maddy's own age, a fellow who said he was considering the priesthood. Not long after they started sort-of seeing each other, Michael told Maddy there was no way he could introduce her to his family if she wasn't willing to pretend she was still Catholic. She was fine not having to spend time with another crazy Catholic family and the sisters always took her back in on the holidays when the dorms closed, so she didn't need Michael or anyone to put her up when one normally needed some family. Michael and

Maddy had gone very slowly through the bases, finally fucking when she convinced him one night, over a fair bit of vodka punch, that screwing an atheist wouldn't count in the eyes of his family or a seminary. Apparently, he thought it would also not count in his God's eyes?

It had all been clunky and awkward – Michael had a tendency to yell out, when he came in her, "I love you, Madeleine Shanks!" as if he had to prove something to the universe about the spiritual purity of his cum – but Paula focused Maddy on the idea of feeling in control of her own needs.

"You know, you don't have to tell him you love him just because he yells that he loves you when he orgasms," Paula said. "If someday he says it without an orgasm, we should talk about that."

He never did.

Paula reassured Maddy that it made perfect sense to keep doing gymnastics – that it was not a toxic relic of her life. Doing gymnastics, Paula said, would let Maddy make clear to herself that The Jerk controlled nothing in her mind, her body, or her life anymore. She was her own person now and she need not cede any history or any territory of her anatomy to him. Not her vagina, not her abductors, not her mouth, not her abdominals, not her brain. She should retake them all.

Maddy had already had something of that sense before meeting Paula, so she had kept up her gymnastic skills, partly with the help of one of the sisters. But she was glad that Paula agreed gymnastics was hers and not his. That nothing was his in her life.

Then came that lovely day, the day she got the acceptance from Indiana University to do a Ph.D. in History of Science and Medicine, when she knew she had to break up with intelligent-but-dull Michael, when she knew she would now go off to Indiana and be truly free – free not only of The Jerk, but of the whole Church of her father. She fucked Michael one more time, wincing a little when he yelled, "I love you, Madeleine Shanks!" – and then excitedly showed him the letter from Indiana and told him that was it; they were through.

She put her clothes back on and went for a run, a run through the streets of Georgetown, past the million-dollar Georgian houses with their magnolias and boxwood and lilies, and as she could feel Michael's semen start to drip out of her, down the inside of her thigh, it felt okay, and not bad – not black the way it had felt when The Jerk's semen leaked slowly out of her, the oil of seed that would leave her with steel wool and barbed wire growing out of her uterus. Michael's semen dripping out of her did not yet feel as it would someday, with Colin and Giovanni – like old-fashioned hot fudge dripped on full-fat vanilla ice cream – but it was perfectly okay. Not bad.

With the letter from Indiana, a full-ride deal to a Ph.D., well, the sun felt so brilliant, the world so open, the opportunities so plentiful. Perhaps someday she would even own a house, even a house with a porch and old windows and a garret like some of the houses in Georgetown! Perhaps she would make enough from a tenured job someday. She could sell the billboard for the down payment and get a mortgage.

And no matter how little money she would have, sex would now be free. And in a world of Ph.D.'s, the sex would surely be smart. *Sex would be free and smart!*

Sex had become just like the public library.

She could not stop smiling.

Just before she left Georgetown, as if she needed to confirm the library card worked, she finally hooked up with a philosophy professor she'd been flirting with for the last few weeks. It did not feel quite right – and she never told Paula about it. But this guy knew a lot better than Michael what he was doing, and he came with none of the guilty affection that saddled Michael. He didn't care if she was never going to call him again.

And this, of course, was the trajectory that had eventually led her to Giovanni, to the pleasures of being fucked so nicely by Giovanni against a tree in the woods and fed raspberries by him on a sunny blanket, all in a sweet dress that he had picked just for her.

So why did she care that he had dumped her? She had the memories. She even had the dresses.

Sure, there was the awkwardness of having him on her committee. And maybe his bizarre claim – that she wasn't ready to give a talk at Penn's department? – maybe he never would have said such a thing if he hadn't felt awkward about having had a sexual relationship with her. But she didn't need to have the sour note of the ending cause her to feel dissonance about the whole relationship, did she? He had been mostly lovely. It had been mostly lovely.

Much better than that guy with the beard in Paris.

So much better than that one-night-stand with the famous historian of science from Cambridge at the annual joint meetings.

But here she was, in bed with these men and every other guy she had ever slept with, thanks to Giovanni's rude final way.

What an asshole.

She knew what Liz would say was the solution: *Back up on the horse, Mad Girl!* Which meant finding another horse.

But Maddy was afraid her horse standards were getting higher and higher, and so the horses were getting harder to mount. It wasn't just that guys in the age-range she preferred were often partnered. It was that she had come to have certain expectations about being treated well, of having a feeling of actual intellectual connection, something that felt real....

She felt suddenly ridiculously sentimental about her friendship with Liz. It was the kind of friendship she had never had before – the kind of close friendship she could see herself maybe developing with Wolf, if she was going to know him long enough. The kind of connection that could sub in comfortably for sex at night and make Maddy not care all that much about getting laid, not in the short term anyway.

She hadn't expected to miss Liz so much during this time away from Bloomington. Yet here Maddy was, sentimentally missing the rituals of coffee with Liz, beers with Liz, runs with Liz, weepy funerals for pet rats with Liz. This feeling was just so ironic given that it was their mutual *lack* of sentimentality that began their friendship.

They had met in a rare cross-disciplinary grad course, on feminism and scientific practice, and they hadn't talked to each other outside of class for the first few weeks. Liz seemed to be skeptical of anyone in the humanities, even in History of Science. But then one day, one of the other students invited everyone in the seminar to his impromptu engagement party and Liz and Maddy found themselves there in a polite three-way conversation with another woman. It was shortly thereafter that they realized they ought to be friends.

At the party, the third student had been telling Maddy and Liz about receiving a call from her parents that day. Her family home had had a significant flood of the basement, and several boxes of the woman's childhood possessions were ruined. This woman was quite upset, going on and on about the loss of drawings she had made as a child, the ruining of yearbooks from her schooling, and the like.

Maddy could see Liz was faking sympathy about as earnestly as she was. When Liz said, as a way to get out of this conversation and this boring-yet-loud party, that she had to leave to go check on the rats at her lab to make sure a new feeding system was working, Maddy asked if she could score a ride. Once in the car, she confessed to Liz that she didn't really need a ride.

"I am just struggling to understand what kind of school produces yearbooks in *elementary school*," said Maddy while buckling her seatbelt and Liz said she'd been wondering the exact same thing.

"Some expensive private girls' school, I imagine," said Liz. "Her teeth look expensive."

From there, the conversation had quickly turned into an analysis of this third woman. Was her expansive sentimentality just a form of narcissism? Or simply the sign of a happy, wealthy childhood of the kind that Liz and Maddy had both managed to avoid?

The two of them got into a joking competition about who had retained fewer objects from her past. Maddy won, but by a much smaller margin than Maddy expected. Liz remarked how it seemed odd that someone like Maddy, studying history, didn't care if objects recording the past were lost.

"But I *do* care if the history is *important*," Maddy explained. "I would care, for example, if these woman's elementary school yearbooks might someday tell us something genuinely interesting about someone genuinely interesting. But the possibility seems remote. Few people are interesting in early childhood. And frankly I don't think she will ever be interesting."

Nearing campus, Liz invited Maddy to come to the lab with her to meet her colony and to see what a modern small mammal operation looked like. Maddy had only read about the early rat and mice labs that had been used for the study of behavior and had only seen this kind of lab in photos and she found it fascinating. From there, they'd gone to the Irish Lion to have some dinner and keep talking. They were both mostly out of steam when Maddy asked Liz how she knew she was a lesbian.

"In my experience," said Liz, "any woman who asks me that ends up coming out about a year later. Shall I mark the calendar for you and prepare your coming-out party?"

"To be honest," said Maddy, "I was asking because I have trouble imagining what that would feel like. Feeling that desire."

"Not into the delights of pussy?" asked Liz.

"Very much into my *own*," Maddy laughed. "Not interested in *yours* even though I like you. If you were a man, I think I'd have a terrible crush on you by now. But there's something in me that is specifically attracted to the masculine package even when it is in my best interest to step away."

"Wow, I think you really *are* straight. You sound like an articulate version of my female rats. You have a sense of inevitability about heterosexual mating. Were you a rat, you would be pregnant in no time."

"Which is why the I.U.D. was invented, thank you very much," answered

Maddy. "But seriously – what makes me attracted to men when they are often so much trouble?"

Liz answered glibly that sex didn't think with the brain.

But Maddy pushed her, asking her as a mammalian researcher to help her understand desire.

"Well, we know remarkably little about human sexual attraction," Liz told her. "But we can guess that it has something to do with some combination of auditory, visual, and olfactory stimulation – that there is some kind of combination of what you are seeing, hearing, and smelling that turns you on, when you are turned on. You like the smell of a man during sex, yes?"

"If I like the man," Maddy answered, "then yes, I like his scent *a lot.*"

Liz was starting to ask her why she'd have sex with someone she didn't like when Maddy interrupted.

"Wait, do women have a particular smell? Like, if a woman comes straight out of a clean bath, with no fragrance in the bath water, and no soap, does she have a smell?"

"Yes," said Liz. "Definitely."

"Do you like it?" asked Maddy.

"I realized one day, after studying rats for a long time, that I like the smell of the women that I want *so* much, I can't even *imagine* being attracted to the smell of a man," answered Liz. "It would be like being sexually attracted to a rat. I don't mind how most of them smell – men and rats – but their odors do nothing for me in terms of genital engorgement."

Maddy nodded.

"Aren't straight people just so strange?" Maddy asked.

Liz asked Maddy what she meant.

"Well, you presumably like your own genital package and you like the *same* in your lover," she explained to Liz, and Liz nodded. "Well, that makes sense. But by comparison straight people like me, we like our *own* genitals but we want nothing of the kind *in our lovers.* Gay people make way more sense!"

"Yet your kind has it well over my kind in the self-replication department," Liz noted. "You all are efficient breeders. Especially your natal tribe – the Catholics."

Before becoming friends with Liz, Maddy had not thought about the way the Catholic Church functioned like a reproductive pyramid scheme with putatively celibate men at the top effectively issuing dictums to breed and tithe, to keep it all going.

These conversations with Liz had helped her understand so much....

She sighed now, pushed herself back into her pillow, and felt her ribs with her fingertips. She noted with a little pressure where the ribs met her sternum.

Had Michael become a priest? It was funny now to think of someone like Michael or Father Tad as part of a reproductive pyramid scheme.

Maddy thought back to her conversation with Father Tad on the bench at Rittenhouse Square at the start of that long day that had ended with Giovanni dumping her. After thinking on it a while, Maddy understood why Father Tad had told her about Wolf's wife – to drive home just how important it was for Maddy to drop the subject of Wolf and his marriage, to leave him alone and not get tangled up with him sexually. Liz was right that so much of the job of the priest was to organize sex according to the needs of the church – and Father Tad had been doing just that, understanding Maddy to be dangerous in the Catholic scheme, dangerous to Wolf and the houseful of virgins. (As if Maddy would be interested in wasting her time and energy trying to corrupt Catholics.)

But hearing from Father Tad the story of Wolf's cheating wife had not simply startled her into unexpected guilt. It had also fascinated her.

Wolf had been left in such a strange position. Just as he had found out the truth about his marriage, he'd been stuck with a brain-dead spouse. No doubt the doctors and nurses had pushed him to disconnect his wife once the scans and the passing months had made clear she would not recover. Wouldn't knowing she had cheated on him make him more inclined to let her go? Most people would think it was at least time to move on and would feel justified in doing so.

"Has he forgiven her?" Maddy had asked Father Tad while they shared the slice of lemon poppyseed cake from the paper bag in which Father Tad had delivered it.

"I think so," said Father Tad, unzipping his jacket to relieve some warmth, revealing his clerical collar in the process. "He and I had many long talks when we met, not long after the accident, and we prayed together for a long time. He understood after a few months that what he needed first was to forgive himself for his own anger – his anger at her and his best friend. Once he did that and found some peace, he found it easier to forgive her, too."

"And the reason he doesn't just let her die of some infection? Why doesn't he choose to see whatever infection comes along as God's will and let her go?"

"I think," Father Tad explained, "he does not want God thinking he is exacting revenge on her. Of course, the Lord would see into his heart and know whatever his real motivation was. In any case, I think he feels that treating the infections is not contrary to God's will."

She did not answer.

"Tell me about *your* accident, please?" he said. "Your family's?"

Maddy cleared her throat and adjusted her sleeves, straightening the seams to line up with the drape of her arm. She realized as she did this that this was a gesture Sister Mary Grace used to make – clearing her throat, adjusting her sleeves – just before she broached an indelicate subject. How funny that Maddy had picked it up.

"Something happened that day that set my father off. He packed my mother and my sister in the car and ordered me in, too. But I refused to go. He ended up driving into a highway embankment on the way. I don't think it was on purpose or anything. My sister and my father died in the crash, apparently of a fire. My mother died of blunt force trauma."

Father Tad said nothing in response except to mutter something in Polish. Maddy could tell it was religious.

The way he looked up and returned her gaze made her eyes suddenly well up. It was one of those weird moments where she wasn't feeling sorry for herself – she was sympathizing with the good person who was in pain over her own pathetic situation. She was sympathizing with his pain.

What a strange thing her female brain could be.

"You had no other family to take you in?"

"Only the most distant," Maddy explained, "people I had never met. I was fifteen, and the West Virginia sisters had offered through the – "

She almost used Liz's term: the rosary mafia.

"The sisters had offered, through the Church channels. There were extenuating circumstances that made me inclined to like the idea of a place that was far away among women, where incoming phone calls and letters and visitors would be closely monitored."

Father Tad's eyebrows went up.

"You are thinking," she said, "that that doesn't sound like me. I am rather independent and strong-willed. And I have always been. My mother used to tell me that I came out of the womb not needing anybody. I guess my sister had been a needy baby by comparison? Anyway, at the time of the accident, at the time of the funeral, at that moment, the convent offered me a form of protection from a man – from a particular man – someone who had in essence caused it all."

Father Tad said nothing and Maddy looked around the park, settling her gaze on a couple of two older men playing chess at a small table, looking almost like an old married couple.

"It's good Wolf has you as a friend," said Maddy, seeing in the chess-playing pair the bond of Wolf and Tad – seeing herself and Liz in them, too. How lucky Wolf had been to find Father Tad and how lucky Maddy had been to find Liz, a woman her own age whose experience had to some extent mirrored her own: a life of feeling sexually misunderstood by her family but capable of enjoying sex in spite of the consistent message that one's female anatomy was somehow all wrong, disruptive, a betrayal of one's tribe. Wolf and Father Tad must be bonded, Maddy thought, in their crazy joint celibacy, celibacy in both cases borne of unrequited devotion to their God.

Wolf, Tad, and God – a truly dysfunctional love triangle.

"May I ask you," said Father Tad, "did you want to go to the sisters after the accident? Or was it not your choice?"

"It's hard to say from this temporal distance," Maddy answered. "It was all kind of a blur at that point. The diocesan priests, they wanted me locked away somewhere. West Virginia was very far away."

She paused, thought about what Paula would say – *you have nothing to be ashamed of, Maddy* – and then continued:

"Listen. I'll tell you what happened, if you promise not to tell anyone else, including Wolf."

Father Tad nodded.

"What my father found out that day was that my gymnastics coach was screwing me. This all happened at the Catholic school I was at – it was the diocese's school – and when someone at the school found out about it, he told my father, and my father flipped out and he crashed the car and, well, the school and the diocese did not want the scandal of all this coming out, especially since it had led to my family's death. So the priests and the school needed me gone. When the priests mentioned in front of me the sisters in West Virginia as an option, I realized something – that The Jerk – I mean, I realized that my coach could not get to me there. That was their thought. That was my thought, too. So it was decided."

She pulled the last bit of cake out of the bag between her fingertips but did not eat it yet.

"It was strange, in retrospect," she said. "When I was in that relationship with the coach, I fantasized that he would somehow help me escape from my father. He would help me escape my father and then I would escape from my coach, next. That's what felt like it was justified – that he was going to be my off-ramp from the highway? It doesn't make any sense. I didn't have a plan but he felt like a way out somehow. Maybe because I knew my father would throw me out when he found out. If he found out."

She brought the cake near her lips but then paused.

"Once my father was dead, I realized very clearly that I didn't want to be with my coach at all – I didn't need him anymore as a way to get away from my father. I didn't like what he was doing to me. I wanted to get away from all of it, from my history, from him. From what he was doing to me. And I knew the sisters would not allow a man into the convent, certainly not a man who wasn't a priest and who had sexually abused a girl. I knew they would not even let him send me letters or call me. They would screen people trying to reach me and if he tried, they would stop him. So, I realized this would be like my own little army of female Swiss guards at my own little Vatican for a few years. I could start my life over. Study and figure out what to do next. They would help me get to college. And they would protect me. They *did* protect me. They *still* sometimes protect me when I ask them for help. They are how I got to Wolf. You know, Wolf's house."

He nodded silently again, and she ate the last little bit of cake. For a moment neither said anything. Father Tad drank down the last of his coffee as Maddy did the same. She reached down into her backpack and pulled out a stapled set of photocopied papers.

"Listen, Father, I don't suppose you could tell me what this says?" she asked.

Father Tad could see that it was an article in Polish from a medical journal dated 1892. It told the story of the physician-author's trip to Philadelphia and his viewing of a specimen of a cancerous testicle taken from an esteemed society woman. She had died of testicular cancer.

He read the first couple pages in silence, then flushed red and looked up at her.

"I'm not just playing with you, Father," Maddy said, with a mischievous smile that seemed to belie her claim. "I have to give a talk soon on the specimen that was taken from this woman, and I know that this Polish doctor was a specialist in hermaphroditism. He writes in the piece, I think, not just about her but about the syndrome. I say that based on what another author who referenced the text said about it. We now know what causes the condition – now it's called androgen insensitivity syndrome. Today, we know it's genetic, that it runs in families. But they didn't know that back then. They just knew from the autopsy that she died of testicular cancer, that she appeared very much to be a normal woman all her life, but she turned out to have no womb and no ovaries inside, in spite of living thirty-two years as a woman in the upper class. An infertile, quite attractive woman. With testes."

He handed her back the papers.

"Yes, the article says that she was infertile and quite beautiful," he responded. "That her shape was so womanly, but she had no body hair. And her external and internal parts were as you say. How could this all have been?"

"Sex doesn't always turn out like you expect, Father. Androgen insensitivity syndrome is a remarkable condition. The hormone receptors are lacking to respond to testosterone. So you get genetic male embryo who comes out of the womb a baby girl, and she grows up into an infertile woman. She has no body hair, and she has some male organs inside, but basically she ends up as a woman. Because of the lack of response to testosterone."

"You don't have it, do you?"

"No, no indeed," Maddy said. "I would not be this short, nor would I be quite so cranky once a month if I had that syndrome. Women like her grew tall and did not menstruate. As far as I know, I was born with nothing interesting. Quite dull, really, just a typical female."

She almost offered to show him her armpits to prove she had hair there, which a woman who was androgen-insensitive would not. But she had shaved her armpits for the plan of seeing Giovanni.

"I'm afraid," Father Tad said, with a friendly-enough grimace, "it makes me a little uncomfortable translating it line by line for you. I would help you if I thought you had no other options. But John's young colleague, Wes, he was raised bilingual, Polish and English, and he can probably translate it for you well enough. I can lend you a Polish-English dictionary if that would help."

"Wes, of the blue eyes?" asked Maddy.

Father Tad nodded. They all understood that Father Joe wasn't wrong about Wes's eyes. They were a beautiful blue, a summer-flower blue, a Van Gogh blue.

"He will be at John's birthday party next week, I'm sure. I invited him. John doesn't like a lot of fuss, but he lets me throw him a small party at his house once a year. Oh, you should be there, too, since you'll still be there, presumably."

Now in her bed at Wolf's place, she felt her ribs again, and thought again about the river-skating dream. It made sense now – when she'd gone back to bed, the bed Wolf had so neatly made, after talking to Liz about the nightmare and after working for a while, she had left the local classical music station on the clock radio playing softly to orient her away from the source of her nightmare.

The Blue Danube Waltz in the skating dream had surely come from the radio, leaking through to her in her sleep. Her brain had simply chosen the nearest river to match that river waltz. And instead of waltzing, she was skating.

But why ice skating?

When she was about fourteen, she had tried figure skating. She was very good at it. But The Jerk had stopped her from pursuing it. He didn't want her spending time with another coach.

She closed her eyes now in the hope of bringing back the Blue Danube dream. She moved her fingertips from her ribs to her eyelids.

-12-

Maddy only had about fifteen minutes alone in Shirley's office to do what the National Institutes of Health clerk had asked of her. Shirley would then be back to ask Maddy if she had collected her thoughts and was ready to give the talk upstairs. Maddy didn't want to be in the middle of the fax to the NIH clerk at that point. It would just be awkward to be discovered by Shirley to be snooping around the unpublished work of a prominent physician who had not only arranged the relatively prestigious talk that Maddy was about to deliver but who was going to give Maddy and Shirley dinner at his home afterwards.

The NIH Freedom of Information Act clerk had received Maddy's request and then emailed Maddy to ask her to call him. He revealed in his email only that there appeared to be a small problem with her FOIA request. But what problem could there have been? Her request had been so short and straightforward.

As soon as Shirley had left Maddy alone, Maddy had shut the door and used Shirley's phone to call him, hoping he would still be there this late in the day. When he answered and she told him who she was, he explained to Maddy that she had indicated in her written request that she had wanted all of Dr. Wilhelm's annual grant reports from January 1, 1864, forward.

The request had been assigned to him, and he was thinking she meant 1964 forward? Or did she mean some other date?

"Oh, gosh, yes," Maddy answered. "I'm sorry, I'm usually in the nine-teenth century. I meant 1964 forward."

"No problem," the clerk answered, "if you can just fax me over an adden-dum indicating the correction."

He gave her the fax number and confirmed the street address where she wanted the materials sent to her.

"I should address it in care of John Wolf?" he asked.

"Yes," she said. "That's my landlord."

"It's so funny," he said. "I used to live right in that neighborhood. On Waverly Street. I can't quite picture the house you're in."

"It's just a classic brick rowhouse. Nothing memorable. I'll bet the area hasn't changed much."

"Probably not. That part of Philly doesn't change. Except for the cracks in the sidewalks getting bigger. And some of the houses getting a little nicer and some getting a little more down in the tooth, I guess. Listen, do you want all of the addendums to all of his grant reports – all the published papers attached and the c.v. copies and all that? A lot of it is likely to be duplicative and there will be a ton. I don't get to decide what to send you, exactly...but you also didn't specify if you wanted the main reports or the whole packet for each – like I said, there will be a ton of duplication of ma-terial you're probably not interested in. And I can get it to you faster if you don't need everything. And there's less likely to be a charge."

Maddy wondered if she could just tell him what she wanted. The rule in the field of history, she had long ago learned, was to always treat a librarian or an archivist like one's therapist – just get to the point of why you're there.

"Are we supposed to play cat-and-mouse?" she asked the clerk. "Would that mark me as a pro in this game? Or can I please just tell you what I'm looking for?"

"Sure, you can tell me," he said. "We don't usually keep an eye out for specific content you're seeking. We're just supposed to follow your request the way it's written. But if you tell me, I suppose I can scan the attachments to the main report, and if I see something relevant then I'll attach the whole package."

She explained that she was interested in the history of Dr. Wilhelm's specimens – anything about the people they had come from, what he had learned from those in particular, how he spoke of them. She said she was doing comparative history, this series of specimens collected by Dr. Wilhelm and practices of his predecessors a hundred years earlier (not a total lie?) and that she didn't need his published papers because she had easy access to those. He asked her a little more and told her the subject sounded interesting.

"To be honest," he added, "I try to look up what eventually happens with various FOIA requests I answer. I like to see what people – scholars and journalists and whoever – have done with the material I send them. Makes one feel like one's job is not a total waste of time and taxpayer expense. Although so many requests I answer never seem to come to anything.... Anyway, just fax me the correction and I'll be working on this request next, right after I send another one out tomorrow morning. Yours shouldn't take too long. Pretty straightforward and there won't be much if anything that needs redacting, I expect."

She hung up and thought about how to make sure in her haste that she did this version of her request exactly right. She had left in her possession only three sheets of her university's departmental letterhead from Indiana because she had brought only four in total with her to Philly. (Her standard list of what to bring on a research trip included a couple of sheets of letterhead, just in case.) She could always ask the departmental secretary in Indiana to send more but that would take a week, and she might have to explain what she was doing with it all.

She did a test run of her request addendum on plain paper on Shirley's printer and then, seeing that it looked okay, she printed it out on letterhead. She signed it and sent it off using Shirley's fax machine. As soon as the machine seemed to be done with the transmission, she called the clerk back to confirm its delivery. He said it looked good.

She hung up the phone just before Shirley walked back in.

"Ready?" asked Shirley.

"Yes, indeed," said Maddy, using her fingers to check the integrity of the bun of hair on her head. "Ready."

She couldn't stop thinking about what the FOIA response might show. She shouldn't be spending time on this tangent – it was so important to stay focused entirely on the dissertation at this point. That's where other people went wrong and ended up never finishing their PhD's. Tangents (professional or personal) could lead to delays, which could lead to funding running out, which could lead to having to get a job that made it impossible to have the time and energy to finish. Some people just didn't realize how important it was to stay so completely focused, to work at least a little every day until it was done. Finishing her Ph.D. meant holding everything together just so, like the bun on her head.

...

"For the translation of this next text from Polish to English, I am indebted to Officer Wesley Larsen," Maddy told the audience. "So, if I get any major organs wrong here, please blame the Philadelphia Police Department, not me."

A chuckle went through the room as Maddy advanced to the next slide. The mention of his name roused Wes from the thoughts he'd been having, which were only sort of connected to the content of Maddy's presentation. If he was honest with himself, he was mostly thinking about how hot Maddy looked in this conservative-librarian get-up, her hair pulled up, just a few strands hanging down, curling at the ends near her jawline. All she was missing was a pair of cat-eye glasses on a rhinestone chain or something.

As Maddy walked a few steps to and fro at the front of the museum's small auditorium, continuing her lecture, her calves looked to him so good in those heels – feminine and strong, obviously the legs of a woman who was runner – and, he knew from their conversation, the legs of a gymnast, too. She had asked him about the gym Wolf had been taking her to, whether Wes could take her to the same place if Wolf wasn't free, so she could do gymnastics.

Wes glanced over at Wolf, seated next to him. He couldn't figure out why Wolf was looking more and more intense, the way he looked when he was working step by step through a case that bothered him. What was up with that? Maddy was doing a fine job from what Wes could tell – so it could not be that Wolf was worried that she was bombing. She seemed to have the audience of doctors in the palm of her hand, to be delivering her material with confidence.

Wes was glad that he and Wolf had taken Maddy up on the offer to get them into this presentation so Wes could see what she did with the text he had translated for her. He had been very curious to see whether other people would be interested in what she was interested in. These people did seem to be.

Maddy had asked Wes at Wolf's birthday party if he'd help her translate something from Polish and when he said sure, she pulled him into a corner of the living room to show him the photocopies. She said Father Tad thought it'd be better that Wes do it.

As soon as Wes started reading it, he cracked up and told her it wasn't the kind of thing you'd ask a priest to translate, now, was it?

Wes told her he wasn't sure about a few of the – uh, medical terms – and at that Maddy disappeared quickly upstairs and came back with a thick Polish-English dictionary and told him she'd just look up with him what he wasn't sure about. She said Father Tad had lent the dictionary to her.

When he told her to look up one word and it turned out to be mean uterine cervix, she asked him if he didn't know what a cervix was, and he said, blushing, he just didn't know the word in Polish.

"Have you not had sex in Polish?" she asked, laughing at him and taking another swig from her bottle of beer.

"I had it in Polish once," he admitted to her, taking a drink from his own, "with a Polish girl my mother wanted me to marry. But this here, this was not a word I needed to get the job done. I'm not saying I don't know *what it is* – I just didn't need to name it in Polish right then, at that time, at that particular moment."

He could not believe he just told her that, but it made her smile and laugh.

Wes asked Maddy why the woman being described in the article didn't have a uterine cervix, and Maddy explained that if you didn't form a uterus – which girls don't if they have this condition – then you didn't form a cervix.

"Can't have a fingernail without a fingertip," she said plainly. Although then she cocked her head and held a finger to her lips like she was thinking maybe in fact you could.

Wes kept translating aloud, getting to where the author, still describing the absence of the cervix, described the woman's vagina as being like a sock – simply ending at the top rather than leading to a uterus.

"So, you know the Polish words for *vagina* and *sock*," Maddy nodded at him, amused. "Those you know."

"Now, vagina and sock, those sometimes *do* go together," he answered. "But I myself prefer a vagina without a sock."

"Who doesn't?" she asked, laughing out loud.

He had had to put his head down for a second not to appear like a fool from the look on his face. That just made her laugh at him more and poke him on the elbow.

"You're very pretty," he said, looking up at her. (He had learned this was a good thing to say, especially if a girl might believe him.)

Maddy shook her head at him side to side and rolled her eyes a little, like he was hopeless. But she was still smiling.

When he got to the part in the old medical journal article about the woman not having any hair in her armpits or her pubic region, he paused from his on-the-fly verbal translation and looked up from the paper to Maddy's face.

"Yes," she said, anticipating his question. "I do have hair there."

"That's fine," he said. "I mean, that's cool."

"And it grew there on its own," she explained further. "I don't have a merkin."

"What's a merkin?"

"A pubic-hair wig," she explained.

"Get outta here! Those exist? That's a real thing? An actual thing?"

"Yup," she said. "Believe it or not, fashions keep changing about what people like down there, on women anyway. It's all kind of stupid, if you ask me. A natural body is nice no matter how it comes, right?"

And here he was trying to formulate a joke to highlight what she had just said, but before he had the chance to, she realized what she had just said and started giggling, a little like a kid.

"Um, that's not exactly what I meant to say!"

"Uh huh," he said. "Well, I was just going to agree with you. Your observation seems to me correct. Quite correct."

At the end of the party, Wolf was supposed to give Wes a ride home in Wes's car because Wolf needed to borrow Wes's car while his own was stuck in the shop waiting for the mechanic to install some part he had ordered. But after working on the translation together, Wes and Maddy decided to convince Wolf to let Maddy give Wes the ride home. She could bring Wes's car back to Wolf. Maddy told Wolf she was happy to do it and added that if she didn't drive now and then, especially in a real city, she'd lose the hang of what Liz had taught her when Liz helped her get her license.

When they got to Wes's place, several miles away, it was dark out. He said he'd invite her in except his mother was probably already in her nightgown. He asked her if she felt confident about the way back and she said yes, she'd been watching carefully on the way over.

"You know which streets are the one-ways near Wolf's?" he asked.

"I can figure it out," she said. "There are probably signs that say 'one way,' right?"

"There are. We point them out to people when we pull them over for going the wrong way."

Then there was that pause. And then there was that kiss he put on her cheek. When he brushed the tip of his nose against her cheekbone as he pulled away, she let out a little sigh that sent all the blood in his head to his groin.

"Thank you," was all she said.

"Happy to serve," he answered.

The skin of her cheek had been as soft as baby hair.

Now, remembering all that, listening to her go on about another specimen in the museum's collection – What the hell? A seven-month fetus with two heads, did she say? – he was having the same problem with his blood being redirected.

Well, maybe she would call him later for a ride home from the doctor's house after the dinner as she had asked Wes if she could. She wasn't sure how she was getting back home otherwise, she said. Maybe then....

Wes looked again at Wolf. His brow just kept furrowing harder. But Wes knew better than to ask Wolf later why this was. Wolf never wanted to explain anything in a line of thinking until he caught something and was ready to pull his line out of the water. Asking him what he was thinking just got you the brush-off, or worse, a sort of short verbal smack across your lips. No thanks.

-13-

Maddy felt as if she had broken into one of the most incredible private history of medicine libraries in the world. *Were* there ones better than Dr. Wilhelm's?

Granted, his collection of works played directly to her interests – anatomy, teratology, and pathology with texts stretching back to – good lord, to the sixteenth century? At least.

Perhaps someone interested in the history of epidemics or the history of pharmacology or very specifically the history of soft-tissue surgery – perhaps that kind of historian of medicine would not find this nearly so thrilling. But to Maddy, the scene was astonishing. The idea that one person would own this many works in the history of anatomy....

Jakob Ruff, *De Conceptu et Generatione Hominis,* 1554.

Johannes-Georg Schenck, *Monstrorum Historia Memorabilis,* 1609.

The oversize edition of Paré's collected works.

She could spend her days simply reading from one shelf to the next. Yes, she'd have to stick to the languages she knew but there were plenty of texts in those tongues. Within a week of living here, her Latin would necessarily be much improved.

And the architecture – the furniture –

She dared to creep over as quietly as she could to the panel of switches near the entry door to turn on more lights, so she could see it all better. As the room lit up with the shine of the two crystal chandeliers, she looked around with wonder at the built-in bookshelves – mahogany? or cherry? – the ornamented moldings, the Persian rugs. About half the wall shelves had leaded glass doors, the other half being uncovered. The shelves went all the way from within a foot of the floor to within a foot of the ceiling – a coffered ceiling, which had to be at least fourteen feet high. A series of rolling library ladders set into a polished brass rail made it possible to reach the volumes on the upper shelves. Lower down, free-standing cabinets throughout the room held more shelves of books and on top of each of these cabinets, polished marble tabletop slabs served as pedestals for folio volumes laid out.

William Cheselden, *Osteographia, or The Anatomy of the Bones*, 1733.

Albinus, 1749, with its exquisite drawings comparing the skeleton of the human to that of the magnificent rhinoceros.

The marble edges of these cabinet surfaces were ever so gently worn in places, as if someone had been leaning up against these cabinets for years, looking through these books.

Alone in Dr. Wilhelm's library with the room insulated from any outside noise by the closed, weighty velvet curtains, she ran her fingers along the bindings, feeling the weaves, the leathers, the embossed titles. He seemed to have virtually everything she could think of. The complete set of Geoffroy Saint-Hilaire's treatise on teratology; multiple editions. Sims on congenital tetanus. Neugebauer on the forms of hermaphroditism. Spemann's work on experimental development biology. What appeared to be a near-complete run of the first centuries of the British Medical Journal and The Lancet?

She was so enthralled, she did not hear Dr. Wilhelm come up behind her. She startled when he asked her what she thought. She turned around to face him, her mouth hanging partly open.

"It's astonishing," she said. "Astonishing."

He looked pleased at her reaction.

"Joining the two houses together made it possible to create this room," he explained. "The engineering was a little tricky in terms of opening up the wall, but it turned out to be possible. I'm not sure anyone will ever want to buy this house with a library taking up most of the first floor. But then I didn't create it for sale."

"Magnificent," she added. "All of it."

He bowed a little in acknowledgment. She wasn't sure how to react. She looked at him and realized he would be a few inches taller than her were he laid out for dissection on one of these marble-topped shelving units. But he was bent now from age, and so he seemed about her height. His frame held maybe thirty pounds more than a doctor might want to see on a man his age, no doubt the result of eating well. She knew his birthdate from looking up his work; he was now seventy-three. His work was still going full-tilt and showed no signs of slowing. The room showed what he had done with the monetary rewards for his work.

"I have had a number of very good book buyers keeping an eye out for me over the years," he explained, going over to the switches to turn down the lights to a more comfortable level. "They know in what I might find interest, interest enough to buy. Would you care to see my *Fasciculo de medicina*? I've got a 1522, the Italian."

She just nodded. He went to one of the cabinets in the end of the room farthest from the main doorway and she followed him. It was a cabinet Maddy now realized was more modern than it first appeared. It had a climate control feature to keep the humidity and temperature to the books' liking, to keep them healthy in old age.

He opened the cabinet door, unlocking it with a brass key from a set in his pocket. He removed the book, laying it carefully on a bookstand on the cabinet's top. The stand would prop the volume open at an angle comfortable for its ancient spine. Maddy was familiar with this kind of tool; such a stand always struck her as rather like the bolsters a kind nurse would put under your knees if you had to lay on your back on a gurney for a long time.

Dr. Wilhelm opened to the iconographic illustration of the *Fasciculus*, of the anatomy scene – the lecturer seated well above, the men below earnestly cutting into the dead body, their attention focused on the dissection table. Then he turned the pages carefully to show her the other classic illustrations of the text – one explaining with pictures and words how to diagnose disease by sampling the patient's urine (the color, the smell, the taste), another showing how to bloodlet to relieve various symptoms and perhaps save a life (or so they thought).

He turned now to "Wound Man," an image Maddy had only ever seen in reproductions. It showed a man comically subjected all at once to being beaten, shot through with arrows, and stabbed with a knife – all the assaults packed into one single drawing in the interest of teaching how to treat various wounds.

Shirley came suddenly and noisily into the room with Dr. Tate, another distinguished member of the museum's medical society. Like Shirley, Dr. Tate had been invited to this little post-lecture gathering at Dr. Wilhelm's home, perhaps to round the number out to four. Shirley had told Maddy in a quick aside earlier that Dr. Tate was a very prominent neonatologist at the university, a man who shared Dr. Wilhelm's passion for the history of medicine. Maddy had guessed Dr. Tate to be around fifty, though she found it a little hard to tell. (His ethnicity threw her off, as she had learned anatomic age cues while being around mostly white people.) His accent sounded West Indian to her.

"Dr. Wilhelm, Ms. Shanks!" cried Dr. Tate. "Shirley and I have successfully procured the libations! Come and have a refreshment."

He carried on a silver tray four full martini glasses, each perspiring a little.

"But not near the books!" Maddy blurted out, and they all laughed at her.

Dr. Wilhelm moved to put away the *Fasciculo* and gestured to them all to sit at the sofa and armchairs gathered around a coffee table in the center section of the grand room beneath the apex of the coffered ceiling. Sitting down on the library couch – an old-fashioned tufted settee she thought would have looked perfectly at home in Versailles – Maddy looked up and saw now that the ceiling section above them contained an elaborate painting of the Zodiac. She immediately understood it as a reference to medieval medical texts that linked the Ptolemaic universe to the body of man, connecting the immortal stars to the fate of mortals in the center of the world. Dr. Wilhelm must have commissioned it.

"Enjoying Dr. Wilhelm's collection?" Dr. Tate asked, setting the tray down on the table and handing Maddy one of the drinks. "Quite nice, don't you think?"

"It's astonishing," she said again. "I cannot begin to imagine living in a house with all these gems."

"Come now," Dr. Wilhelm answered her, taking a sip from his glass, "many are fairly ordinary texts. I've just been collecting a long time."

"But it's the whole collection!" Maddy exclaimed. "The compilation!"

"It's quite something," agreed Shirley. Then she turned to Dr. Wilhelm to ask, "Will Sergey be joining us for dinner? I didn't see him at the lecture."

"Dr. Goncharov is seeing a patient for me this evening," answered Dr. Wilhelm, looking up briefly to the grandfather clock near the main entry.

"Too bad," said Shirley. "Anyway, Maddy, I knew you'd like to see it. I hope you didn't miss the eighteenth-century medicinal cookbooks or the surgical field reports of the Union Army. Or that marvelous section with the popular eugenics manuals."

She pointed to an area across the room from her.

"Not terribly rare or expensive, those," said Dr. Wilhelm.

"True, but I still think the eugenics-for-the-masses tomes from the '20s and '30s are particularly fun," replied Shirley. "I mean, they're fun if you forget that it all led to the Nazis."

"Many of the early eugenics manuals are from your Indiana, Ms. Shanks," Dr. Tate added, leaning back comfortably in his armchair and crossing his legs. "Your state, Indiana, it was the real early leader in the movement to breed better humans. But you probably know that."

Maddy nodded. She was spending a portion of her conscious energy trying to sit up straight on this squishy couch.

"Better cows, better corn, better humans!" said Shirley. "A state-fair state on a mission of scientific breeding."

"The goal was perfectly *reasonable*, of course," Dr. Wilhelm noted, getting up to walk to the open-shelved section of the room to which Shirley had pointed, to find and retrieve a particular book. "No reasonable person would think it a bad idea to make sure every baby is born healthy – free of physiological or anatomical defect, free of disease, free to have as good a life as possible. Born with an untroubled body."

He brought back a book bound in red cloth and handed it to Maddy. She read the faded printed title: *Eugenics and You.*

She looked it over seeing it was a "marriage manual" from 1928 meant primarily to teach young men how to pick a good wife – one who would produce healthy children. She could see from the copyright page it had been printed in Indianapolis. The inscription inside the front cover indicated a mother had given it to her son shortly after publication as a gift.

She flipped gently through the pages, finding an illustration showing with simple line drawings and a few words what distinguished a suitable woman from an unsuitable one where mating was concerned. The unsuitable woman was dressed like a flapper and the text noted the various faults of her skinny frame. Maddy understood that her short bob and angular nose were meant to mark her as trouble.

The suitable woman, by contrast, came with big hips, ample breasts ready to satisfy a hungry babe, lush blond tresses, and a classically attractive face. She was dressed in a long skirt, sensible shoes, and a neatly buttoned-up blouse. This was a girl you could bring home to mama.

"I've certainly seen a lot of books like this at flea markets and antique stores in Indiana," said Maddy. "It's always a little startling to come across them, next to the old tractor catalogues and copies of Dickens."

"Eh," said Dr. Wilhelm, "I think we forget the proportion of good sense that came with the whole movement. We just emphasize the pathology in the history of civilization, not all the moments of normal societal development. The Progressive Era was a period of embracing science for the public good and this was part of that zeal. The problem wasn't teaching people the basics of where skin and eye color came from or teaching them the value of good nutrition and of avoiding the transmission of disease – whether sexual or inherited. The problem was the Nazis turning it into an ethnic cleansing campaign – an outright genocide. My mother's side was Jewish, but I can still distinguish what might have been reasonable in the American Midwest from what turned into tribal madness in parts of Europe. We don't condemn all of chemistry because some tyrants have used chemical weapons to slaughter the innocent."

"Truly," nodded Dr. Tate, "no one objects today to the notion of women trying to be as healthy as possible before and during pregnancy."

He took the book from Maddy and flipped through the pages, chuckling at some of the images.

"But helping women stay healthy before and during pregnancy," objected Maddy, "is surely different from the state promoting – rewarding – so-called better breeding."

"Ms. Shanks," asked Dr. Tate, leaning forward and holding the book closed between his hands, "surely you aren't against the government's decision to push folic acid in wheat as a public health measure with the aim of preventing neural tube defects like spina bifada in the general population? Folic acid added to wheat has prevented thousands of babies being unnecessarily born with neural tube defects."

"Quite right, Dr. Tate," agreed Dr. Wilhelm. "Ms. Shanks, you can't think that a life with spina bifada is *easier* or *better* than a life without. Or that the mother's life is easier or better if she has a child born to her with a neural tube defect that will require hospitalizations, surgery – that might lead to the child's death. The government is right to try to ensure women give birth to healthy children by pushing folic acid into the human food supply."

Maddy wasn't sure what to say.

Shirley brushed some hair off her cheek, took another sip of her drink, and said in a quiet voice as if to no one in particular, "Today, if an obstetrician does *not* offer a pregnant woman a genetic check to see if the fetus has a trisomy, he's often considered to be guilty of malpractice."

Maddy made a mental note of Shirley's use of the male pronoun for an obstetrician; Shirley did seem quite comfortable in the male-heavy orbit of Dr. Wilhelm.

"Ah, yes, good point!" said Dr. Tate. "The whole 'wrongful life' concept – where a woman sues her doctor for the birth of a child with Down Syndrome she says she would have aborted had she but been offered the test and known the child would be born with Down's."

"I suppose," Maddy began slowly, putting down her drink to try to collect her thoughts, "I suppose it's not unreasonable to try to *prevent* disease – although we have to wonder whether abortion can be thought of as disease prevention? It prevents more than just a *disease*, right? But we still ought to be aware of how these approaches can end up at the social extremes."

"My dear," said Dr. Tate, "you are speaking to a gay black man! I am certainly aware of the historical extremes of the belief that some genetic or anatomic types are inferior to others. But it's easy to forget that even the worst ideas sometimes grow from ones that begin as not half-bad."

"Modern American democracy is a good example of that," said Dr. Wilhelm, and Shirley and Dr. Tate laughed.

At that moment, the man Maddy took to be Dr. Wilhelm's butler came and invited the four of them to the dining room upstairs. Shirley gathered up the cocktail glasses on the tray and handed it to the butler. Leaving the library, Maddy took one more glance over her shoulder.

. . .

As politely as she could, Maddy declined again more wine. She was already a little tipsy and still determined not to embarrass herself or Shirley, even as Shirley was veering into the territory of having had too much.

Maddy could hardly blame Shirley for being a little drunk; new wine kept coming with each course, each new wine matched very pleasantly to the new dish set before them. She was trying to memorize what she could ascertain about each course to tell Wolf all about it later. But, she thought to herself, she would have to describe it to Wolf in a way that sounded like she was gossiping with him, not criticizing his own cooking through implied comparison.

She could barely concentrate enough to enjoy the flavors and textures here – she felt so out of her league. All of her energy was being spent on using the right utensil and saying the right thing. Perhaps later she could relive it in description and enjoy it with Wolf that way.

She had spent the last twenty minutes politely asking Dr. Wilhelm about his work, mentioning what she knew he would consider his most significant findings from the last several decades. He seemed very pleased she knew so much about it. At one point, Dr. Wilhelm had his butler bring him pen and paper so that he could draw for Maddy the way a spinal column could malform under the influence of a particular genetic syndrome.

"Do you suppose," Maddy asked, "whether someday you – I mean physicians – will be able to diagnose the presence of the genetics for some kinds of dwarfism in the embryonic stage and to intervene, to promote typical development in the fetus and beyond?"

"At this stage," he answered, "it is difficult to see what such an intervention would look like. We are not talking about anything like a simple nutritional deficiency on the part of the mother or an enzyme lacking in the fetus, or anything of that sort. But prevention would certainly be the goal."

"And does the dwarf community" – she almost paused to correct her language, and then decided there wasn't much point in this setting – "do they all agree that is a worthy goal?"

Dr. Wilhelm did not answer immediately, so Dr. Tate jumped in: "People need to understand that prevention of a disease is not meant as a condemnation of the identity, a diminution of the worth of the people now living with that disease. Preventing dwarfism doesn't devalue people who are dwarves."

"What you say makes sense," answered Maddy, rearranging the napkin in her lap to lay more in line with the rectangle created by her thigh bones. "I'm just thinking of what Dr. DesJardins said when I met him a few weeks ago about stigma being culturally specific, about trying to help the community of little people understand that."

"You met Dr. DesJardins?" asked Dr. Wilhelm, and Maddy nodded.

He poured Shirley and Dr. Tate a little more wine.

"Well," said Dr. Wilhelm, "Dr. DesJardins is fortunate in that he doesn't suffer much from his condition beyond stigma. He must put up with a world designed for adults who are significantly taller. And that creates challenges for moving around – as he would tell you – setting up a functional home, driving a car, using a public toilet. Trying to find romantic partners. But he does not suffer from the physical pain and disability that many other forms of dwarfism entail."

"That's true," said Maddy. "Although I suppose his midline defect could cause him some serious physical trouble in the long-run."

"Maddy spotted his cleft lip scar right off the bat!" cried Shirley, as if bragging about a favorite student. "She has a good eye."

"His is surely an interesting body," said Dr. Wilhelm. "The combination of the dwarfism and the midline defect suggests a line of inquiry – one we've been pursuing in the lab."

"Dr. DesJardins has gone and gotten the programming community to invite Maddy to give a talk at the annual meeting in Washington," Shirley announced with haste in her voice.

Maddy wondered if Shirley was moving the conversation along to keep Maddy from mentioning what Dr. DesJardins had said about having a physician-researcher at the Cleveland Clinic interested in his "celebrity bod."

"She'll be giving a history talk," added Shirley. "So you will see Dr. Wilhelm again there, Maddy, next week in Washington. He always goes to answer all the community's medical questions, encourage people to come see him at his clinic."

Dr. Wilhelm rang the small brass bell positioned near the top of his plate and the butler came in to take away their plates from that course. It had been centered on a lovely cut of pork tenderloin, herb encrusted and served over some kind of fruited, herbed puree. Was it parsnip with apple? With a side of bitter greens, balancing it so perfectly. An upscale version of a good Germanic dish. Maddy wondered what would come next.

"What are you planning to cover in your history lecture at the conference?" Dr. Tate inquired.

"I haven't decided quite yet," Maddy answered. "Probably something about representations of the condition in medical texts over time." She turned to Dr. Wilhelm and pulled the conversation back: "Dr. Wilhelm, I suppose Nicholas DesJardins' risk of the heart problem is higher given his midline development issue?"

Dr. Wilhelm pivoted his gaze to her somewhat sharply and asked her what she meant.

"Well, I read in some of your papers about the increased risk of death from heart problems in the population," she explained. "That is how Margaret Lovisa died, yes?"

Dr. Tate put down his fork and looked up at Dr. Wilhelm in what Maddy thought was a significant way. Did Tate, like Maddy, find the way Wilhelm kept Lovisa a little shocking?

"I found interesting," Maddy continued, to politely fill in the conversational gap, "I found interesting that you had located that text from 1888 – Schlesinger, yes? – the pamphlet? The one documenting the index case of heart failure in two brothers with dwarfism. Index cases, plural, I suppose, with two brothers dying of the same thing."

"Yes," said Dr. Wilhelm. "A good find, that text – supported my own findings. That text, Schlesinger 1888, it showed the record of heart problems, the comorbidity of heart failures and dwarfism. Showed there was a record of the problem before I noted it."

Maddy thought to herself that only a doctor genuinely interested in the science and the history of medicine would be happy to discover that a predecessor had found something interesting before he himself did. Most would want to take credit for the "index case" – the first documented case of an interesting phenomenon or pathology. But Dr. Wilhelm was happy to find verification of his own findings in the historical record and let Schlesinger have the priority claim.

"Do you have it?" asked Maddy.

"Do I have what?" he asked.

The Butler brought in a tray of fresh plates and a serving bowl of salad. He began to apportion out the greens onto four plates and to distribute them among the four of them at the table.

"Do you have Schlesinger 1888 – the pamphlet linking the heart defect to dwarfism?" asked Maddy. "Incidentally, why was it published by Schlesinger as a pamphlet and not a journal article?"

"I think perhaps he was trying out the idea before he published it in the peer-reviewed literature," said Dr. Wilhelm. "Seeing how it played."

"An odd approach," answered Maddy. "I would understand if what you'd found had been a manuscript....The pamphlet must have been the last thing he published, based on the date. Anyway, do you have Schlesinger 1888? I would love to see it."

"No," said Dr. Wilhelm. "I did at one time. But it was lost. In any case, it was just a text – no images. Not very interesting as a document."

"It was lost in the fire, correct?" asked Dr. Tate in a helpful tone. He began to eat his salad.

"Yes," said Dr. Wilhelm. He pushed his own salad about on the plate but did not eat any yet.

"Dr. Wilhelm's library suffered a small fire," explained Shirley. "A year or so ago. There was a power outage and Dr. Wilhelm had a candle to check on the books, to see whether he had to start the generator to run the climate control and he stumbled, and some of his works were out – "

"It was a small fire," Dr. Wilhelm cut in. "I was able to use an extinguisher quickly to put it out. We lost only a few texts. And they were insured. It gave us an opportunity to improve the fire safety system in the house. In the long run, a blessing."

"But what a thing to lose, that pamphlet!" said Maddy. She put down her fork and knife for a moment. "I mean, given the direct connection to your own work, that must have felt a great loss!"

"It was not terribly valuable," answered Dr. Wilhelm now drinking a little wine and bringing a forkful of salad to his mouth.

"Fortunately," explained Shirley, "Dr. Wilhelm had given photocopies of the work to some in the community, so the text itself – what Schlesinger had said – that was preserved. I mean, we still know what it says even if we don't have it on original paper."

"It isn't the only copy of the pamphlet anyway," said Dr. Wilhelm. "Of course it would not be the only copy."

Maddy asked what other collections contained it. Dr. Wilhelm answered that he wasn't sure, but he was sure there would be a few.

"And if it comes on the market again, I will simply purchase another copy," he said.

"Yes, well, it may not be monetarily valuable," Maddy said, trying to be a sympathetic guest, "but I'm sure you found it historically and scientifically very valuable. To your work, I mean – to your publications on – "

Dr. Wilhelm rose suddenly, went to the library, and returned with a volume of the *Transactions of the Pathological Society of London.* He opened it to a particular page and handed it to Maddy. She could see the date on the top of the page: April 23, 1897. It was an article about a stillborn specimen, born with shortened limbs, a hare lip, and a genital malformation.

"I see," said Maddy. "The index case of dwarfism with midline defect?"

"I believe so," he answered. "I have shown it to Dr. DesJardins. He found it of interest, of course."

She was trying to understand why he had bothered to get up to show her this just now. She handed him back the volume, and he closed it and leaned back to lay it on the sideboard.

"May I ask why it was a police officer who translated the Neugebauer for you from Polish, about the lady with the cancerous testis?" he asked, not looking up at her but focusing on his plate now.

"Just a local friend of a friend who can read Polish and who happened to be available," Maddy said, smiling a little. Dr. Tate and Shirley smiled back at her. "I found out through the friend that he's a native Polish speaker, so I asked him for the help."

"Will you be needing his help again?" asked Dr. Wilhelm. "For more?"

"I seriously doubt I'll need help with Polish translations again," answered Maddy. "Not too often I run into one I need. But he's picking me up later."

"Why is that?" asked Dr. Wilhelm, with one eyebrow up.

"He came to the talk and I told him I would be having dinner here and he offered me a ride home – I expect he wants to hear how the talk went. And maybe he's worried about my walking home, what with the serial rapist and all."

She didn't really think the rapist was Wes's concern. It just seemed like gossipy small talk of the kind one could share at a table of this sort, and she had the sense changing the subject wouldn't bother the host. He seemed embarrassed by the conversation about the fire. (Perhaps he thought it marked him old and clumsy?)

"*You* are not worried about that – the serial rapist?" blurted out Dr. Tate. And then, as if he had accidentally insulted Shirley by not suggesting she should also be worried, he turned to her and asked, "Or you, Ms. Anseed? Worried?"

"The cost of living in a real city," said Shirley, shrugging her shoulders. "There's always something one could worry about. And the lions don't usually try to take down the giraffes. They go for the gazelles, right? Are you worried, our little country gazelle?"

"I'm actually from New York, not Indiana," answered Maddy, a little defensively. "So, I suppose that means I have the *good sen*se to worry about a serial rapist?"

She stuck her tongue out a little at Shirley. Shirley gave her back an annoyed look.

"I will admit," Maddy continued, "there's less to worry about in Indiana than Philly or New York, or so it feels on the average day. But it's not like this guy attacks women on the streets. He attacks women in their own homes."

She realized from their reaction that maybe they didn't want to be reminded of such an image.

"Now *that's* frightening, if you ask me," said Maddy. "And this coming week, I'm going to be stuck home alone every night while my landlord is gone. So I admit I'll be thinking about it. And it's creepy. He's not a murderer, but it's creepy. This guy, he shows up in a black ski mask with sunglasses, so you can't see him, and with a knife – he binds the victims' wrists

134

and ankles with electrical tape. Threatens them if they scream – "

"That's enough detail, darling!" cried Shirley, holding up her hands. "Now you're going to have to have your officer friend give *me* a ride home, too."

"I can drive you home after dinner, no trouble," said Dr. Tate. "You, too, Ms. Shanks, if you like. I am happy to drive you both home."

"That's okay," Maddy answered. "I told Officer Larson I'd take him up on the offer of the ride. I'm sorry, Shirley. I didn't realize anything could scare you."

"The human *form* never does," Shirley said, putting her hands in her lap and cracking her knuckles audibly. "But human behavior, now that's another thing. It's one reason I much prefer the dead."

-14-

The passenger cars jerked forward when the engineer released the break. The train slowly began to pull out from the station. The sudden movement of air through the coach now enabled Maddy's olfactory bulbs to pick up the traces of that distinctive deodorizing spray Amtrak used in its passenger cars. It smelled to her like some combination of chlorine bleach and rotted melon. She wished she had thought to bring a little lavender oil to dab under her nose.

Standing on the platform, Wolf held up his hand briefly to give a sort of wave to Maddy through the scratched-up window. She thought it looked a resigned salute more than anything else. She held up her hand briefly in return and watched him turn to head home.

She thought about Wolf's confession to her on the walk to the station, that he was torn about her going to Washington for a few days. On the one hand, he had said, he didn't much like the idea of her going to be with an unfamiliar crowd in another city when she was still jumpy and sleep deprived following the attack at home. On the other hand, he had said, it would finish out the week of him working nights, so he wouldn't have to figure out what to do about not leaving her home alone again.

"Maybe you could just move in with Wes and his mother until we find you another place?" Wolf had said, as he had been walking her to the station. "He seems to be happy to be around you, and I would bet he would give you his bedroom and he would sleep on their couch a while if I asked him."

"No, thank you," she had answered flatly. "And I don't see why you're worried about leaving me home alone again. It's not like whoever it was is going to dare to come back again. Not after you chased him."

"We still don't even know how he got in."

"I can latch the doors with the chains when you're not there. You can just call me if you're on your way home and I'll unlatch the door when you get there."

"I'm not comfortable with it – with you being home alone. We need to find you another place. You can still come over and eat dinner with me, Rabbit. And we can talk. Like we did last night. You don't have to worry about that."

"Let's discuss it when I get back from D.C.," Maddy had said. "I have to focus on work right now. So do you."

They had just hit the point of the Market Street bridge where the tall windows of 30th Street Station started to come into view. She had had on her backpack and he had been carrying the suitcase he was lending her for the trip. (Her own suitcase was too big for a trip lasting just four days.)

"You'll be back to working days when I get back from Washington, right?" she had asked.

He had nodded.

For a moment neither of them had said anything. As they kept walking, Wolf had checked his watch and sighed.

"Tell you what," she had said. "I'll call you from the hotel tonight to tell you that I'm fine."

"That would be good."

"It might be late."

"That's okay. I'll be up. Wait, I'll be working. Just call the desk and leave me a message saying you arrived at your destination. I mean call and leave me a message that you're safe when you're in your hotel room, not just to D.C. They'll get the message to me."

He had looked at his watch again, even though they had plenty of time.

"Hey, Rabbit, do remember to latch the door when you're in the hotel room, will you? And put the 'do not disturb' sign up so no one tries to knock and get you to open the door."

"Wolf!" she had cried out, in frustration. "I'm sorry. But listen, you're going to have to just calm down about it. I'm fine."

"You might not have been fine. I'm changing the locks while you're gone. I've lent people keys over the years, and – well, I'm changing the locks while you're gone. You and I will have them – you and I will have the new keys – but just us. And we're going to keep them on our persons. At all times."

"Even when I'm in the bath? Sorry. Joking. Sure, yes."

"And you'll latch the doors when you're home without me, Rabbit. And even when you're home with me. That's how it's going to be."

A city bus had roared past them, kicking up dust. She had waited until the noise had subsided to answer him.

"Here's an even better idea," she had said, the dust settling on the road and sidewalk. "You take a leave from your job and become my personal bodyguard while I'm here, like the last two days since the intruder. And you be my cook. You can also iron my clothes if you feel like it."

He hadn't laughed.

"My point, Wolf, is that I'm used to taking care of myself. I *did* sort of take care of myself in this instance – remember? You said I did a good job."

"It could have been a lot worse. We don't even know who this guy is – I mean, he's not the guy we've been looking for, so we don't know what he might have..."

She had peeked over the dirty stone railing and looked down at the Schuylkill. This was right where she and Wolf had been ice skating to the Blue Danube Waltz. It was all so much quieter and darker in the dream. So much more peaceful. And not just the river. He was so much calmer.

"I mean, it might have been – "

"Yes, Wolf," she had said, suddenly leaning toward him and grabbing his free left hand in her right. She could tell it had startled him. "Who knows what he might have done? But someday, someday I'm going to die! No way out of that."

She had squeezed his hand and in response he had quickly tightened his grip on hers. His sudden hard grab of her hand felt almost involuntary. But it also felt to her like she could move safely in any direction holding on to it, anchored to it. Go down on one skate, one leg out in front of her.

"Until I die, Wolf, I'm planning to *live*. You think there's a life beyond. I know this is all I've got."

She had released his hand and let hers fall back down to her side. She had noticed from the corner of her eye that his was stuck at the angle at which she had left it.

...

She pushed the button to recline her train seat a few inches, rested her head against the seat, and tried to make out the characters in the windows of a New Jersey Transit train riding along right next to theirs, going a couple of miles an hour faster. A man in a suit on his computer. A child about seven years old, kneeling on the seat to see out the window. A bearded backpacker and his girlfriend, asleep on each other.

Maddy's train was picking up speed and the conductor was coming down the aisle to collect the tickets. She held hers up, to be ready.

"Washington?" asked the conductor, and Maddy nodded. The conductor adjusted her cap over her cornrows, punched Maddy's ticket, and gave it back.

Finding herself without Wolf for the first time since the attack, Maddy involuntarily started to play the scene from the other night in her head again. She figured this fugue of the memory – going over it again and again – was inevitable. Paula had taught her that this sort of repetition of a traumatic moment was not a sign of an obsessive inability to let go but rather the work of a healthy brain trying to work out what had happened to feel in control and to try to prevent it from happening again.

Wolf wasn't supposed to be home, having been on the night shift. She would have been home alone if not for some bad Chinese take-out ordered by someone at the Roundhouse. He had come home without warning, dashed in past her working at the kitchen table, run to the bathroom, and thrown up what was left in him.

Maddy had cleaned up the bathroom while he had cleaned up himself. She had felt his forehead and had told him he had no fever, so that meant it was probably all over.

"Really bad food poisoning comes with a fever," she had said. "You'll feel better soon."

He had felt so poorly, he made no protest when she followed him up to his bedroom on the third floor. He had walked into the room like a zombie, fallen down into the bed almost silently, rolled on to his side, and yanked a pillow over his head.

She had found herself caught at the vestibule. It had marked the first time she had seen his bedroom, a low-ceilinged space on the third floor. A king-size bed – how had they gotten a bed that big up here, up those narrow stairs, around the bends? Maybe it was a split mattress.

Thinking about that for a moment, she had felt way too close to his unfathomable marriage. She had suddenly wanted to go lose herself alone in the bath. But she had kept looking as she had the one time she had managed to get into the cloistered part of the convent. It reminded her exactly of that. Wolf's bed had an old-fashioned bedspread, with a knobby weave. The bed was so neatly made, military-neat, just like the nuns'.

Maddy had finally walked over to him, pulled off his shoes, and put them under the bed. She went downstairs to get him a vomit bowl, a dry washcloth, and a glass of water, and came back to put them all on the nightstand next to him. She had had to move aside the copy of *Cooks Illustrated* she had given him on his birthday. (She had gotten him the current issue and ordered him a one-year gift subscription. "How thoughtful," he had said, unwrapping it, "and how very self-serving, literally." She had laughed and pointed him to page 23 – a recipe for pork empanadas.)

She had quietly struggled with the switches to the various lights as she had tried to figure out how to leave enough light on that she could come back and help him quickly if he needed it, but not so much light that it would bother him as he tried to sleep. As she switched various lamps on and off, she had kept looking around furtively. Odds seemed good she would never be in this room again. The only thing that had surprised her was the reading area he had set up near the front dormer windows. It held a slipcovered armchair with an ottoman, a low pine bookshelf full of books, and a small white side table to hold a drink and a lamp.

She had wondered how often he was up here reading as she worked at the desk in her room just below him. She had turned on the lamp on the table near his reading chair to see what the bookshelves held. The selection was much like what she had found on the first floor – mostly histories, mostly military and biographical. But here, there were also a few older Catholic theological texts, a travel guide to Rome, and what looked to be second-hand copies of various classic cookbooks – *Mastering the Art of French Cooking* and *The Joy of Cooking*. He also had what appeared to be a near-complete run of the books of M.F.K. Fisher. She had felt so viscerally excited by this find. When he was feeling better, she could tell him what she herself had learned from Fisher about how to save money when cooking. Like using water in which potatoes have boiled as the basis for a soup and cramming full an oven with various dishes when you bother to turn it on, to save on the gas bill.

She had reached under his pillow and felt his forehead one more time before leaving. It was still not hot, just a little sweaty from the effort of throwing everything up. She had pulled a blanket off the closed wooden chest positioned at the end of the bed, unfolded it, and laid it over him. Then she had gone down to the kitchen to get her work, to bring it up to her desk in her room. From the second floor, with both of their doors open, she could probably hear him if he stirred or called. She had felt glad – in this, her latest convent refuge – to feel a little useful while also to be able to stay up as late as she wanted working on her studies.

How much time had elapsed before the stranger had entered her room, she had no idea. How he had gotten into the house and come up the stairs without her hearing anything – again, she had no idea. She had been so lost in work. All she knew was that she had turned in her chair at some point – turned from facing the window, writing on her laptop, writing an outline of the fourth chapter of her dissertation. And there he was.

That he would be just as Wolf had described him had completely disoriented her: the black ski mask with the sunglasses; the knife; a roll of black electrical tape slung over his wrist. For a split second, she had thought perhaps it was Wolf playing a joke? Testing her? But no, Wolf was too sick to play around, and this was not remotely funny.

Her second thought had been that she must be simply dreaming. She must have constructed this figure – this figment – from Wolf's descriptive words and her own lingering and perfectly normal fears. Yes, this figure was just made up, made up of old words and background fears, like the simple houses she made up as a child from popsicle sticks and glue.

This, she later figured, was why she had not called out, why she had said nothing. Because it had seemed too unlikely to be anything more than a disorienting fictious hiccup of her tired brain.

He had held up the blade of the knife level with her eyes and had motioned that she should get on the bed. When she had merely frozen, he had whispered clipped two-word orders to get on the bed – "there, bed" – and to put her hands together behind her. She had stood up, aware now that her heart was trying to leave her body. Her pupils had felt rather as if they had been blown out. Her ears had been ringing.

She had had just enough blood going to the thinking parts of her brain to calculate that to bind her wrists, he would need both hands – and that would mean he'd have to temporarily take the knife out of one hand?

So she had laid down on the bed, face down, and waited just until she felt the tape go once around her wrists, and just as he had started to go around one more time, she had used all her strength to turn over and kick as hard as she could at his groin. At the same time, she had summoned her voice and let out a scream – "Wolf!"

(Why hadn't she added "Help me?" She could practically hear Liz say again, as she had before, "Is it so hard to ask for help, Maddy?")

The intruder had lunged forward and tried to cover her mouth with his gloved hand. He had looked around, clearly wondering if there was some-one else in the house. She had tried to get her teeth into his leather-gloved hand, all the while kicking with her feet and her knees and screaming. It had seemed rather soon like he might be ready to give up and flee? But she could not be sure and thought if she just kept screaming, perhaps finally Wolf would rouse and help her.

"Wolf! Jesus Christ, Wolf!"

At the sound of Wolf finally answering – first weakly – "What?" – and then immediately more as if he were alarmed – "Rabbit, are you okay?!" – at the sound of him beginning to come down the stairs, the intruder deter-minedly grabbed his knife and the roll of tape and took off, dashing down the stairs.

From her room, Maddy could see Wolf almost tumbling down the stairs, third floor to second, then second floor to first. She could hear them both emerge from the back of the house, out the kitchen door, and head down the alley – ejected from the house as if vomited by the house, she had thought. Had the house caught the food poisoning, too? Could it not digest these men? Would it digest her?

She had tried to get her wrists out of this stupid tape, to get out of the all-consuming house – it was at most, by her mental math, just *two fucking rounds* of tape, so why was it so goddamned hard to pull off, why was it twisting so and becoming harder to pull off, why did it cut into the flesh of her wrists but not give?

She had gone to the top of the stairs, and sat down fast, scooching her way down, step by step, afraid that if she stood and stepped her way down, she would surely fall, and just as she reached the bottom, the tape had finally come undone, and Wolf had come flying back in the house and grabbed the phone and was dialing, and she had thought he looked so grey that perhaps he was going to throw up again.

She had felt so useless – here he was, feeling not at all well, but he was doing all the work, chasing the intruder and calling the police – and she was so useless again. A useless convent boarder. So, she did all she could do to help. And that was to throw up for him. She moved quickly over to the sink and just started throwing up. And some part of her brain had told her this was good – she was at least getting that out of the way for them.

Only it was not Chinese food. It was that white bean and lamb cassoulet that Wolf had left her to have for dinner. It had tasted better on the way down.

...

The house full of cops for an investigation had felt nothing like the house full of cops for poker. They had asked her the same questions over and over again, and she had told them the same things over and over again – what she could ascertain of his height and build, what she could remember of the knife and the gloves, of his words and his clothes, that he hadn't said much but it seemed like maybe he had a foreign accent. She wished she had taken a linguistics class so she could have written down in formal linguistical notations what she heard before she ended up so uncertain of what she had heard, because they had asked her too many times. They had tried to find any loose hair or useful footprint and had made her give over her clothes in an evidence bag. (She had been glad she had been wearing her old sweat-pants and not her favorite jeans.) They had tried to get her to give up one more detail she had not on the first five run-throughs. Wolf had eventually had to tell them to stop. It had reached the point of feeling like a berating.

One of them, a plain-clothed cop she didn't know, had finally said to Wolf, "It wasn't him. Wrong build. Wrong words. Wrong gloves. Wrong tape."

"I know," Wolf had said.

"Wrong tape?" Maddy had asked.

"Black," Wolf had answered. "This guy used black tape on you. The guy we have been looking for, he uses – "

But the cop Maddy didn't know had cut him off with a "Hey! Wolf, no."

"Copy-cat?" Wolf had asked aloud, as if to no one.

Copy-cat? Someone who knew enough to make it look sort of like he was the serial rapist but didn't know enough to know these cops would knew he wasn't?

Who would have known what this guy knew, Maddy wondered? Someone who knew the guy, or a victim of the guy? A nosey reporter? A cop?

Maddy had suddenly wondered if she should tell Wolf the creepy way Manny had come into her room that night of poker. He would have expected Wolf to be working the night shift that night.

But she hadn't said anything, not wanting to make more trouble just now. After the other cops had finally all left, Maddy had flopped down on the couch and asked Wolf how they were supposed to go to sleep after all of that. Wolf had sat down in the armchair in the living room, next to the couch, looking so completely spent. His head had been in his hands.

"They've torn my bedroom apart," she had said.

She didn't like that it came out like she was whining about some incompetent maid.

"Wolf, I don't want to sleep down here in the living room with you all the way up on the third floor. And I'm not sleeping in your room." (She had thought she'd better add the last bit, to make clear what she wasn't asking.) "Would you please sleep near me tonight? I know you don't feel at all well, but – "

"Of course," he had said, quietly. "Of course, Rabbit. But do you think you could give me the couch?"

"Of course," she had said, and she had rushed upstairs to get pillows and blankets from his room for both of them. She had moved the coffee table and set the couch up for him while he went upstairs to pee and drink more water. She had made herself a place to sleep on the floor, right next to the couch. When he had come back, he had knelt down next to the couch. She had wondered for a minute if he was going to pray. But it soon became evident that he was just kneeling to put his gun under the couch.

He had turned off the lights and laid down on the couch, on his side, facing out.

"Come on," he had said, tapping the blankets she had laid for herself on the floor.

She had laid down with her back up against the couch, still in the jeans and sweatshirt she had put on after the police asked her to give over her clothes. She had pulled the blanket up over her. He had draped his hand over the side, resting it on her shoulder. Lying next to him like this, with him a foot above her, she had been reminded of when she was little and would plaster herself against the base of her parents' bed, on her mother's side, when there was a particularly violent electrical storm. The storms on the Island could grow so intense.

"It'll be okay tomorrow," he had said, rubbing her shoulder with his thumb in a weary fashion. "We'll change your room around tomorrow."

"Why?" she had asked.

"We'll put the bed against the other wall, facing the window. And we'll move the desk to where the bed is now, to face the door when you're sitting there."

"Why?"

"We'll change – I have different blankets for the bed. We'll use different blankets."

"Why?

"So it all feels – different. It'll be okay."

"Okay," she had said. "Okay, Wolf. Thank you."

She had started imagining her room set up the way he was describing. It would be okay – having her desk face the wall instead of the window. Less distracting. And maybe he would let her put a bulletin board above the desk while she was there. It would make organizing the dissertation outline easier. But mostly she would be able to see the door while sitting at her desk.

"I'm so sorry, Rabbit," he had said unexpectedly, just as he was falling asleep.

She wanted to ask him what he was sorry for. For taking the couch? For holding on to her shoulder, as if he couldn't quite trust her not to run? For not catching the intruder? For men in general? (Wolf was just the kind of man who would apologize for his whole sex.)

But she hadn't wanted to stop him from rest by asking him to explain. His hand had gone limp as he fell into sleep. She had laid there awake in the near-dark for a long time, trying not to think about what might have happened if he hadn't been around. Trying to ignore the residual taste of stomach acid in her mouth. It had the flavor of grapefruit juice gone bad.

She had realized too late that she should have put on her pajamas and brushed her teeth. Those would have given her body the cues that all was sort of normal again, and it was okay to go to sleep.

Wolf's hand had twitched momentarily from some dream, tapping her neck as if he was flicking something off his fingernails onto her skin. Maddy had sat up, picked up his hand, and tucked it in next to his body. Then she had again lain down and pushed herself up next to the base of the couch. And she had again wondered if she should have said something about Manny.

-15-

The day after the intruder, they had recreated her bedroom just as he had said they would, and he had come to ask her, as she had climbed into bed and adjusted her pillow, if she felt like everything was okay now.

"No," she told him frankly. "But I appreciate all you've done for me today. You're like a one-man convent-full-of-nuns."

At that, he had smiled and sat down at her desk, as if it had been an invitation. The way he was soon taking visual note of all of her things on the desk struck her as so familiar because it exactly reminded her of the way she could not seem to stop herself scanning her surroundings all the time. Soon he saw the draft pages from her dissertation writing, printed pages organized into small stacks by chapter. Each batch was bound together by a pair of paperclips, one on the top and one on the right side.

"You can read what's in those manuscript pages if you want," she said to him. "It'll read better after I rework it, but you might as well tell me if it's lousy now so I can fix more. It's draft work for my dissertation. I've been printing it out at the museum."

He took her up on the offer and silently read several pages before reaching to pick a pencil out of her canvas pencil case and jotting what she figured must be a correction of a typo. He kept reading a while longer, marking a little something every two pages or so. After about ten minutes, he looked up to see she was looking at him, lying on her side.

"It is interesting, Rabbit, what you have been finding," he said. "And it is well written. I find very interesting how you're laying out the story of individual people you can only know about through the medical texts about them. Like photo albums – you've collected the snapshots of them through the texts. Like this man who was born with one arm and a deformed ear. You've followed him from France to Belgium back to France through the primary sources. And so you've been able to match the drawing of him made in the Belgium doctor's clinic back to the story of him from the French doctor. It's as if, because they had something odd about them, their histories are kept alive through the eyes of the doctors."

She bounced her head up and down in a satisfied nod. No one else had read this yet and it was gratifying to see he found it rather fascinating, as she did.

His presence that evening, the night after the intruder, the day before she would head down to Washington for the conference, it did deepen her breathing, relax her bones. He had dragged her all over town on foot that day, ostensibly to get every ingredient he needed to make a lasagna – the right tomatoes, the right oregano, the right noodles, the right cheeses. He was cooking this because he had asked her what was her favorite comfort food – he had said that, since he was taking the day off to stay home with her, he could make whatever she felt like – and she had blurted out, "Lasagna! With garlic bread!"

She had realized somewhere along the way – somewhere between the right chop meat and the right ricotta – that he had dragged her out and around on this long journey to try to wear her out, physically and verbally, so that she might sleep later. Miles of walking, miles of him asking her how she was thinking about the attack the night before, miles over which her story of the night before cohered. It had cohered safely into the past tense. In between the verbal prods, he had asked her bits about her life history and had told her a little about his own: He had grown up in New Jersey and moved to Philadelphia because of his wife's job. He and his wife had met via a mutual friend whom she had been dating at the time. His own parents now lived near Boston, near his sister and her family. He didn't see them much, nor his wife's family except when he ran into them sometimes at the hospital....

She first thought that his method of talking about nothing in particular with her, while occasionally gently verbally poking at her about last night – that this approach was aimed at trying to find out more to use for the police department's search for the man who had invaded his home.

But no, she finally realized; that wasn't what he was primarily doing. He was pulling out the threads of her memory of the frightening things that had happened last night – things that over coffee in the morning she had still been talking about in the present tense, illogically – and working to get her to turn it into a small bit of past-tense fabric in the long ream of her life history. He had been helping her see it wasn't much of anything. Yeah, so, a guy had broken in; he had threatened her; she had successfully defended herself; nothing really bad had come of it.

After hours of this, she had told him she knew what he was doing.

"You're making me realize last night is over, and it was just a little something in the story of a life."

"Is that what I've been doing?" he had asked. "I thought we were just talking."

"Well," she had said, "whether you know it or not, you've been helping me compose myself."

He had smiled at her verbal pun.

She had said that she appreciated it but asked him if they could please go to the gym for an hour, before he started cooking.

"Of course, Rabbit, if you don't mind having a snack when we get back and then a late dinner."

"I don't mind that at all," she had said. "A full stomach helps with sleep."

At the gym, he had watched her for a little while as she worked on various maneuvers on the rings, moves that he knew would try her biceps and her abdominal muscles. He noticed that she had looped a series of cloth headbands around her wrists, as if the headbands were sweatbands, to cover the marks on them left by her struggle against the electrical tape, so no one would see.

When she had seemed fine on her own, when he could tell that no one was going to trouble her, he had gone to go lift weights on his own. He had come back a half-hour later to find her on the mats doing what looked like a little bit of ballet, lost to some piece of music in her head, dipping and spinning, a look of intense concentration on her face – no performance smile.

A few hours later, lying in her bed full of dinner and a little wine and seeing a chunk of her dissertation draft in his big hands felt – well, it felt to her like Liz must have felt the time when Liz had handed Pumpkin over to the one vet she trusted, to help figure out why the little rat seemed to be sneezing all the time, as if he might be ill with a bad respiratory problem Liz said rats sometimes got.

Wolf was slowly turning the pages, reading carefully, not skimming.

"Can I ask you something, Rabbit? How come when you gave your lecture at the museum, you didn't get into what your dissertation is about – where the specimens came from? Why did you make it sound like a talk just about – about – "

"About heroic medicine?" she asked.

"Yes," he answered. "I'm not familiar with that term, 'heroic medicine,' but, yes – you made it sound like medicine is *just* heroic? All noble? All you talked about was stories where doctors and scientists successfully figured important things out from research on people's bodies. Forgive me, but it was rather like a comic book, as if doctors wear capes. To be honest with you, Rabbit, it troubled me a little. It sounded, well, *obsequious*. Not like you. It was not what I expected, because what I was expecting was a lecture about the kinds of things you've been telling me about your dissertation research – the power struggles, figuring out who had control in various relationships between doctors and people with – what is it you call them?"

"People with unusual anatomies."

"Right," he said. "I expected you to talk about that, the issue of who had control before and after death, of the unusual anatomies. Who had the say."

"Yeah, but the museum's head curator, Shirley Anseed, she is worried that if the doctors in the museum's medical society know what I'm looking at, at the history of specimen acquisition, they'll think I'm there to call their collection unethical. To try to do repatriation. And I need access to the collection."

"Well, isn't that ironic."

He shook his head a little.

"What do you mean?" she asked.

"They have control of the bodies and the texts about the bodies. That's what you're documenting – right? How they won, in history? And so *you* now have to do what they want for *you* to get access, for *your* research about how they got there. So you're figuring out how to have power over them, to get the bodies and the texts for *your* work?"

"Huh," she said. "I hadn't thought of it that way. You're right. That is ironic."

Neither of them said anything for a moment. At least he hadn't specifically observed aloud that she'd essentially been lightly whoring herself up that evening of the lecture in order to maintain her access to the museum's stores. But Wolf was right that she had been trying to maneuver Dr.

Wilhelm to make sure she could get what she needed for her research so that he wouldn't stand in her way – admiring his library, asking to see the Schlesinger 1888 text to impress upon him that she'd been reading his work and knew what he'd documented in the literature.

Wolf had gone back and read a few pages over and then asked her, "Doctors have a way of thinking they own it all, don't they?"

"Police aren't the same – thinking they should control the body? I mean, around crimes? And scientists. And historians, for that matter, as you just pointed out – thinking they should have control of all the texts anyway. Aren't we all the same? *Don't* cops think they own everybody's body?"

"No," he said, but he cocked his head as if he wasn't quite sure. "I don't think so, Rabbit. I mean, we have to investigate when there's a crime, obviously, but our goal is to get bodies back to the right people. Let victims get on with their lives. Let innocent people have their lives back. Let families have back the bodies of murder victims, accident victims, as soon as we can. At least I do. But doctors…"

"You're thinking of something with your wife?" asked Maddy, sitting up a little in the bed, pushing the pillow behind her lower back.

"Yes," he said. "Just how one of the nurses warned me that they – some of the doctors – how they want her organs. They figure she's not coming back, that her brain is gone, and they can use the organs for someone else."

"How do you feel about that?" Maddy asked, genuinely curious.

"You will think I'm an old superstitious fool for saying so, Rabbit, but I feel like she ought to keep it all together. For the resurrection, I suppose."

She was about to say something and he cut her off.

"I mean, listen, I know that can't really matter – God isn't going to deny people who are organ donors a chance at complete resurrection. That would be absurd – theologically absurd. God would not punish generosity. But it's just, well, I feel like she should have all her parts stay *in her*, not be in somebody else. I can't explain why it feels like that's the way it should be. It's not like I don't believe in organ donation. I have signed an organ donor card for myself, for heaven's sake! But I feel as if she should be whole and I should not dole out her parts."

"I understand your feeling," said Maddy. "If we speak of a person as if they are *not* somehow associated with their bodies, their body parts, what does it mean to speak of a person? How much can you take away before it isn't that person anymore? So, I think you and I meet there, Wolf. Perhaps it's just instinct, not rationality. But I think you and I have the same sense of personhood – that it requires the body of the person somehow?"

She was picturing Margaret Lovisa, in the jar.

"Wolf, isn't that why we hope for a *resurrection* of the *body*, and not just an afterlife of the soul? Because we picture people truly being with us again, as the ones we have known?"

He made a small noise of agreement and took to reading silently again. She watched him turn page after page, and she found herself hoping he would stay all night, right there, reading and talking to her. She wished she had written more so that he might stay longer.

He got to the last page in the section he had been reading, neatened the pages as a stack, secured the paperclips back on it, put it down, and picked up another stack.

This one he started reading aloud – just loud enough for her to hear. She recognized it as a meditative section she figured would be in the introduction or the conclusion of her dissertation, if she kept it. It was a series of pages where she was trying to work out an idea.

Archeologists have long appreciated how the lived history of a body may adhere to that body into death, how a life is literally inscribed on it as if Life were writing down a record of itself on the tablet of human form.

Access to calcium, to fluoridated water, to dentistry, or lack thereof – these particulars of a life in a particular civilization become quite literally part of the person, through formation and preservation of the teeth. We can look in the teeth later and see the person's history, at least to the extent we can obtain clues about how long a person lived on the earth, what she ate through those days, whether she had access to the luxuries of primitive or modern dental care.

Similarly, a fatal blow, be it caused by a medieval weapon or the steering wheel of a modern car, will leave the mark of a particular society's existence on a body. The final sentence of a person's life story may be writ small or large – depending on the cause of death – on the head, the spine, and – if we have soft tissues left – on the large internal organs or on the skin.

In this sense, the body becomes a manifestation of its time and place in human history, and so it becomes a monument to its own life. It is like the plant that absorbs its very particular location as it grows, recording for a moment in its absorption of soil elements and air where exactly it grew, dating itself by the carbon. So it is when the human body is formed in prenatal and postnatal development by its little world. The body absorbs its world and turns it into a record, like the tree that petrifies by becoming constructed of the minerals that surrounded it.

Perhaps because the body provides at best an imperfect record – a goosebumped, moist page on which Life tries to write of itself – historians have preferred literally written texts: unchanged words on flat pages. But we should still look to every possible source in our quest to understand a life of the past. Too often, we forget that the flesh may give us direct textual records where writing will be at best indirect, filtered through the limiting sieve of a language and of a mind.

Some records left in the body represent the general marks of a particular civilization; they are indiscriminate to social strata. Everyone who lived in an area with chronic famine, for example, will have their bodies record that cyclic malnutrition. These localized generalities will be of interest more to the archeologist than the historian who wants to know mostly about particular lives.

Some bodies, though, will record the specifically personal as it existed in the social. When we look to the body itself as a record of a life lived in that body, we are vividly reminded of how some social inscriptions on the body are specific to assumptions made about an individual's class, race, gender, maturity level, and more. There are assumptions made about a particular person's rights, worthiness, ability, value that will, in effect, reify and amplify social distinctions that are otherwise assumed to have their basis simply in biology.

So, the person who is poor will wind up with a body more broken, more stooped, less repaired, because of the specific social assumptions and rules about class. In turn, that more broken, more stooped, less repaired body will be seen as evidence of its original relative unworthiness. Poverty and wealth are seen to prove themselves in bones and teeth and flesh. Similarly, the person who is enslaved will have the marks of slavery impressed upon the body by the master, as if somehow this is merely fate.

But all this, all these reified social distinctions, have nothing to do with genes – not in any simplistic, one-to-one, direct way – and everything to do with culture, with contingent power, with the lingua franca, with the fact that the human form allows itself to become a tablet of social dogma.

In human life, the word may be made flesh.

Wolf paused for a moment here, as if to consider for a little while what Maddy had written. The way he looked around the room made it seem almost as if he had heard a strange sound. Then he continued reading.

So much of the experience of living in a body is the experience of living in one's culture. It is not that there is no natural biology, independent of culture; of course there is. Some of us are born male, some female, some with four limbs, and some with fewer, or even more. But that biology will inevitably be molded, like clay, by the potter that is one's culture, one's kin, one's little world.

The woman pressed into a corset or into foot-binding will have her skeleton permanently reshaped — and not just the part subject to the constriction, not just the ribs or the feet, but all the other parts as they try to compensate for the local deformation of the skeleton.

The enslaved person whose bones are broken through cruelty and never properly reset will become even unto death an artifact of slavery.

The traditional religious peasant woman might see and feel her breasts stretched into the shape of bananas under her culture's collective belief that her job on earth is to receive a man and bear him as many sons as possible, whereas the modern, independent, godless woman of wealth and status might have her apples preserved as plump and round, free of the tug of babes on the stem.

The charming American myth, that anyone can become anything through will and determination and hard work, it fails to recognize not only the natural history of any human body — what teratology, pathology, injury, and the normal ravages of development and aging will bring — but also disregards the social histories that will be sometimes recorded in flesh —insults, demands, values, and bonds. Stories of who was lovable and unlovable, who was a source of honor or shame.

Wolf read in silence for a little longer. Then he paused and told Maddy in a soft voice a series of anecdotes about at-first unidentified bodies he had had to deal with in his work, bodies that had left clues about who they had been, how they had died. He spoke of a woman whose hands were stained a peculiar kind of orange; a man identified by a serial number on his artificial hip; a child whose hair and fingernails showed signs of extreme malnutrition.

He told her these stories not so much as if he was speaking to her. It was more as if he were reminding himself of what he had seen that accorded with her meditation.

"I have thought in such circumstances about what it is we can detect from the body in terms of a crime or a possible crime – cause of death, for example, when we look to see how a person died to try to figure out if it was homicide or manslaughter, or suicide, or an accident, or natural death," Wolf told her. "But I had not much thought about the way that in every life, the story of our lives is being written down on us over the course of the whole life."

He read a little longer silently, then aloud:

By coming to own parts or all of many bodies — of many persons — the medico-scientific men of the nineteenth century coalesced their own social power. A single physician or anatomist had but one body of his own and had to live with whatever limitations it came and whatever limitations it acquired through its movement in the world. Each European or American medico-scientific man had but one body of his own to start, as do we all.

But such a man could come to "own," to control, many more persons, and to accrue a kind of army, socially speaking.

The standard image of the strong army is the image of every body alike, marching perfectly in step as if all clones. But for these medico-scientific men, it was the diversification of the bodies in their private armies that gave them real power – intellectual, professional, social. One didn't want an army of clones; no, no. One wanted a captain with acromegaly, a lieutenant with situs inversus, a private with achondroplasia.

As they accrued these armies, increasingly it would be these medical doctors, these surgeons general, who would decide what each anatomical attribute meant – who would determine which forms of normality were "scientifically proven" to be tied to which social norms – female: passive and emotional; male: active and rational. It would be these men who would decide which supposedly detrimental biological attributes would be mitigated, erased, celebrated, or stigmatized.

Wolf said nothing for a while, holding the small stack of paper silently in his hands.

"It's still rough," Maddy said quietly.

She could see Wolf going back and reading a few sections again.

"At some level what you're saying is obvious, Rabbit," he said, "because of course what a person experiences in their body depends on their social position, their life circumstances. And of course the body records life. But you're also pointing out that there's a way in which the human body becomes a Catch-22 if you're not a person with a lot of power. A physical disadvantage is magnified by social beliefs about the physical disadvantage. You're right. It's like you can't win. Like for black men."

"Yes, but there *is* change sometimes in culture for *some* people," she replied. "I mean, a hundred years ago as a female I couldn't get a Ph.D. and live independently like I do – well, I mean like I *will.* I would have been much more restricted a hundred years ago out of assumptions about the female anatomy. That changed. Liberation came. I could not, a hundred years ago, have had so much control over my body, sexually, reproductively, or as far as my ability to travel, in terms of what I eat, how I strengthen my body with running and the gym. And there is healing, too – physical liberation from some of life's writing. For some of us, there is healing from the scars caused by an oppression. Sometimes you can heal, and more and more we can heal because the world around us enables it by enabling healthier flesh and medicines and therapies and all."

She thrust out her arms.

"My wrists will heal soon, Wolf."

She kept holding them out in front of her and looked at them in the dim light that enveloped her bed. She was thinking about how these scars would not derail her from her plans.

"If I don't die tomorrow or the next day, the writing of the assault will be erased. I will act to write over it. You've already helped me today start writing over it."

He came over, sat down on the bed next to her, and held her wrists gently between his forefingers and thumbs as if they were delicate samples of something – crumbly cheese; a fragile flower; thin, antique glassware. His fingertips were warm and she thought for a moment it felt as if he were stroking her, even though his hands did not seem to move.

Yes, the marks that had been left there by the electrical tape would be gone soon. The memory of the attacker leaning his weight on her to bind her wrists was also already beginning to soften, those neurons being blunted and quieted somehow by the process of brain regrowth, reorganization. Just as the skin of her wrists was healing, so was her brain – something she counted on in her life, this way the body had of healing itself in the face of waves of harm.

But that kind of healing from assault never came without the deep fatigue of an inflammatory response. Mildly inflamed – that's how her psyche had felt since the night before. And that kind of psychic inflammation always evoked the ghost of The Jerk.

She figured it about eight years now since The Jerk had been in her. And in that span of time, in that time in which she had been free of him, not only had her uterine lining sloughed and grown anew maybe a hundred times, but she assumed that by now, so, too, were many of the cells in her vagina and cervix replaced. What his seed had touched was gone, like him. There were just the neurons in her head that he would not leave. And how strange that was – no one would ever be able to read what he had written there, unless she read it to them. Yet there he still was, inscribed on her flesh, a history she had never asked to be written into. He felt sometimes like the seed of a cancer, hiding in an organ and waiting to metastasize. Like an encapsulated tuberculosis, waiting for a moment when her immune system weakened, to take over her lungs and choke them with blood.

"You know what you said when we went to the gym this evening?" Wolf asked. "It makes sense to me now."

"What did I say?" she asked. "I don't remember."

"You said, 'Wolf, I need to go to the gym, to own myself again.'"

"Did I say that?"

She was truly surprised.

"Yes," he said. "You said after the assault last night, you needed back the feeling of owning yourself."

How was it she had been using that language all along – using it for years to refer to her recovery from The Jerk – and never realized that she was working on that very issue in her dissertation – the question of who owned what body? The Jerk had always called her "my little Madeleine" as he fucked her and she hated it – the possessive. The electrical tape the night before, it was nothing compared to the feeling of being accidentally chained to a man like The Jerk. But how was it she never connected this – the quest to own her own body – with her dissertation research?

She must have looked disturbed because Wolf suddenly said he did not mean to rattle her.

"It was just," he explained, "that what you said – that you had to own yourself – made me realize why you were troubled by the idea of my wife – my wife's condition – suspending my own life. You said, the night you and I had that linguine-argument and you had that bad nightmare, you said that my wife was suspending my life, that she was controlling my body. Because *you* think of the goal in life as self-ownership. Self-ownership of the flesh."

"What do you mean?"

"For me, marriage is about giving my body and myself over, in love, letting someone else have control. Because I believe ultimately that by giving myself over to a sanctified love, I give myself to God. But you, Maddy, you think of salvation as owning *yourself*."

He didn't mean it as a criticism, merely as an observation. She could tell by his tone. But why was he suddenly using her name, calling her Maddy, instead of his own name for her? It felt especially strange since he was still holding her wrists. It was as if he had transformed for a moment from the Wolf she knew to a merely kind officer of the law come upon a woman who had stumbled at the curb. He was helping her up, like a stranger of no real interest. She felt suddenly ashamed of this whole stumble, of what he knew about her. She thought she might be turning red in the face.

He laid her wrists and her hands down in her lap and clutched her hands in his for a moment. It felt to her, that paternalistic clutch, completely up-side-down. Such a clutch ought to feel like one was pulling one closer. But this squeeze, this condescending squeeze, felt like a push away. It felt like the dismissal by a man who thought himself more clever, more righteous, than her.

She pulled her hands back and tucked them under the blanket.

He looked suddenly guilty.

"I'm sorry. I should not have made that observation to you. I didn't mean to disturb you."

She would not meet his gaze. But she could feel him make a small movement that felt to her like he was now very uncomfortable.

"Rabbit, I don't want to leave you to try to sleep when I've upset you. What can I read you that would be less troubling than hearing your own words from me? Tell me."

"No, Wolf," she said, trying to find words that would relieve him without feeling like she was selling herself out. (Damn it, there was that metaphor again?) "I just hadn't thought about it. I mean, there are all these people around me in the humanities working on their own identity issues, and I prided myself on working something that had nothing to do with me – so it's just – well, it's just – "

"You *have* been passed around a lot, Rabbit," he said. "You've been passed around a lot in your life. I understand why you want to feel like you own yourself."

She wondered if she should tell him about The Jerk. So that he would understand. Should she tell him? So that he understood?

She pulled her hands out from under the covers and rubbed her eyes. She thought about how it was that the reason he could undergo this sudden transformation from warm familiar to cold stranger was that they had reached the point of the warm familiar. She reminded herself that she and Liz were known to undergo such swings. It was just a matter of finding the place of meeting again, wasn't it?

"Would you read to me from M.F.K. Fisher?" she had finally asked. "I saw her books up in your room last night, when I was helping you get to bed after the food poisoning – before the intruder showed up. I saw you had *How to Cook a Wolf.*"

"You do know that book is about World War II and how to survive by cooking and eating sensibly, cooking and eating thoughtfully, right, Rabbit? It's not about how to cook a wolf."

"I know!" she had answered, almost yelling, embarrassing herself. "I know. The wolf is a metaphor for Hitler, for the war," she had said more quietly. "The sisters had it at the convent and I read it, twice. Once in the winter and once in the summertime. I just wanted to tell you that I had learned, reading that book, how to save money on food once I was on my own. I thought it was funny you and I have both read that when no one else I know has read it. But you know, Wolf, most people just read it for the writing, for the prose that conveys such an appreciation of food. But I got tips from it that I used. Like never leaving space in the oven – filling it up if you're going to turn it on, so you don't waste money on the heating of the oven."

"Making crackers out of leftover bread, roasting walnuts," he had said, "using the extra heat of the oven."

"Yes!" she had answered, almost as if in desperate relief, as if she had found a fellow expat just when she needed one.

"Of course, Rabbit," he had said. "I can read that to you. To us both. I would be happy to."

He had gone upstairs and come back with the book, sitting down and asking her to please lie down and please try to fall asleep while he read.

"The plain fact is that if you don't sleep," he had said, "and you get thrown off your dissertation schedule, I will never forgive myself for having locks that let him come in while you were here."

She had not answered but pushed the pillow aside and laid down flat on her stomach, pulling the blanket up to her waist. She had bent her right arm around her head, leaning her wrist on her crown, and tucked the other under her chest, her wrist lying in the space between her breasts.

He had soon found the pages they had been talking about, about cramming the oven full, and so he began to read.

Another thing to do while the oven is going is to put a pan of thinly sliced bread that is too stale to use anymore. It makes good Melba toast, if you watch it so that it does not get too brown. If you want to, you can soak it first in water or watery milk with a little sugar in it, or even a little salt and pepper, to make zwieback that is very good indeed with soup or tea. (These petty tricks seem somewhat more so when gas flows through the pipes and firewood is available and electricity actually turns on with a button. But in each one of them there is a basic thoughtfulness, a searching for the kernel in the nut, the bite in honest bread, the slow savor in a baked wished-for apple. It is this thoughtfulness that we must hold to, in peace or war, if we may continue to eat to live.)

Or you can roast some walnuts in their shells, and eat them while they are still pretty hot, with fresh cold apples and a glass of port if possible, for one of the desserts most conductive in this world to good conversations.

She had let out a little laugh.

"Hey," he had said in what she thought sounded like a happier voice. "Try to sleep."

He had continued:

While these various shortcuts to economy are simmering and fuming in their borrowed heat, you can be roasting a large joint of beef, which will seem expensive beyond reason when you pay for it but which will last a long time if your family is of normal size and appetite. Potatoes can be baked around its pan, about an hour before it is done, and if their skins are oiled and they are pricked when they are taken from the oven they will not grow soggy and may even be used after they are cold, if they are good potatoes, for a casserole or a salad....

-16-

It seemed impossible not to think about what Ambroise Paré or Isidore Geoffroy Saint-Hilaire or Charles Darwin – or Josef Mengele, for that matter – would have made of this scene. For here were a group of people who through the ages would have been marked alternatively as marvels, tragedies, manifestations of sin, inborn errors of development, and symbols of racial degeneration, simply having coffee in the lobby of a big-chain Washington hotel. Coffee with cream. Coffee with milk and sugar. Coffee black. Taking care of their squirrely kids. Looking over visitor maps marked with the monuments and museums. Looking down to their chests now and then and turning over their conference badges to make sure that their names faced out. Greeting each other excitedly after a year apart. Just generally being human.

Maddy had figured the conference would *look* like this: average-sized persons mixed in with many whose short stature had come from achondroplasia, iatrogenic stunting, pituitary dwarfism, and the like. She knew what the people would *look* like. What she hadn't expected was how it would *feel*. Specifically, what she did not expect was her own reaction: an overwhelming feeling of gratitude for being included.

She needed particularly to thank Nick DesJardins. But also the programming committee. Also the woman who had sent her the conference materials, and the man who had checked to make sure she was getting the discounted rate at the hotel, and whoever left the conference bag and badge for her at the hotel desk.

She had to wonder if she would have felt this way – overwhelmingly grateful – without the assault three days earlier, an event that had left her feeling in need of the company of basically decent people. (There were sure to be a few assholes here as Nick had warned, but she could already tell they were mostly decent people.) But the more she thought about it, the more she thought she would have felt this way even if the intruder had never entered her room. Sitting in this ill-shaped hotel lobby armchair covered in ugly, tourist-resistant fabric, Maddy grew consciously aware that her gratitude to this group stemmed from a generally unfamiliar feeling: the feeling of being normal.

It wasn't a feeling borne of *contrast* to these people; it was *not* that she felt normal because they seemed abnormal. No. Her sudden sense of normality came from a feeling of sharing their experience. In talking casually to the people here, in watching them, she had seen plainly that these were people who went through their days feeling often like she did – like they could manage *just fine*, thank you very much, yet they were constantly being quickly judged by strangers as too small, incompetent, and of suspicious, unclear provenance. Being made to feel out of place. That, she realized now, was *exactly* what she felt so much of the time when she was among strangers: this tiresome disjuncture between their apparent perception of her as small, young, classless, homeless, incompetent, and inscrutable, and her self-conscious reality of her own solidity, her own resilience – her right to be there.

Her eyes now felt a little wet from this unexpected wave of gratitude for the way their group presence felt like empathy. She sniffed a little, hoping no one saw her. Her emotion could easily be misinterpreted by anyone who might see it – misinterpreted perhaps as pity or anxiety or loneliness – read as something other than this momentary feeling of being implicitly understood.

She pulled a tissue out of her backpack, blew her nose, and shoved the tissue into the pocket of her pants. Just then, Nick waved at her from across the room and Maddy waved frantically back. He came over and sat on the edge of the coffee table in front of her chair.

"All good?" he asked, and she nodded.

He smiled broadly and held out a fist. She bumped it lightly with hers.

"Thank you again for arranging for me to be invited," she said. "It's been a very good experience, and the timing – it's been a very good experience already and it's only Day One of the meeting. I am truly in your debt."

"Hey, you're the one here working for us without getting paid!" he answered. "We should be thanking you. I saw you talking with Bess McFarlane earlier?"

Maddy said yes. She told Nick that she had found Bess's story – of accidentally conceiving a late-life pregnancy, twins no less, and of being told to abort to save her own life, and opting not to – well, quite intense. Bess had told Maddy she had *osteogenesis imperfecta*, a genetic disease Maddy knew causes the bones to just keep breaking, as if one were a crumbly cookie. Bess was small not because her bones didn't grow, but because they just kept fracturing, one after another.

Bess used a fancy electric wheelchair to get around, a device that gave her a height advantage over some that were here because she could raise her chair level to comfortably talk with people at various levels. Her machine, she told Maddy, was the equivalent of a posh S.U.V. where motorized chairs were concerned. She showed Maddy some of the bells and whistles. Clearly proud of the story, Bess told Maddy that she and her husband had thought there was no way she could get pregnant, and then she did at forty. And then, when it became evident she was pregnant with *twins*, the specialist obstetrician assigned to her told her she would be risking her own life with the pregnancy. Said she should abort. But Bess and her husband were "strong Christians" and decided it was God's will and they would see it through to whatever end came.

"And with God's help," Bess told Maddy, "the twins did alright. And, obviously, I made it, too."

Both her children were born with the same genetic condition, Bess said, and now they were four years old. She told Maddy she left "the little scamps" home with their father while she came to the meeting. They lived in North Carolina, and she had driven herself up.

"Bess can be intense," Nick told Maddy. "A whole lot of God."

Maddy laughed and told him she could handle it.

"I'm used to a whole lot of God."

"It'll be a different scene from Bess's world tonight," Nick told her, looking around the room. "The meet market gets going later, at the bar."

Maddy asked him what he was talking about.

"The meet-up market. The dating scene. Starts later – this is one of the places little people can meet each other. Plus, the young folks know the bartenders will be too embarrassed to ask for their IDs – the kids always go to the bartenders who try to proof them, 'Oh, you think I'm a child just because I'm a little person?!' – so they use it as an opportunity to drink and carouse."

"It never occurred to me this would be so much like an academic conference," Maddy confessed. "The same thing sometimes happens at night at the hotel bar. Only everybody is of age."

She did not add that she felt more at ease here than at many academic gatherings, where she often felt socially inept and of a lower class, terribly aware of not being born to the intellectual bourgeois.

"Of course, not everybody partners within the community," Nick explained. "My wife was about your height, and we met at an art gallery opening. But here, it can be easier to find romance, a partner, someone who has the same household needs in terms of what's where."

Maddy nodded in understanding.

"If you're looking for love, you might come hang out with us all tonight," said Nick, winking at her.

She wasn't sure if he was serious – whether she would be welcome and whether he thought she would be seeking dating opportunities here.

"I'm not looking, but thanks," she said, adding quickly, "I'm not partnered, but I'm also not in the market. Focused on finishing my degree."

He asked her bluntly if she thought she could see herself dating someone a foot or two shorter than her.

"Just curious," he added.

She told him honestly that she doubted it.

"Couldn't see yourself loving a little person?"

"Loving?" she asked. "Sure. But love is what I get from friendships, not from dates."

He squinted a little, evincing curiosity.

"Confidentially," she explained, figuring that since he was a psychologist, she could explain this, "I came out of a traumatic sexual history. At this particular point in my life, I like keeping loving relationships and sexual relationships separate. Sex for me is about bodies feeling good – about getting laid."

"And you have a taste for a particular kind of body."

"I think everybody does?" Maddy answered, hoping he wasn't going to feel insulted by her response. He did not seem to be. "If I want sex from a short person," she added, in a joke-whisper, "I just masturbate."

At that, Nick roared with laughter.

At that moment, a young woman with nearly translucent skin came over to see Nick, greeting him warmly. The way she walked, twisting her body with each step forward, suggested to Maddy hip dysplasia. She catalogued it in her brain without really thinking.

...

Maddy took off running as fast as she could out of the back door of the hotel. She ran down the long grassy hill, down and away from Connecticut Avenue, so fast she almost stumbled, making a beeline for the trail she knew she would find close along the shore of Rock Creek.

Finding the path, she turned fast on her heel, heading southwest, toward Georgetown. In about a mile, according to the map, she could cross the creek via a low footbridge. Then she would pick up a paved drive near the back of Dumbarton Oaks' walled garden, putting her right near R Street – the old neighborhood she had run sometimes in college. She was wondering if that house with the black shutters near R and 31ˢᵗ would still have that big oak desk in the turret window that she always envied. Would the room still be painted electric blue?

Liz had called while Maddy was lacing up her running shoes in her hotel room. She apologized for calling so early, but Maddy said it was fine – she hadn't slept all that well and was getting up to exercise anyway.

Maddy had figured Liz would call soon. Starting the morning after the intruder, Wolf had kept suggesting Maddy call to talk to Liz about it. But Maddy had figured that if *she* told Liz, Liz was going to make a bigger deal of it than it needed to be – whereas if *Wolf* called and told Liz, he'd explain it in that dry, descriptive police prose, the kind of language that made everyone a two-dimensional character, flat and a little dull. He could turn everything into a finished-and-done history. He'd make clear it was over. Wolf would tell Liz that Maddy was fine. He would tell Liz that he was mostly calling to explain that he'd sent Maddy to D.C. a day earlier than originally planned, and that he had asked her to stay a day longer, to make sure she wasn't home alone at night again this week.

And maybe in telling Liz all this, Wolf would realize what he was saying to Liz was true: Maddy was fine. She hadn't been hurt. Nothing was wrong.

When she called that morning, Liz didn't ask Maddy if she was really fine. She asked instead how close Maddy was to wrapping up what she needed to do in Philadelphia.

"So, when are you coming home to Indiana? It's been – what – a month and a half? You said a couple of months?"

"It won't be forever, Lizard," Maddy said. "Two or three months, I said."

Maddy didn't feel like telling Liz that she would be a lot closer to wrapping up in Philly if she hadn't wandered off into Dr. Wilhelm's work for quite so many days, if she hadn't decided to come to Washington in part to see what the little people community seemed to think of him. (She had been trying to find a subtle way to ask some of them about Margaret Lovisa but never could come up with a method that might not lead to awkwardness.)

"So when, Mad?"

Maddy answered by telling Liz she would be back to work in Philly in just a few days. She was giving her talk at the conference late the next day, and the day after that, with the conference officially over, she would go up to Bethesda on the train to the National Library of Medicine and do a little work at the History of Medicine Division and then go back to Philly.

"But you did work at the National Library of Medicine *last* year," said Liz. "Why do you need to go there again?"

"It's always good to check in with the major libraries when you're in town," answered Maddy. "Renew the contacts and the friendships. And there's a text I can't seem to find in the indexes that I'm thinking they can help me find." When Liz didn't answer, Maddy added, "It's Schlesinger 1888 – it's a case history of two brothers with dwarfism who both died of heart problems. Significant pamphlet but no one seems to know where it is in terms of public collections."

Liz asked again when she'd be coming back to Indiana and Maddy said perhaps in a few weeks. Maddy asked after her palm tree and then Margie and then Liz's rats and research, as if they hadn't talked just a few days ago, just before the attack. It was a stilted conversation. Maybe having Wolf call her had been the wrong thing to do.

The path above the creek suddenly offered a division into two – a trail that went up the embankment and one that went down. Maddy took the left option, heading down. She figured the trail going up would just lead back up to the streets, and down would take her closer to the creek, to wherever the bridge was. She slowed a little to manage the tree roots and the sharp rocks sticking out of the dirt of the path here and there. The brush and trees and ferns felt a little too dense here, but they opened up as she drew close to the water. A man was standing near the edge and Maddy's heart picked up for a moment from coming suddenly upon him. Then she saw he had a dog with him. The dog was wading through the creek, drinking the water and looking up at his master. Of course, this man was just here to walk his dog. She had been a little stupid to try to calculate his height and weight, as if this might be *him* again.

She pondered for a moment what she had also pondered before – how much could she tell about the build of the intruder? She felt she could be confident that he was wiry and tall. Wolf had said the same thing: that he seemed tall and thin, maybe six-foot-five, maybe160 pounds. The way he moved suggested he was not very old, but perhaps not very young. Not a youth.

Beyond that, who knew.

He wasn't much like Manny's build, when she thought about it. And he hadn't smelled of cigarettes. He had smelled of something else. Not quite the smell of the Amtrak disinfectant. But something – something similar?

. . .

Maddy didn't notice Dr. Wilhelm in the audience of her talk until it was over. It was only as the last members of the association who had stayed to speak with her were filing out of the room that she noticed him, sitting near the back near the exit doors, making notes intensely in a leather-bounded folio.

She stacked up her laptop and her pages of notes and walked over to him.

"Dr. Wilhelm? I didn't realize you were here."

"Miss Shanks," he said. "Why don't you sit and we'll talk?"

He stood up and pulled two chairs into the side aisle of the room, freeing the chairs from the stiff, front-facing rows set up by the hotel staff for her lecture.

"It is kind of you to come to my talk," she told him, sitting straight up and feeling nervous. She was reviewing in her head what she had said, wondering if he might disagree with anything she had presented.

"Your approach is an interesting one for the audience," he answered, closing his folio in a formal fashion and looking up at her.

He adjusted his seat to face her more directly. She felt as if she was in an oral exam.

"I gather you were trying," he said, "to suggest that stigma is culturally specific, that in some contexts a person with dwarfism can have quite a lot of power? Or has *had* such power in times past. You don't think you overplayed it a little?"

She asked him what he meant. She leaned over to put her laptop and papers on the floor next to her seat, sat back up, crossed her legs, and clasped her hands together around the front of her knee. She was trying to avoid a defensive posture and this was the best she could do.

"You don't think," he asked again, "that you made it sound like a fantasy world could exist, where being born with dwarfism would not put you at a disadvantage socially? Leaving aside the physical problems – which you seem to have left aside."

"I hardly think one needs to remind this population about the anatomical and physiological problems that come with some of the conditions, but I mentioned Schlesinger 1888," she answered, defensively. "And your lab's research."

He ignored her and continued.

"You met Bess McFarlane?"

Maddy nodded.

"You know her twins were both born with osteogenesis imperfecta."

"You must be very interested in that condition," she said trying to turn the conversation to his work. "You must find it very helpful as a condition to study for your research?"

"Yes, well, I have one," he said.

I have one? He must have meant a specimen.

She cleared her throat and he looked her dead-on in the eyes.

"Perhaps my message came across as overly optimistic," she said, using her fingers to push her hair behind her ears. "But I think history gives us reason to think – to know – that the experience of people with unusual anatomies differs depending on context. The same is true for all women, for that matter."

"But you have to agree that being born without the challenge – the social and the physical challenges – is better than being born with."

"One isn't born *with* a social challenge," she answered, "one is born *to* a social challenge."

He threw his hands up in the air for a moment in a gesture of exasperation.

"You are one of those people who thinks you don't notice race?" he asked. "You think you didn't notice that Dr. Tate is black?"

"Of course, I do," she said. "But what I do with that is culturally learned."

"The human brain is always going to register difference, Miss Shanks. It's a core survival mechanism. Normal people have it – the ability to spot difference without thinking. And where human anatomical abnormality is concerned, it's going to register as a *problem* first and foremost. There's a *reason* all parents count their babies' fingers and toes when they are born."

She wondered for a moment if her mother had done that with her.

"Okay," she said, "let's say there will always be a social challenge with these conditions. Let's say the human brain is such that it will always see these conditions as fundamentally wrong in some fashion. Does that mean it's better to be born without any anomaly? I don't know. That's an empirical question, one that would be hard to answer because of all the variables. Perhaps one learns to cope better than a person born with a simple body."

Dr. Wilhelm made a guffawing sound and shook his head a little.

"Dr. DesJardins suggested this approach, hmm?" asked Dr. Wilhelm. "He suggested you take your talk in this direction?"

Maddy nodded.

"Nicholas DesJardins has a very romantic view of history that I struggle to share. There's a reason so many people here support my work, and it's not just because of their physical pain. They don't kid themselves."

She did not know how to answer.

"In any case, Miss Shanks, I'm surprised to see you at the conference."

"Why is that, Dr. Wilhelm? I told you I would be here."

"Because," he answered, "Shirley told me something had happened and you said you might not be coming after all. She told me you have not been to the museum in several days, but she said you wouldn't even tell her why. It must have been something disturbing?"

Maddy looked at his visage, trying to figure out what his expression was. Continued exasperation? Mere curiosity? A kind of criticism?

"A friend of mine – a good friend of mine – had a problem in Indiana," Maddy answered, "and I thought I might have to go back. But she is okay now."

"I think you may be irritating Miss Anseed, taking up office space at the museum yet not showing up to work there and being evasive about why."

"Shirley hasn't said anything to me like that," answered Maddy. "It's only been a couple of days."

"Dr. Tate was charmed by you at dinner at my home, you know? And so, the next day, I asked Dr. Goncharov, my assistant, to look up your work. He then gave me your publications and your c.v. And then I told Shirley I thought we had been a little misled about your interests. Would you say? You're primarily interested in *specimen acquisition*?"

Maddy didn't answer. She saw him looking at her hands. She was just about to pull them back into her lap when he leaned forward, grabbed her by the palms, and pulled her arms toward him, exposing her lower arms from under her jacket sleeves. The red and purple marks left by her struggle against the intruder's tape showed clearly.

"What happened to your wrists? Miss Shanks, did you try to hurt yourself? Is that why you've been absent from your dissertation work?"

"No! Of course not," she answered, pulling her hands back and folding her arms.

"Is that why you've been gone a few days then?"

"I was walking a large dog on a leash," Maddy responded, coming up with the only story she could think of, "and I had the leash around my wrists to hold him and he tried to take off."

"Must have been a very large dog," answered Dr. Wilhelm, with evident skepticism. "In any case. You should know I heard from a number of people who were here in the audience that they found your lecture rather – well, insensitive. They stayed after to mention it to me."

"What do you mean?" asked Maddy. She was struggling to keep from sounding worried or angry. "The feedback I got from the people who asked questions and made comments seemed quite positive, Dr. Wilhelm. You must have heard the person who said I should come back next year if I have more material and the support that was expressed in the audience for that?"

"They were being polite, my dear!" he said, tipping back his chair a little and looking at her over the top of his glasses. "You don't know this community like I do. I can tell you they will be very polite to anyone who shows up, but that doesn't mean they will want you back."

Maddy felt startled by this. What had she done wrong? Surely she hadn't done a bad job – so many people had said enthusiastic things after the talk, beginning their questions or comments with a statement of gratitude for her presentation.

"Dr. DesJardins seemed very satisfied with my talk," she told him, bending over to pick up her things so that she could leave, get away from this barrage of criticism that seemed to come from nowhere. Was Dr. Wilhelm just jealous that her talk had been well received? Was he just angry that she was working on specimen acquisition and might pose a political threat to the museum's collection when she published her work?

"Well," Dr. Wilhelm replied, pushing his chair back and standing up, "Dr. DesJardins may not be representative of the general population here."

"True," she answered. Then she added, "I guess that is why *he* is willing to consider seeing another specialist."

At that, she stood up and faced him. She could see from his surprised expression that he didn't know what she meant.

"What are you talking about?"

"Nick hasn't told you? There's a specialist at the Cleveland Clinic who he's thinking of switching over to. He told me and Shirley he might want to give that fellow's group access to his 'celebrity body' instead of your team."

Maddy started to walk towards the door.

"Is that right?" Dr. Wilhelm said in a rhetorical tone, following her. "Shirley hadn't mentioned it to me."

"Of course not," said Maddy. "No one likes to deliver bad news."

No one except someone feeling spiteful, she thought to herself.

"Excuse me, Dr. Wilhelm, I have a phone call to make."

. . .

"Why didn't you tell me you were going to be in town!" exclaimed Booker Alton, Maddy's favorite librarian at the History of Medicine Division.

She let go from their friendly hug and told him the trip to D.C. was a little unexpected and she wasn't even sure she'd have the time to run up from Washington to Bethesda for a visit.

"Well, I'm so glad you did. Perfect timing – I can show you my work on the latest special exhibition – on the history of anesthesiology."

"That sounds great," she answered. " And I'm so glad *you* are here. You are truly a sight for sore eyes."

There was nothing like being with a librarian who knew you. And she would always feel particularly grateful to Booker, who had done all he could to help her out last year, including disregarding the division's policy and letting her order as many items per day as she wanted from the desk instead of stopping her at the official limit of twelve. He had understood she was there for only a few weeks and on limited funds. When in the middle of that trip it had snowed eight inches overnight, Booker had even come in specially to open the library doors for her, when no one else in the D.C. area would be going to work. Chatting during their sack-lunch breaks, they had discovered that they shared the experience of having happened into a field neither of their families would ever have expected. Booker came from a long line of D.C.-area African American public servants, but his family members had been State Department staff, Secret Service agents, public works engineers, and judges, not humanities scholars working in libraries. They couldn't understand any more than her family would have why one would get an advanced degree in medical history – although, Booker told her, his family regularly joked that maybe it was the name he had been given.

"I'll tell you the truth, Booker," Maddy said to the librarian. "I had a scare a few days ago in Philly, and I thought it would be good to be among old friends."

"You want me to pull Abelmarth 1874?" he asked jokingly.

She elbowed him.

"You know I meant you. Although I wouldn't mind spending time with Abelmarth 1874, if you've got him handy."

He chuckled at her. Then he asked her what the scare had been. He wasn't too surprised when she said she'd rather not go into it. Maddy had always had a way of being a little private about her life.

"Booker, I was wondering, too, if you could help me find a text I've read about but not located, a pamphlet from 1888 by Martin Schlesinger – documenting deaths from heart failure of a pair of brothers who were dwarves?"

"Of course," said Booker. "Never heard of it, but happy to try."

He walked over to his computer with her and began plugging in the information she gave him.

"Odd," he said. "We don't have it – I mean, that's only a little surprising – but it doesn't even seem to be in *Index-Cat*."

"Let me check the paper copy," said Maddy. "Maybe somehow Schlesinger 1888 just didn't make it into the digital Index Cat yet?"

"Doubtful," said Booker, "but worth a look."

She walked over to the shelves holding the *Index-Catalogue of the Library of the Surgeon-General's Office*, a series of big volumes bound in green. Starting in 1880, John Shaw Billings, the father of medical informatics, had overseen the cataloging of all medical texts, organizing a great bibliography of the library of the Surgeon General by author and by subject. It was a project that ultimately led to PubMed, the online catalogue. In the last few years, the system had been reaching backwards, absorbing the old paper indexes and making them available in computer searchable form.

She pulled and checked the *Index-Catalogue* volume in which Schlesinger 1888 should have been listed. She quickly found Martin Schlesinger's other publications. But not this one. She checked the subject heading listings. She also could not find the pamphlet listed there. Meanwhile, Booker tried looking in a later series of the *Index-Catalogue* to see if maybe it had just been picked up later and not yet transferred to the digital Index-Cat.

"It's possible," he said to Maddy, "that it just didn't get picked up because it was a pamphlet," he said.

Maddy nodded, but they both kept pulling more volumes to look for it.

Finally, Booker went back to his computer and tried searching for it in other libraries' databases.

"Ah ha!" he told Maddy. "New York Public has a copy! There we go. You could try ordering a copy of it through Interlibrary Loan if you don't want to make the trip up – they can probably photograph it and send it to you."

"Great," she said. "Can you print that information off for me? And then we can go see your special exhibition and I can take you to an early lunch, so we can catch up? I want to hear about whatever you have in the works in terms of the next exhibition. But I have to grab a train back north in a little while, so we'd have to go soon."

"Sounds great to me," Booker answered, "so long as we go Dutch. The topic of the next exhibition is the history of lobotomy, so it's the perfect topic for conversation over victuals. Let's get noodles."

-17-

Out the window of her seat in the Amtrak coach car heading back to Philly, Maddy watched a set of emergency vehicle lights go flashing by on a nearby road. She could just barely hear the siren through the double panes of the foggy window, over the low rumble of the train. Red lights. Must be a firetruck. Or an ambulance. She yawned and wondered to herself again why there had been an ambulance parked with its lights off outside the conference hotel when she had gone back there to retrieve from the bellhop station the suitcase Wolf had lent her, on her way from the library in Bethesda back to Union Station in Washington. The bellhop had told her he didn't know what the ambulance was about. But then, he had said with a shrug, big hotels like this often have people fall ill given the numbers, given people binging on food and drink at such places. That's right, she had realized: simple epidemiology.

Now, this train was already two hours late. Stupid Amtrak. That would mean it would be at least nine-thirty before she made it back. Would Wolf be there to meet her train at 30th Street? Before she had left Philly, he had made a note of which train she would be taking back. If he was planning to meet her train tonight, would he have had the sense to check by phone to see if it was late so he wasn't stuck hours waiting for her? And what if he wasn't there and he wasn't at home and he had changed the locks?

She'd have to figure it out when she got there. She ought to have tried harder on the train to get a little shuteye, to have tried to make up for the lousy sleep ever since the intruder, to have some energy in case she got stuck at the station a while. But she had felt too out of sorts to fall asleep easily. She yawned again and stared out the window.

"Wilmington!" the conductor called, leaning into the car. "Wilmington, Delaware, five more minutes, God willing!"

A little laughter rose up in the coach car at the conductor's expression of frustration at the delays. In theory, Maddy knew, Wilmington put them a little less than a half-hour outside Philadelphia. She glanced at her watch and saw it was 9:05. Her stomach was grumbling. She was now out of the food Wolf had packed her for the four-day trip – peanut butter sandwiches; apples; walnuts. Wait – apples and walnuts! She smiled to herself. He must have been making a purposeful reference to reading her M.F.K. Fisher in that bag of food? It hadn't occurred to her until just now. She remembered how, as he had been reading to her from Fisher about apples and walnuts, she had fallen asleep for just a moment and then woken up to ask him how he had kept the bread from getting soggy.

"Rabbit?" he had asked quietly. "Are you talking in your sleep again?"

"No, I'm talking about the garlic bread. How come it wasn't soggy, like it is sometimes when people make it? Like when they make it at bad Italian restaurants?"

"I toast it in the oven a little first, sliced, and then add the garlic and butter. It keeps it crispier."

"Ah ha."

"They also use bad butter, the cheap restaurants," he added. "And pre-processed garlic, probably. You know how I feel about garlic that isn't chopped right before you want it. Now, go back to sleep."

She wondered – when she got home from the train tonight, would he be too tired to stay up and talk again? She wanted to tell him about what had happened at the conference, maybe even tell him about what Dr. Wilhelm had said about her lecture – that some of the audience members had been offended by it? It just sounded so wrong to her, she wanted to bounce it off Wolf and have him ask his good questions.

She wished that her lecture hadn't been slotted in as the last presentation block of the little people conference. Then there would have been more chance for her to ask around afterwards, to find out if Dr. Wilhelm was

174

right in his reading of the reception of her talk. Maybe she should have plunked down the forty dollars to go to the conference banquet held at the hotel ballroom just a couple of hours after her talk. Then she could have causally talked with people there, to figure out whether what Dr. Wilhelm had told her about the reception of her talk was true. She could also perhaps have mitigated whatever trouble he might cause at the dinner by talking about her to those at the banquet.

Nick DesJardins had told her earlier in the day that there were a couple of tickets still left for the banquet. He had even offered to buy her one. But she had told Nick she had already arranged to see an old friend that evening. She hadn't explained that the old friend was Abraham Lincoln – that she had planned to reenact a ritual she had when in school at Georgetown. On Sunday nights, when the dorm cafeteria was closed, she would get a cheap falafel sandwich at the take-out place on M Street and walk down to The Mall to the monuments, mostly to see Lincoln, to remind herself that even if she were lonely, she was truly free.

The first time she had visited Abe, she had pulled out of her shirt an envelope of folded papers and held it up to the statue, to prove it to President Lincoln and herself: a judge had ruled her free. Sister Mary Patrick had helped her find a lawyer who had ultimately secured for Maddy the paperwork that guaranteed that she counted in the eyes of the law as a legally emancipated minor. While she knew that her state had never been anything like that of an enslaved person, she relished the thought that no longer could she be legally – and sexually – controlled by another just by virtue of her biological age. What was in that envelope entitled her to direct access to birth control, abortion, the police, and more. She might be seventeen, but she was no longer under anyone else's control, not even remotely.

But how disorienting now, eight years later, to learn from Wolf the seemingly obvious connection between the way she framed her own sexuality and the subject of her dissertation: who owned whose body. Was she free if this issue of bodily ownership somehow still obsessed her – obsessed her enough to write a book on the subject?

Had it been Paula or Maddy or Liz who had originated Maddy's talk of "owning myself"? Given that before Maddy had even met Paula she had gone to Abe to announce she was now free, given that she remembered distinctly how much she hated The Jerk calling her "my little Madeleine," perhaps she had come up with that language herself.

The train came to a halt with Maddy's window directly facing one of the signs that said "Wilmington" in blocky letters. She watched as a handful of people disembarked and boarded and then felt the train start to move again.

Wolf's conception of sexuality certainly did stand at odds with hers. He spoke of sex as giving himself over – a kind of loss of self-integrity in terms of one's borders, a melding of one person into the next. But for Maddy, the pleasure of sex came from how it *marked* and *reiterated* her anatomical borders. How it showed her where she stopped and started, where she ended and the rest of the world began. How it reminded her she was her own person.

This, she figured, was the reason she found herself sexually attracted to men who were a good bit bigger than her, taller and muscular, not smaller, not softer. Their size and the resistance their bodies put up against hers – well, it was the dialectic, wasn't it? That wonderful, sweaty, erotic dialectic that told her where she was and who she was. Just as one could not be a mother if one did not at some point have a child; just as there could be no black if there was no concept of white; just as the poor were only poor if someone were rich: just as every identity required one in opposition to cohere: so Maddy derived from sex with a strong man a better sense of who *she* was.

That bright distinction between the skin of his lips and the skin of her neck.

That electric feeling of his lower abdominal muscles against her flank.

The sculpting stroke of a finger tracing around her areola.

She shuddered and smiled for a moment, remembering one time in winter during a wicked cold snap when Professor Butterfly stopped over to her place, the feeling of him coming into her with him still cold. She had let out something of a delighted whelp, feeling more than ever the yin and yang of where he in his cold ended and she in her warmth began.

"Colin! Your cock is as cold as a flagpole in a fucking blizzard!" she yelled.

"Oh, sorry!" he had said, laughing.

"This must be why butterflies don't mate out of season?" she asked, grabbing him a little harder and focusing on the extraordinary feeling of the way his corona bumped over her rugae, like pearls run over the chin.

"No," Colin muttered as he tried to breath normally, "it's the life cycle, you silly human."

"Philadelphia next, in about fifteen minutes!" the conductor cried. "Philadelphia will be next."

Maddy cleared her throat involuntarily, as if she had made an indelicate remark causing the announcement of her stop. Just as well she hadn't gone to the conference banquet as she had the sense Nick DesJardins was looking to maybe get her into bed and it was going to feel awkward having to turn him down. She couldn't blame him. He was a year past losing his wife and no doubt looking for a new relationship, or at least sex. He had said Maddy was about the height of his wife – his type? But Maddy couldn't see herself having sex with him. Did it make her a bigot that she didn't want to have sex with a man significantly smaller than her? Or was she, in fact, maintaining reasonable control of her sexuality by recognizing the shape and the limits of her desire and heeding them?

She wondered to herself for a moment what Wolf's touch would be like during sex. She vaguely imagined herself being her dissertation in his hands; him reading her. Did he give himself over fully with abandon when he had had relations with his wife? Or did he move, as he did with Maddy the night before she left from Washington, from a tender touch of her wrists to seeming distant – calling her Maddy instead of Rabbit – a little self-righteous about how he was making love to God?

Well, it didn't much matter. She would never find out. His company was good for the *intellectual*, that was clear. And the intellectual could be very satisfying.

Maddy, you're intellectualizing.

Paula had said that to her during one of their sessions, and when Maddy had asked her in return what that meant – "intellectualizing" something – Paula had explained that Maddy had been trying to convert a raw emotional feeling about something into a colder rational thought.

"I see. So, if I'm intellectualizing, is that a good thing or a bad thing?" Maddy asked. "Is saying I am intellectualizing a criticism or a compliment?"

Paula had let out a chuckle.

"No, really," said Maddy. "I don't understand. Are you criticizing me or complimenting me when you say I'm intellectualizing?"

"Well, usually in psychological therapy, saying a patient is 'intellectualizing' is meant as a criticism. It means you're avoiding emotional or psychological work. But in this case, I think I meant it simply as a description of what you were doing, Maddy. You like to intellectualize."

"It seems to me," Maddy had answered, "that it's a good way to deal with things – intellectualizing. Not only does it take away the emotional sting, I get insight out of it. Double bonus. What's wrong with that?"

"Nothing," said Paula pensively. "Absolutely nothing. Maddy, have you thought about pursuing a Ph.D.?"

...

She emerged from the train, her backpack over both shoulders, Wolf's suitcase in her hand, never expecting Wes. She felt so completely relieved to see him – to see that she would not be alone in making her way back to Wolf's house. And she could not help but notice that Wes's pretty eyes widened prettier as soon as he spotted her.

"Maddy!" he yelled and slalomed his way through the other people on the platform until he reached her.

He took the suitcase from her and held it between his knees so that he could free up his hands to take her backpack, too. He slung that over his shoulder.

"What are you doing here, Wes?" she asked, smiling involuntarily at him.

"Wolf told me to come get you because he had to get to a show that is starting soon – Bobby's. You know Bobby?"

Maddy shook her head no.

"He's playing at The Postman's tonight. It's a bar. They have some small shows and Bobby got a gig. Anyway, Wolf said I could take you there, or if you're tired, I should take you home. What's your pleasure?"

"Let's go see it," she said. "I mean, you'll come too?"

"Yes," he answered, "for sure. Bobby's got the goods, and he's a nice kid. Hey, Wolf told me about the other night – the intruder. You doing okay?"

"Yes," she said, "I'm doing okay, thanks."

He started walking a little ahead of her to get the door for her. She quickly sized him up and confirmed what she'd been thinking: he was a little bit shorter and definitely broader in the shoulders than the intruder. (When would she finally stop sizing up every man this way?) And now, she noticed, he had quite a nice ass. She wouldn't mind her hands on that.

They had walked just a few blocks away from the station when Maddy realized what she wanted. Wes had been asking her all about her trip in a most solicitous way and, well, with the way his ass had looked when he was in front of her, and with the way he was talking now, and with the way he was carrying the ten-pound suitcase as if it weighed less than a pound...

"Wes, would you do me a favor? Would you duck into the next dark alley with me, and kiss me?"

He stopped suddenly and looked at her, surprised.

"Uh – do you usually invite men into dark alleys for kisses?"

"Hell no," she replied, laughing. "But I'm not usually assured of having very nearby a handsome and chivalrous policeman whom I know personally."

He switched the suitcase from one hand to the other, reached down and took her hand in his, and started walking again. He directed her into the first dark space that presented itself on their side of the street. He quickly put Wolf's suitcase down next to him, wrapped his hands around her cheeks, anchored behind her ears, and bent over and kissed her right on the lips. Within a couple of seconds she was deep into that delicious dialectic, his tongue finding the inside of her lips, hers finding the inside of his cheek, one of his hands on the back of her head, stroking her hair, the other on the small of her back.

She found herself pressing her crotch up against his thigh, now wrapping one of her legs around his, feeling the heat of his leg against her, through his jeans and her jeans and whatever panties she had on under those jeans – was it the pink ones with the subtle pinstripes or those awful beige ones? – and oh, if she could just rub just right, maybe –

"Christ, you feel fantastic," he said.

She laid her head down on his shoulder and wrapped her arms around his shoulders and closed her eyes and he held his leg still while she lost herself in the motion, in the thought that he was the ride-on pony at the supermarket and she had enough pennies in her pocket to go on forever.

...

They got to The Postman just before Bobby had to go on. The place immediately felt to her like a classic old East Coast bar – an accumulated pile of mahogany and patched Naugahyde, mismatched Tudor-style lamps hanging from the ceiling and, on the walls, visual references to local sports heroes. The air felt full of the noises of familiarity – clanking bottles and real laughter.

Wes introduced Maddy to Bobby and told her he would go find Wolf to put her stuff down at their table. After a little bit of friendly chatter with Bobby, Maddy bought Bobby a beer and herself a vodka tonic, and then she found the table with Wes and Wolf and a couple more of the guys from the poker game, Neller and Crappy. She could not help but notice that Manny wasn't there.

When Wolf saw her, he stood up and took her forearm in his hand and they exchanged a kiss on each cheek. This was something no one in the Midwest ever seemed to do – give a friend a smudged peck on each cheek – and it made her feel immediately back home. This was the right way to come back to a good friend. And his face smelled just like Wolf, too – a little garlic, a little Head and Shoulders, finished with a human fragrance specific to his pores. She wasn't sorry to have had a little bit of Wes, but she also wasn't sorry to be home to Wolf, who wouldn't want her on his thigh.

Neller introduced Maddy to the woman he was with (his wife Sally) and Maddy sat down in the chair Wolf had saved for her next to him, with Wes on her other side. As she sat, Maddy's foot bumped into something soft that suddenly moved under the table. She sprung back and looked under the table. There was a dog – a white German shepherd. It poked its head out to see Maddy.

"Maddy, this is Hunter," said Wolf giving the dog a scratch on the head.

Hunter held a paw up to Maddy and she shook it.

"Pleased to meet you, Hunter. I'm Maddy."

The dog laid down, leaning lightly against Maddy's calf. His warm, living weight felt reassuring in a primal way.

"Hungry?" Wolf asked.

"Starving," she said.

He reached down into a grocery bag on the floor and pulled out a small casserole dish with a glass lid. He put it on the table in front of her, took off the lid, and handed her a fork.

"The lasagna!" she said.

"And I think it's still warm enough," he answered, feeling the side of the bowl with his open palm. "I saved a piece of it for you."

"I hope you're going to share that," Wes said to her, bumping his shoulder into hers. "It smells delicious."

"Maybe," she said, and she tasted a little bit of it. Wolf had spooned on a little extra scoop of his tomato sauce, to keep it moist. She felt almost as if she hadn't eaten in days.

At the mic, the manager was introducing Bobby and the crowd was starting to settle down in response.

"Alright," said Wolf, "which one of you knuckleheads bought him that bottle of beer?"

"Wasn't me, Wolf!" said Neller.

Crappy and Wes said the same.

"Not me neither, Wolf," Sally chimed in.

"Um," said Maddy, "was I not supposed to buy him a beer? He asked me to – said he'd pay me back later."

"He's underage, Maddy," said Wolf, rolling his eyes. "He didn't ask you to buy it because he didn't have the money."

The rest of the people at the table laughed at Maddy.

"Miss Shanks," said Crappy, pulling out a pen and grabbing a napkin, "I'm going to have to write you up. Now, what is your address?"

Bobby launched into his first song, a piece he introduced just by saying that it was a little something he had written. His fingers picked off the notes on the guitar as he started to sing about a girl and a swimming hole. Listening to him sing and play, Maddy stopped eating for a moment.

"He's good!" she said, surprised.

They all nodded at her, all except Wolf, who sat there looking nervous for Bobby. Wolf kept scanning the crowd to see the reception. As he could see it was going well, he seemed to relax a little.

"Hey," Maddy whispered into Wes's ear, "how do you all know Bobby?"

"His father Robert was a cop," Wes whispered back.

He used his fingers to take a little bit of lasagna noodle and ate it.

"Christ, that's good," he whispered to Maddy. "Let me have the rest of it?"

"Maybe in a minute, after I've had more," she said. "Wes, what happened to Bobby's father? Why do you talk of him in the past tense?"

"You didn't know? He was in the car with Wolf's wife."

"Oh," said Maddy. "Oh."

"Hunter was Robert's dog," Wes added, a little more quietly. "Bobby's been keeping Hunter. Since his father Robert died in the crane accident. Wolf insisted."

Hearing his name, Hunter popped up momentarily. Maddy rubbed him behind his upright ears, and then went back to eating and listening and glancing at Wolf's face. He was nodding along to the song, as if helping Bobby keep the rhythm from twenty feet away. Not that Bobby needed any help. He was genuinely good – he had written a good song, sweet in melody and words. His voice, his face, and his guitar playing didn't require any charity. The song ended and Wolf looked relieved to hear the crowd's sincere clapping and happy murmur.

"Kid just needs a haircut," Wolf said to no one in particular.

Maddy looked down to see the dish had disappeared. She turned to see Wes finishing off the last of the lasagna.

"Hey!" she yelled, a little too loudly. "What the hell?"

Wes smiled at her and shrugged his shoulders.

"You didn't even eat it slow enough to appreciate it!" she told him, the annoyance in her voice evident.

"Shush," Wolf said to her. "I'll make you something when we get home."

...

"I think Wes was hoping to spend some more time with you, Rabbit," Wolf said as they walked the mile from the bar back to his house.

Maddy was wearing her backpack, carrying the grocery bag in one hand and holding Hunter's leash with her other. Wolf had the suitcase, occasionally shifting it from one hand to the next.

"If Wes was hoping to spend more time with me, the shithead shouldn't have finished off my lasagna," she answered grouchily, adjusting the backpack on her shoulders.

Wolf grunted at her as if to imply she was being unreasonable.

"I do feel badly taking Bobby's dog, Wolf."

"I told you," Wolf replied, "Bobby is allergic and he doesn't need Hunter anymore. Plus, he's starting to go on the road for his music and he can't take Hunter with him. He's fine with it. Didn't he tell you the same thing?"

"Yes," said Maddy, "but I assume you put him up to it."

"I'll feel better if you have Hunter with you when I'm not home," Wolf said, reiterating what he had told her earlier.

Maddy wasn't sorry at the idea – having a retired police dog temporarily would be great. But she couldn't help but feel she was making Wolf's life too complicated, even if for just a little while.

It was dark now and the streets were mostly quiet. She liked the feeling of being out so late in the night air. With Wolf and Hunter as her unobtrusive companions, the world felt open and free, like they could go in any direction she pleased without much consideration. It reminded her of the times she would sneak out of her bedroom window, after her parents were fast asleep, and wander their neighborhood quietly in the middle of the night.

"I'm hungry," she said, without realizing she was even thinking it before she said it.

"I promise I'll make you something when we get home," Wolf said. "How about some sausage and eggs?"

"Which kind of sausage?"

"Fennel," he answered.

"From D'Alio's?"

"Yes."

"Okay," she said, realizing too late she had said it in a tone that made it sound like she was doing him a favor. "Would you mind if I grab a bath while you cook it? I would like to get the smell of Amtrak off me."

"Not at all," he answered. "I know you like the sausage well browned, so it'll take a while."

"They must put a little sugar in it, the way it caramelizes so nicely?"

Wolf nodded. Maddy looked at the way Hunter was trotting along with them. He was strong and healthy – he would be a good dog to take running. He seemed to know how to keep the right distance and he was good at pacing himself to stay in step with his human.

"Listen, Rabbit. Father Tad did find you a place. So I'll have to figure out what to do with Hunter when you go."

They were just turning a corner, passing a bodega closed for the night. Hunter's nose went up in the air a little as they passed the store. Wolf waited another fifty feet or so for a reply from Maddy, but she didn't answer.

"It fits the bill," he said, "the place Father found. It's not too far from the museum. It's a family. The kids – four of them – they are aged seven to twelve, and they go to bed early and they sleep through the night. The room for you would be small, just a twin bed, but it has a desk in it. There's a bath you can use after the kids go to bed."

"It sounds like a horror show," she answered.

He didn't respond.

"If it's what you want, Wolf," she sighed.

She was so tired now, it seemed like there would be no difficulty falling asleep tonight. In fact, she was so tired, she realized, she felt a little like crying. She wondered if she could take Hunter to her room with her tonight – if that was what Wolf had had in mind.

"I know you said I can still come eat with you if I'm staying somewhere else, Wolf, but it's not just the food. Talking to you about my work, it helps. It helps me stay on track."

"We can still talk about it over dinners," he said. "I should tell you, by the way, I read the rest of your dissertation draft, the parts you printed out. I think it's very good. I mean, I know you have a lot left to finish, to research and write still."

"So, I could still screw it up. That's what you're saying."

"You know that's not what I meant, Rabbit. You *are* in a bad mood, aren't you. I'm sure you're exhausted. And I'm sorry Wes ate what I brought for you."

He tried to put a hand on her shoulder, but she moved away. With the shift in her gait to the side, Hunter looked up at her.

"And I'm not in your field of study," Wolf continued, "so me judging your dissertation would be a little like you judging a criminal investigation." She wondered if he had picked up why she had been looking at late-twenti-eth-century texts. "But I think your committee and the other people in your profession will find it very good."

"No one will read it besides the committee," she said.

She sighed again. They were nearing his house and she felt suddenly like she was being too much of a shit, given all this kindness. It was like at the convent. But she wasn't a teenager anymore.

"Anyway, Wolf, thank you. For reading it, and for saying it's good. Because I know you don't bullshit me."

"How was the trip?" he asked.

"Fine," she said, saying nothing more.

Now they were just about two blocks from his place. Maybe she would tell him more – much more – about the trip over the sausage and the eggs? But right now she was stuck on the idea of having to pack and leave his place to go to this other place, as if somehow she had done something wrong. She had no energy to unpack what she'd taken to Washington, no less to wash her clothes and pack up everything to move. And now she was wondering where this dog she had just met was going to end up. Everything suddenly felt like too much.

"Did you get to go to the National Library of Medicine, as you were hoping? To see your friend, the librarian – you said his name was Booker?"

"Yes," she said, but again said nothing more.

"Tomorrow will be a normal day," he said as he put down the suitcase and put the first key in the first lock of the alleyway door that led to his kitchen. "You'll go back to work at the museum tomorrow morning, and I'll go to work on the day shift. I was thinking of making a mushroom risotto for dinner."

Again, she didn't respond. Wolf put the second key in the second and third locks, opened the door, and turned on the lights for them. Hunter entered the kitchen and looked at Wolf for a command. Wolf unhooked his leash from his collar and told him to lie down. He pulled the lasagna dish from the grocery bag to put it on the counter and then moved to get Hunter a dish for water.

Maddy was trying to figure out if she should spend the money it would take to just rent a small apartment for the next few weeks, for the time she needed to stay to finish her work here. How much could it possibly cost?

She had saved hundreds of dollars thanks to Wolf not charging her for food or rent. But those two extra nights at the hotel in Washington – added after the assault, when he asked her to go a day early and stay a day longer while he finished working the night shift – *that* had cost her a small fortune. Almost five hundred dollars more than she had planned, with the extra night at the hotel and the train schedule changes. Nevertheless, she was still way ahead on her budget for this dissertation research trip to Philly, thanks to Wolf. Maybe it wouldn't be that hard to find a little place that would be furnished and ready, with a small kitchen or a kitchenette? Maybe they would let her keep the dog, and then she could give Hunter back to Wolf when she was ready to leave Philadelphia? With the dog, she could probably sleep okay.

"Tomorrow will be a normal day," Wolf said again.

She wasn't sure what he was trying to achieve with this prediction, this incantation, this declaration about a normal day. She was trying hard to have it not feel like a criticism of the abnormality she had brought to his days and nights.

Wolf put a dish of water down on the floor for Hunter, who came and drank five laps from it. Wolf went back to the back door and locked it, doing now what he always did – putting his keys, his wallet, and his gun on the counter. Maddy was thinking about how accustomed she had become to his household rituals like this one he had when coming home – how it had felt so familiar. And now she would leave it because of the break-in? It didn't seem quite fair....

Wolf went over to near the stove, broke off a small piece from a loaf of bread, and walked over to her.

"Try this – it's an olive loaf," he said, bringing it to her mouth.

"Wolf!" she yelled suddenly, pulling away. Hunter stood up at her cry.

"What?!"

"Why does your hand smell like that?" She pulled his hand to her nose and smelled it more carefully.

He pulled it back and smelled it.

"Oh, it's the hospital's disinfectant soap," he said. "I went to see my wife, when I knew your train was late and I had a little time."

That was it – the smell of the intruder's hands – like the Amtrak disinfectant, just a little less fruity. More chemical.

Her heart was racing. Why would someone who knew Wolf through the hospital break in and come after Maddy? Had he talked about her being at his home? Was it just a coincidence?

She was about to explain her reaction to the smell when he spoke.

"I can understand why, with that smell on my hands, you thought that bread would taste terrible. The bread is good – believe me. I'll wash my hands well with dish soap and some lemon juice and slice you a fresh piece of the bread to go with the sausage and eggs. It'll be perfect with good butter and a side of fruit. I have a good apple for you – a Cortland."

She said nothing. She wanted to calm down her heart and make some sense of all this, before she tried to tell Wolf that his hands smelled like the intruder's.

"Go take your bath," he said, turning to the stove and pulling out his heavy cast iron pan. "Tomorrow has just got to be a normal day, Rabbit. Remind me to give you the new set of keys before you go to work. And we'll get you set up to take Hunter with you. *He* won't be any trouble at all."

-18-

Soon Wolf would be home. He would give Hunter a show of love and start the risotto, and she would have a strong drink. And all of that would mean she could tell him. Tell him what she thought was going on.

She should probably be sure he had a drink first, too, so that he would not immediately disbelieve her.

He had told her last night he wanted a normal day. Was it her fault this again wasn't turning out to be anything like a normal day?

Maddy sat at the kitchen table, her backpack still fastened on her torso, her head now in her hands. Wasn't it a strange artifact of physiology that when the brain became overwhelmed, the head could actually hurt? The brain – that wet bread loaf of nerves in the oven of the skull – it was not supposed to be able to feel itself so well.

Maybe last night she should have told him about his hands smelling like the intruder's. Then there would have been a breaking of the ice of what she now needed to tell him.

Maybe, too, if she had told Wolf last night about the smell, he would have made it his problem – taken it off her – and she would have slept instead of lying awake most of the night thinking about...the possibility? The possibility that the attack had been meant specifically for her. That it had come from someone working with Dr. Wilhelm. That this was the reason the intruder's hands had smelled of hospital soap.

But who was he? It could not have been Wilhelm himself – the intruder had been too tall, too thin, and moved much younger....

By the time she had dragged herself out of bed for breakfast and taken Hunter for a short walk, it just seemed so unlikely. She couldn't remember anyone in Dr. Wilhelm's posse who had the build of the intruder. Yes, she had told Dr. Wilhelm and Dr. Tate and Shirley at dinner that night about what she knew of the serial rapist from Wolf: the electrical tape; the knife; the ski mask with the sunglasses. So, they had all known that much, and Dr. Wilhelm (or Shirley, or Dr. Tate) could have passed the information on to make it look like the serial rapist. And yes, the parts she knew or thought she knew about the serial rapist were exactly the parts that had showed up in her bedroom. And various parts of the act were wrong, the police said – but wrong in a way that matched what she had told the others at dinner.

But what would have been the point? Could Dr. Wilhelm have wanted badly enough to hurt her or to scare her out of town that he would have someone take this risk, the risk of breaking into a cop's house and getting caught?

Of course, Dr. Wilhelm didn't *know* she was staying at a police detective's house, did he?

Wilhelm had known that a man who was a police officer, Wes, had driven her home from his house – and he had seemed concerned, when she had asked a lot about Schlesinger 1888, that she had a friend here who was a cop. But he had probably not known who her landlord was, or what he did. Maddy hadn't told Wilhelm or Shirley or anyone local that her landlord was a member of the police – she had told no one but Liz. And Maddy had said at dinner at Dr. Wilhelm's house that she would be without her landlord, home alone at nights, that week. As far as anyone knew, Wolf wasn't supposed to be home. (And he wouldn't have been but for the food poisoning.)

Had the intention been to hurt her more than just with the electrical tape? Could Dr. Wilhelm talk someone at the hospital into doing something this crazy?

None of this made a lot of sense.

That morning, as she had risen and showered and eaten breakfast and organized her pack including what she would need for Hunter for the day, her thoughts kept swinging wildly from putting the pieces of the attack together with the Wilhelm dinner (and seeing that they fit without any shoving) to telling herself this was just crazy thinking, borne of exhaustion and frustration with how Dr. Wilhelm had treated her.

In the end, she said little to Wolf over breakfast and nothing about having recognized the smell on his hands. She could always tell him later. He gave her the new keys, explained the locks, and suggested she claim Hunter was a service dog for a medical problem of some sort.

"But I don't have a medical problem," she said. Wolf answered that she should just say something vague so they would let her keep Hunter, so the dog could walk her to and from the museum. And she had to admit to herself that given all she had thought about last night, she liked the idea of Hunter going with her.

When she had arrived at the museum, Maddy didn't hang up her keys on the hook in the doorframe of her little basement office. She had originally thought that Wolf had been being a little ridiculous when he had said to her, just after the attack, that he would change the locks and that she and he would have to keep the keys on their persons at all times. But given what she had been thinking about overnight, she kept the keys in her pocket.

She sat down at her desk and put her laptop on the desk. She gave Hunter an order to lie down near her. She had not been back to the museum since the attack, having gone off to D.C. just after it, and it all felt a little unfamiliar, particularly because now Hunter was here. It didn't help that there was a spider hanging down above her desk. She used her dry mug to capture it and take it outside, to shake it into the bush just outside the museum's front door. She told Hunter to stay while she went to do this, and he followed the command, although when she came back, he was standing at the door waiting for her.

She gave him an order to lie down again, returned to her desk and sat for a while, simply looking around the room. She could hear the museum staff moving about, working, but she didn't want to go talk to any of them – especially not Shirley. Even if Hunter was a momentary distraction to Shirley, Shirley was sure to ask about Washington, and Maddy didn't want to tell Shirley about Dr. Wilhelm's reaction to her talk. She didn't want to lose Shirley as an ally. As it was, Dr. Wilhelm was probably going to spoil that relationship. Would he also bad-mouth her in her own field?

Maddy turned her chair and looked up out the window and watched several pairs of feet trod by. What was she going to try to accomplish today? What was she going to be able to do?

She pulled an index card out of the desk drawer and started a to-do list.

Then she got up, walked around past the desk, bent over, put her hands on the floor, and went into a handstand. Hunter cocked his head and looked at her quizzically.

"This floor needs mopping," she said aloud to him, and he came over and licked her nose. "You silly dog, go lie down," she said, and he did.

She held the pose and thought about her list. She had purposefully given herself something fairly rote to start with, something that wouldn't take a lot of mental wherewithal: going through the notes she had been making about which texts she still needed to consult for her dissertation and organizing them into a spreadsheet on her computer to make it easier to print out the list, locate libraries for the texts, and plan how to collect them. She could do that much today. She ended the handstand, went to the restroom to wash her hands, came back, and started into the first item on the list.

After an hour of this, Hunter was asleep and Maddy was yawning furiously. Maybe she should have just stayed home and rested today. But then she didn't want Shirley thinking she wasn't a serious scholar, wasting the space. What Dr. Wilhelm had said.

It was Shirley's sudden cry – a piercing, unnerving exclamation of grief – that tore Maddy out of her fog and woke Hunter up, too. Maddy bolted up and ran down the hall to Shirley's office with Hunter trotting next to her. There she found Dr. Wilhelm embracing Shirley, to comfort her.

The look he gave Maddy suggested he wasn't especially happy to see her, and the look he gave Hunter was no better. But he explained why Shirley was crying.

"I came to personally convey very sad news to Ms. Anseed," said Dr. Wilhelm, looking away from Maddy. "I drove straight here to the museum from Washington this morning. Dr. DesJardins has died. He died yesterday morning."

Maddy felt her salivary glands all contract, her mouth filling with spit. She swallowed.

"Poor Nick!" exclaimed Shirley to Maddy.

Maddy's lack of movement or response and the dog standing next to Maddy all seemed to confuse Shirley.

"I'll be alright in a minute," said Shirley, sitting down in her chair and pulling three tissues out of her box. She seemed to think she should be as stoic as Maddy appeared to be. "Why do you have a dog, Maddy?"

"Possible seizure disorder – but not likely," Maddy mumbled absent-mindedly, saying what she had practiced in her head.

Hunter's nose was twitching nervously at the strange scents of the museum detectable in Shirley's office.

Feeling lightheaded, Maddy sat down very carefully in one of the chairs across the desk from Shirley. She stared at Dr. Wilhelm's face, trying to discern what she could. Hunter came to stand at the chair next to her. She reached out her hand and held his collar, as if for balance.

Now she realized that the ambulance she had seen at the hotel – when she went back yesterday after the early lunch with Booker to get her suitcase from the bellhop on her way back to Union Station – that ambulance must have been for Nick DesJardins. The lights were off because the ambulance attendants knew he was dead. Whoever called it in was sure he was dead. They would not have rushed.

Perhaps the police had been there while she was off in Bethesda, or perhaps they were yet to come, or perhaps they were parked on the other side of the hotel....The police had come, right?

"What happened?" asked Maddy finally.

"He seemed quite well at your lecture and at the banquet," said Dr. Wilhelm. "But then around ten o'clock that night, he called to ask me to come see him, as he was not feeling well. There were some signs – I was concerned. I tried to get him to let me take him to the hospital. But he did not want to be stuck in an emergency room in a hospital far from home, to risk being admitted far from home. Even if I offered to stay with him at the hospital. Which of course I did."

"Of course you did," said Shirley.

"Who found him?" asked Maddy.

"He was in touch with other members of the organization later that night, after I saw him. Quite late, I know, because I called a few of them to let them know he had passed away. They say he told them in the middle of the night that he wasn't feeling well, and they say he told them I had suggested we go to the hospital – but he said he didn't want to be bothered and he would just sleep in and feel better the next day, he was sure. Well, I went to check on him around ten in the morning yesterday, before I was to drive back to Philadelphia. And he would not answer the door. So, I called the hotel staff and the manager and I, we went in, and that is when we found him."

"What did he die of?" asked Shirley.

"Natural causes," said Wilhelm, looking with some disdain at Hunter. "The medical examiner has to rule, but I expect that is the ruling. You know, he seemed very lively but his body had so many problems."

"It's horrible he died alone," said Shirley. "No one was there?"

"He spoke with other members of the group around midnight or one in the morning," said Dr. Wilhelm, "but no one heard from him after that, until I went in with the hotel staff. And by then, he had died."

"And you will get his body," said Maddy, sotto voce.

"No, Ms. Shanks," answered Dr. Wilhelm loudly, with anger betrayed in his voice. "No. He told me he had already promised it to the group at the Cleveland Clinic. That was his choice, of course, and that's how he chose."

Maddy let go of Hunter's collar, stood up, and excused herself, saying she would leave them alone.

"You can stay, Maddy," said Shirley.

"No," said Maddy, meeting the gaze of Dr. Wilhelm. "I think I should go and express my condolences to the other members of the little people group."

With Hunter at her side, she walked out, not to her own office but up the stairs and out the door to the medicinal herb garden in the small courtyard on the side of the museum. She needed to get some air. She sat down on one of the stone benches and stared at the small brass labels at the bases of the plants: feverfew, marjoram, St. John's wort, foxglove, echinacea. Hunter stood near her, his nose lifted in the air as if he was breathing in the fresh air of the garden to dispel the smells of the museum.

Foxglove, thought Maddy, *used to treat congestive heart failure.*

Could Wilhelm have given Nick something to bring on heart failure? But if he did, would Nick have been well enough a few hours later to still be talking to his friends? And would Wilhelm have risked something that might hurt but not kill Nick? Would he risk something the medical examiner might find?

It seemed too unlikely.

Perhaps the truth was that Wilhelm had gone back to Nick's room *after* Nick had been in touch with his friends. Would hotel security tapes show if anyone had been there? But why would Wilhelm bother, if he wasn't going to get the body? And if someone else did get the body, they might find suspicion in the death?

A crow came suddenly swooping down into the garden, landing at Maddy's feet, unafraid of her or the dog. Hunter went very still. The bird looked up at Maddy with its black eyes, expecting perhaps that she would have something in the way of food. The way it stared at her – it felt incriminating.

And then she remembered: When Dr. Wilhelm had been so unpleasant to her in Washington after her lecture two evenings ago, when they had spoken alone in the lecture room, *she* had been the one to inform Dr. Wilhelm that Nick was thinking of switching doctors. *She* had delivered the news that Nick was thinking of leaving Dr. Wilhelm and his clinic and giving the specialist at the Cleveland Clinic access to his body....

Jesus. Had she brought on Nick's early death by telling Dr. Wilhelm that?

But wait – Dr. Wilhelm said in Shirley's office that he knew Nick's body would go to the Cleveland Clinic. Dr. Wilhelm seemed to think he wasn't going to get the body. So Nick's death couldn't have been Maddy's fault, right?

As if the crow had achieved what it wanted, sowing this confusion in Maddy, now it shifted its interests and looked around the garden. Maddy followed its gaze – first to the door through which Maddy had come, then up the side of the wall, to the stone downspouts, then to the small tree behind Maddy.

The corvid's visual mapping of the points in the garden made Maddy remember the last time she had been out in this garden – was it about a week ago? Dr. Wilhelm had come by to the museum, dipped his head into Shirley and Maddy's offices, and told them there was of all things an old-fashioned organ grinder with a monkey out in the garden. The two women had gone out to see, as had a number of the rest of the staff. The man with the monkey wouldn't talk to them – he acted as if he were mute, playing his songs while his primate did a little dance and came up to each of them with a can for coins. With the second song, the monkey banged tiny cymbals together. And with the third, he came back around with his can.

The organ grinder and his monkey – *of course*. That was how Wilhelm had copied her house keys so the intruder-accomplice would have a set to easily break in during the period Maddy had said she would be alone at night. Wilhelm had distracted them all with the organ grinder and the monkey. He had gone into her office and taken her keys and given them to someone to get them copied. This was why, right at the end of the organ grinder's performance, Wilhelm had suddenly shown up with a basket of treats to share with everyone in the garden – chocolate-covered strawberries and candied nuts, saying something about a grant renewal he felt like celebrating. Delaying them further, buying enough time to get the keys copied and back on her office hook.

They never expected Wolf to be home with food poisoning that night. Was the intention to hurt Maddy? Or just to scare her back to Indiana?

Wait.

This was nuts.

A member of the National Academy of Sciences killing patients to get their bodies? She knew that historically there had been cases of medical men hastening the deaths of patients through risky research. Even intentional homicide. But Dr. Wilhelm?

She must be imagining this.

Still, what were the odds that, of the few texts he would lose in a fire that he had supposedly accidentally set himself, one of those texts would be Schlesinger 1888, the text meant to prove that patients with certain forms of dwarfism had died naturally of heart problems, a text supposedly documenting sudden heart failure in dwarfism long before Dr. Wilhelm was ever born?

But if he had faked that text – if he had faked its existence and its supposedly accidental demise – how could there be a copy of it at the New York Public Library, as the online records Booker had consulted at the National Library of Medicine showed?

She would have to go to New York soon and see that text, to see if it was there, to see what it looked like.

But if Dr. Wilhelm thought Nick's body was already promised away, why would he kill Nick?

Maddy stood up suddenly, startling the crow and Hunter. The bird flew up about eight feet and around her, into the tree behind her. She rushed into the side door of the museum and hastened down the stairs to the basement offices with Hunter next to her, just as Dr. Wilhelm was coming up.

"Dr. Wilhelm," she said, pulling Hunter and herself against the wall. "I am glad I caught you. Tell me, who did Nick talk to between the time he saw you and when you found him dead?"

His eyes narrowed. He looked from Maddy to Hunter to Maddy again.

"Dr. Wilhelm, I want to learn what Dr. DesJardins' last expressed thoughts were," she said firmly. "I'm an historian, you know, and these things get lost if we don't record them soon."

"I know that he talked to Bess McFarlane," said Dr. Wilhelm, "because I called to let her know by phone this morning, and she told me she had talked to him in the middle of the night. Sam Minkin as well. Same thing. Beyond that, I don't know."

He started to move past Maddy up the stairs and then turned.

"I thought you were interested in the *nineteenth*-century, Ms. Shanks, yet you seem to have a disproportionate interest in the living."

194

"It is as Shirley says, Dr. Wilhelm," Maddy answered. "The living are just the future dead. Isn't that right?"

He turned away from her and continued up the stairs. She went to her own office and grabbed her backpack, throwing material from her desk into it, and then headed into Shirley's office. Hunter must have been picking up on her anxiety – he was staying close.

Maddy found the curator sitting at her desk, dabbing her tear ducts and blowing her nose.

"Maddy, it's awful," said Shirley, now clicking her tongue and clapping her hands lightly to get Hunter to come to her so she could pet him. He went to her and she rubbed him on the top of his head and around his jaw. "If only Nick has listened to Dr. Wilhelm and gone to the hospital! Perhaps he and Dr. Wilhelm would have averted disaster."

"We may never know if this could have been avoided," said Maddy.

"Well," said Shirley, standing up, "I have to go tell the other staff members who knew Nick. I think later we will all need to go to a very long lunch together to commiserate and remember him. You will come?"

"No, I can't. Can I use your phone?" asked Maddy, and Shirley nodded. "Shirley, you should go home after lunch with the staff – you are so spent by this. Do me a favor and close the door behind you?"

As soon as Shirley left, Maddy had given Hunter an order to lie down. Then she had pulled onto Shirley's desk three things: from her backpack her own research notebook and the stack of business cards collected from the conference, and from Shirley's shelf, the Yellow Pages. She sat down with Shirley's phone and immediately started making calls.

And by the time she and Hunter made it back to Wolf's house at quitting time, she had learned enough to make her realize it was time to tell Wolf.

When Wilhelm said that various friends had "talked to" Nick between the time Wilhelm visited him and he was found dead, he meant that various people had *received email* from Nick. None seemed to have spoken to him by phone. None had heard his voice. In the emails, he had simply said that he wasn't feeling great, that Dr. Wilhelm had tried to get him to go to the hospital, that he had declined, and that he would just rest, so not to bother him.

She had managed, too, to get a remarkable amount of information on the phone out of the hotel manager. (It probably didn't hurt that she strongly implied that she was Nick's distraught sister.) Security had checked tapes for the police and no one had been in Nick's room between the time Dr. Wilhelm came and left around ten p.m. and when Dr. Wilhelm went back in with the hotel manager about twelve hours later.

She figured Dr. Wilhelm must have taken Nick's laptop, used it from his own room, and then returned it to Nick's room. It probably would not have been too difficult to do the latter – for Wilhelm to stick it in his own bag when he was in Nick's room and then pull it back out and put it back when he returned to the room in the morning. The manager would have been distracted by the death and might not notice if Wilhelm put the computer back.

The manager also told her that when they'd gotten to the room, it was very warm – the thermostat was set to eighty – which Dr. Wilhelm attributed to Nick not having been feeling well. The manager and Dr. Wilhelm had cooled off the room by opening the windows and turning down the thermostat before the ambulance arrived.

"Ordinarily we secure a room if someone has died, until the police get there," the manager explained. "But Dr. Wilhelm was his doctor, so this was different. He went with – with Mr. DesJardins, when they took his body."

The manager assured Maddy that Nick had been tucked into bed, looking quite comfortable, like he hadn't much suffered.

Why crank up the thermostat and then cool off the room before the ambulance got there? Maddy knew: to throw off the coroner's reading of the time of death. To push the apparent time of death to after the emails. Another sign of mischief – not that she was feeling like she needed more proof. This was too obvious.

But why would Dr. Wilhelm kill Nick if he thought his body had already been promised to the Cleveland Clinic group? Was he just looking to get some critical tissue sample out of the autopsy, even if the rest of the body went back to Ohio?

Maybe this was all just a bunch of false signs.

But then – the organ grinder. Maddy had thought – when Shirley had left and Maddy pulled out the Yellow Pages – that the difficult thing to do would be to find the organ grinder and his monkey. But it turned out there was but one of these known in the city of Philadelphia and it took just three calls to figure out who he was and how to find him.

When Maddy reached him and confirmed it was he who had come to the garden that day, she told him it had been so enjoyable and she wanted to know who had arranged it because, she said, she was sure it had been done for her birthday and she wanted to thank the person.

He told her he wasn't sure who it was. A man with a slight accent had called him and said he would leave two hundred dollars in an envelope for the organ grinder, that he would leave it under a stone next to the bench in the garden. And sure enough, the money was there when he got there, so he took the money and did the job asked of him. The man who had booked him had asked him not to talk to the people there because, he said, it was a surprise for a friend and he didn't want to give anything away.

"But I guess the surprise is over, so it is okay to tell you all this," he said.

"Of course," said Maddy.

She thanked him and hung up.

As she walked home to Wolf's house with Hunter to her right, she felt a bit like her spine was petrifying step by step. She realized she had had one of those research days where, through sheer bombastic pushing on what she wanted to know, she had figured out more than most people would in a month. Booker had referred to her relentlessness and efficiency at their lunch in Bethesda. He had said it like it was a blessing, a gift. But did he understand it could be a curse?

The sensible person might have made a careful list and gone slowly through it day by day. The sensible person might simply have formally talked to the police to register a suspicion. The eminently sensible person – Sister Ruth, for example – she wouldn't run toward a tidal wave when she was already exhausted.

But something in Maddy caused her to just demand direct and immediate access to knowledge no matter how much trouble it might cause. Of all the stories in the Bible that bothered Maddy, the one that bothered her the most was from Genesis: God forbidding fruit of knowledge. Fuck that. She remembered now that argument with Sister Ruth about just that.

And as for the police –

"A fat lot of good the police are, Hunter!" she exclaimed, confusing the dog walking next to her. "Well, I don't mean you. You're a dog."

Yes, a fat lot of good the police were. After her parents died, the priest in charge of her school had told her he knew about The Jerk and was calling to tell the police about what The Jerk had been doing to her. But never had the police come to talk to her about it. It couldn't just be that they were forestalled in prosecuting him because she had suddenly gone off to West Virginia. They could easily have reached her there. She would have gone back to New York to talk to them if that was what they required. The sisters would surely have taken her back for that.

Never did the police do anything about powerful white men, really. In all these games of justice, the supposed advocate was never working for the victim. The supposed advocate was simply working to consolidate his or her own power.

She would have to be different from them. Yes, it was true this was none of her business – what was happening to these patients of Wilhelm's. But that was the very reason she should *make* it her problem: because she had nothing personally to gain or to lose in this scene. She could adhere to the truth and not protect someone who didn't deserve it.

Yet now, what was she supposed to do with all these threads? Would Wolf think she had just spun a ridiculous yarn? Would he try to stop her from trying to figure out more? And if the police did take it over, would they screw it all up? Would they even give a damn?

Because if there was one thing she knew from history, it was this: any medical care bestowed on people with unusual anatomies was seen as heroic charity, not to be questioned. Dr. Wilhelm would be seen as a hero, not a murderer, unless there was a mountain of evidence to the contrary. And there were those in the little people community who were going to think she was insane if she suggested Dr. Wilhelm had harmed any of them.

Not to mention Shirley.

Maybe she was wrong about him; correlation was not causation.

Maybe she was simply reacting to his unpleasant patriarchal manner, his sexism, his lording of his M.D.

The idea that he would have an accomplice who would have broken in and come at her – that seemed absolutely absurd.

Maybe she was wrong.

As she sat now in the chair in Wolf's kitchen, the backpack strapped around her like a clingy child, the dog near her feet, her head throbbing in her hands, what she knew was this: She had not slept well in almost a week – not since the attack – and she had not eaten anything today since breakfast. She had a terrible headache and a general feeling of vertigo.

Perhaps she should take off the backpack and just lie on the couch a while until Wolf got home.

And now she remembered that Wolf was about to kick her to the curb, to the house of that Catholic family. And they had children. If she was going to be troublemaking of the sort that caused men to come at her, could she be in a house where there were children?

If she went and got an apartment of her own, could she take Hunter with her there? And would Hunter be enough to protect her if someone broke in?

She could bail and go back to Indiana – but then what? Try to figure it all out from there? Or just give up? But if she found out years later that she had been right, and she had done nothing about it –

The sound of the key in the lock startled her and roused Hunter. Wolf came in and shut the door behind him, locking it. Hunter and Wolf immediately greeted each other.

"Hey, Rabbit," he said, seeing her sitting in the chair, her coat still on, her pack still on her back.

He put the mail he had brought in on the counter along with his keys, his wallet, and his gun, just like always. She was worried he was going to look at her – *really* look at her – and then he would see in her face all the trouble, and he wouldn't rest before he pulled it out of her.

But he didn't look at her straight away. He looked through the stack of mail and pulled out an envelope, handing it to her.

"Letter for you, from New York."

"Must be from my billboard lawyer," she said, taking it from him. She did not look at the return address, but ran her finger under the fold, tearing it open. She pulled out what was in it – a handwritten letter on two sheets of wide-ruled notepaper – and started to read.

My little Madeleine,

I was so surprised to find out you are in Philadelphia, only a couple three hours away from me on Long Island. I looked on the internet and found out that your in school now in Indiana and so I called to get your address from the department you are in. I explained to the lady who answered I am an old family friend and she told me your in Philadelphia doing research and they gave me the address where your staying.

Maybe we could meet up in New York City or something while your on the east coast. I am sure you look so different and the same and all.

It looks like your succeeding at your life. That is no surprise to me you know. You always were determined and smart although I know I helped you learn how to focus so you could get things done and all.

(She had forgotten his fucking annoying use of "and all." And forgotten how he did not know how even to spell the contraction of "you are" correctly. Jesus Christ! She had lost her virginity to this moron?!)

I never did get to tell you how sorry I was about your family before they sent you away because Father Paul told me I should stay away from the wake and the funeral so I did. I am sure it was as difficult for you as it was for me to be separated like that out of the blue.

There's a girl I am with now through St. Henry's (your old alma matter, yah I'm still there doing coaching!) and she is a very good little gymnast, very coachable and good at poise and balance especially.

Her name is Katie and I think you would like her. She's 13 now – the same age you were when we first made love. I haven't really had another girl like you but she is a lot like you and I think I could help her to become somebody like I helped you do that. It's taken a while but I have gotten her to let her guard down.

So I was thinking maybe you could send me back a letter to her that I could give to her where you tell her how much I helped you, how much I helped you learn, so she sticks with me with letting me help her and all. I think I can teach her a lot and I think she needs a man in her life who takes good care of her like I took care of you back then. There are boys interested in her because she's good looking but she is way better then them and she needs a man to teach her how to become a lady and all, and with her poise she is quite a little lady as you would see if you saw her on the bars. You know she'll be better off with me than dumb boys.

I'm still at the same address so you can reach me there or here is my phone in case you forgot it.

Norman

She had not forgotten his name, but she had so long taken to simply calling him The Jerk that it seemed somewhat remarkable that that was not now his *actual* name.

She read the letter one more time. The second time it was harder to read because of how the paper was shivering.

"Are you okay?" asked Wolf from a few feet away.

She looked up at him and thought he looked exceptionally ugly just now. His face – it was just plain ugly now. How did he transform like that?

"Are you okay?" he asked again.

The way he said it, with rising alarm but a lowered voice, well, it sounded to her not like a question but like some kind of *conclusion*. A statement of fact: that she was *not* okay. Like the last words the priest says before he closes the coffin lid.

She folded the letter back up and put it in the envelope. The bones in her face felt as if they had suddenly transformed from calcium to marble to porcelain. She left Wolf and Hunter and wandered up to her room, her backpack still clinging to her, and tried to figure out what to do with this communication. This communique. This communion.

Part of her was thinking that she should eat something, because she was feeling so woozy.

And part of her was thinking she should die.

And she was trying to figure out how to reconcile these two things, because obviously one didn't need to eat if one was going to die shortly. That would just be a waste of food. Why eat when the cancer was metastasizing so fast? Why eat when the lungs were about to fill with blood?

She tucked the envelope under a book on her desk as if the letter needed the book to keep it from blowing away. She wandered back down the stairs.

Wolf was still standing in the kitchen, looking a bit like a statue, Hunter looking up at him. Did Wolf think he could not make a sudden move around her?

"What was in that letter?"

She did not answer.

"Where is it?"

She raised her eyes to the ceiling without moving her head, to try to answer the question. But her head seemed to have some kind of quake going on.

"I am sorry, Rabbit," he said. "I don't want to invade your privacy. But you are acting very strangely and I think I have to see what is in this letter."

She did not answer. He left the kitchen and started slowly up the stairs as if he wasn't sure if he should go. Hunter followed him.

Watching them go, she went over to the counter near the back door, took off her backpack, opened the main compartment, and put Wolf's gun in. Then she opened his wallet and took all the cash, shoved the money in her left front pants pocket, and put his wallet back on the counter.

She pulled her new set of housekeys out of her right pocket and put them on the counter, where the gun had been. She did not want to take the only other set he had for the new locks. She headed out the door.

It would have been better to have packed her things properly and taken her suitcase. But then that would have taken more time, and Wolf might have tried to stop her, and she should get on a train sooner rather than later. The suitcase would just slow it all down.

It didn't matter anyway. She would need to get rid of all those clothes because they would just remind her that once she had been pursuing a Ph.D., that once she had been close to having a Ph.D. and becoming a professor, and there was no point in dwelling in the past. There was no point in the dresses from Giovanni. No point in the jackets for conferences.

She thought for a moment about her little palm tree, in its blue pot, home in Indiana with Liz. She felt a little like crying for the thought of never seeing it again.

And Liz.

She started for the station in the usual direction. Buying a ticket at the last minute like this would cost more, but there was no way around that.

But should she go to New York? Or should she just make another clean break, like she had with West Virginia – with Washington – with Indiana – just start over again, again?

Again.

Liz had asked her once what she would do if she found herself alone holding a gun in a desolate alley with The Jerk? In other words, Liz asked, what would Maddy do if no one would ever know what she had done? And Maddy said, well, *that* was easy: She'd just shoot him in the head and feel no remorse.

The answer appeared to have taken Liz back. Which seemed odd to Maddy. Because she thought Liz understood. Why else would she have asked that way?

Yet why was it her job to stop him from doing to some unlucky girl named Katie what he had done to unlucky her? Why should she help Katie? No one had helped Maddy. She had had to save herself. And she had done okay after all.

But maybe Katie wasn't as smart. Wasn't as strong. Wasn't going to be horribly liberated and wonderfully imprisoned with a car crash.

Maddy had the sense she had to be the car crash for Katie. And this time the person who needed to die in the crash was The Jerk, and not her father and her mother and her sister.

The last of the commuters were streaming in and out of Thirtieth Street Station as Maddy got close. They were a gradient flow, she realized. That was what Liz would say, anyway: the commuters formed a dense gradient, like a sugar solution. You could tell you how close you were to the thing you were trying to reach by the density increasing, the intensity of the commuters increasing, the sugar getting stronger.

Sugar being what she needed to take the edge off this headache and this sense of weakness in her muscles. Going to the sugar.

(It seemed no fair to have to give up Liz now because of him. No fair at all.)

Life isn't fair, Rabbit, she could hear her mother's voice say in her head, the way she used to say to her when Maddy would whine about something.

But wait, no – her mother didn't call her Rabbit. That was *Wolf's* name for her. *Don't be stupid. Don't be stupid.*

And she could hear it now – *Rabbit!* – as she pulled open the heavy brass and glass door of the station to enter. She could hear him yelling from a long way away, with anger in his voice, "Rabbit! Rabbit, wait!"

Or was it panic, not anger?

She entered the station just as it was drenched in a gold hue from the evening light, the tall windows framed by the great columns pulling in the last of the day's sun. She walked on past the great winged statue near the door, the memorial to the men and women of the Pennsylvania Railroad who died in World War II – the people who never lived past the time of shoving walnuts and apples with joints of beef and slices of old bread all into an oven at once –

Oh, would she never be in Wolf's kitchen again? Would he never again make her something to eat?

The Jerk did have a way of ruining absolutely everything.

Absolutely everything.

She had reached the great arrivals and departures board. Now it was time to look up at it and decide.

New York? The obvious choice.

Washington, D.C.? New Orleans? Western New Jersey? Even California, if she was reading that board right?

"Rabbit!" said Wolf, suddenly appearing in front of her. The dog was not with him.

She looked at his face briefly. But she did not have the energy right now to read it. It took *such* a lot of energy to read a face sometimes.

She looked back up at the board.

Oh, Boston just clicked away. Too late. Boston is gone.

"Rabbit," he said, "listen. I read the letter. I understand."

She looked at his face again. No, still no energy to read it.

She looked back up at the board.

"Please, give me what you put in your bag – I mean, give me your bag, and I will retrieve it," he said, looking around to see if anyone else was near. "The thing you took from me, from the counter."

This time she didn't bother to look at him.

How did these old-fashioned great departures and arrivals boards work, with the flipping characters? She figured each block must have a full deck with every letter and number, and then each deck just spun somehow until it got to the right character. An electrical impulse probably sent the right amount of energy to spin just the right amount? Or was it done via a timer, a timed spin, where the electricity was sent for the amount it took to get to the desired character in the deck? Did it reset each time to the beginning and then spin to the right letter or number, or did the machine know how to efficiently get from N to G?

It seemed like it must reset first, and then get enough energy to spin to the right character. It would be nice if *she* had enough energy to get exactly to the right spot – if she could just push a button remotely and send electricity, just enough electricity, to The Jerk, to fry him dead.

Then she wouldn't have to take a trip to get rid of him.

Then they would just find his ashen remains and sweep him away.

Katie would get over it. Quickly, probably. Giddily, maybe.

And Maddy would never have to face Katie and explain why she hadn't stopped him earlier. She would never have to tell Katie she knew what it was like to be stuck between your unloving father and a loving creep.

How tiring.

How tiresome.

The train board clicked on. She thought New York would disappear near the top as an option soon. But then, she realized, it would reappear again shortly after that. Lots of trains to New York.

Still, maybe it was time to go and buy the ticket.

She pulled Wolf's cash out of her left pocket and started to count it and then realized he was watching her count his money. Did he know it was his?

She would pay him back, though. She was going to send him the money when she could. She knew that there was a three-hundred-dollar-a-day limit on ATM withdrawals, but if she just did that each day, she would soon have all her money and she could pay Wolf back out of that. And she could find her billboard lawyer and tell him where she was, wherever she was after this, to get the checks to her. So she could pay rent somewhere while she started over.

But, oh. She had wanted *so much* to finish her Ph.D. And with Wolf reading her dissertation, the way he had read her dissertation, it had felt like it was real – that she was going to finish it....

Why did The Jerk make it so that she had to give up this, too? Why must he take everything and everyone away from her all over again?

Perhaps the solution wasn't the end of him but the end of her. She couldn't be responsible for The Jerk, or Wilhelm, or any other problem if she wasn't around anymore.

She could feel the tears starting to roll down her face.

"Rabbit," Wolf said now, bending down on one knee. "Listen to me. You don't have to do this. You don't have to deal with this alone. You don't have to go and help Katie. I will take care of it."

She looked down at him now.

Nope. She still didn't have the energy to read his face.

And anyway, wasn't that the kind of energy expenditure that had gotten her here, in this mess, in the first place? Reading people's faces and having them think she cared. (Having The Jerk see something in her face that made him think he was special somehow? That's what he had said to her, all those years ago. That *she* had picked *him*?)

The noise in her head was starting to become deafening. It wasn't even that it was a *noise*, per se. It was more like a wall of thought, a huge wave of water that was *thought*, coming to press her down and squash her into the floor forever, into the terrazzo. She would be squashed and spilled like a soda knocked out of a hand by a fast commuter zipping by. Mopped up by the cleaning crew later.

"Rabbit, I think what you are doing in your head is catastrophizing."

She did not answer.

"Do you know what that is? When you think everything is collapsing all at once. But it isn't."

She looked at him and tried to remember what he knew and didn't know. Could he legitimately conclude it wasn't all collapsing? Her tear ducts felt like they had collapsed, spilling all her fluids down her face, like a burst water balloon.

"Madeleine," Wolf said very quietly. "Give me your bag."

She looked at him and sighed deeply. The sigh paused her tears.

"I think you should not try to make any decision just now," he said.

"I am just so tired," she answered.

"I know."

"And hungry, I am so hungry."

He didn't answer. He just looked – he looked too sad to her.

"And I want to finish my Ph.D., Wolf," she said. "I want my goddamned Ph.D."

"You will finish," he said. "I know that you will."

What now? What to do with this stupid man sounding so sure?

She sighed again and brought to mind something Paula had taught her. Paula had told her one day, on a day Maddy found herself very low, that one thing Maddy needed to realize was that she had no parents. Paula had said that when she found herself in this state, Maddy needed to consciously realize that she had no parents.

At first, Maddy had thought this was a crazy thing for Paula to tell her when she was already so low that day. But then Paula explained: It wasn't just that Maddy's parents were now both dead; it was that she had *never* really had parents who had it in them to be what parents ought to be. At such times, Maddy needed to know there wasn't ever going to be someone who would take care of her like her parents should have – that even if they had remained alive, chances were good that they never would have gotten the task of parenting right. They were always going to put their faith before their daughter, as that was their understanding of their duties. They were always going to be emotionally incompetent by adhering to their dogma.

And so, Maddy, sometimes you will need to remember it is a time to be your own parent.

What do you mean? Maddy had asked her.

I mean, Maddy, sometimes – especially when you are very low – you will need to treat yourself the way a parent would treat a child. Find the parent in your head and tell the child in you that you are loved – show yourself compassion. Tell yourself to go to bed – take care of yourself as you would a child. Tell yourself to eat something. Tell yourself to study. Tell yourself to get out of bed and try to go outside and run, and if you can't run, then walk. If you need someone to walk with you, ask someone to help you. Let the mature voice in you tell the child in you what a parent would tell you to do if the parent were a functional parent who loved you and had it in her to take care of the child in you. Let the survival voice in your head be the parent to you when you feel small and lost and alone.

What should she do about this man kneeling before her under the departures board?

This is a reasonable man, Madeleine, she said. *This is not a person who is going to do you harm. This is not a man trying simply to get you into a position where he can fuck you. This is someone who can be trusted – he's shown that. Just give him your bag and do let him help you while you are lost, Madeleine.*

She hesitated.

You are lost – you are the definition of lost: you don't know where you are even going right now. You can't help Katie when you are lost, when you are too hungry and tired to make a decision, to think straight. Let him help.

She reached her hands up to the straps over her shoulders and pulled the backpack off of her. She handed it to Wolf. He grabbed it from her like a raptor striking prey. Still kneeling, he quickly opened it, looked around furtively, retrieved his gun, and put it in the holster just above his ankle. He put his pant leg back down again over it.

He zipped up her bag and put it over his right shoulder. He waited to see what she wanted next.

Time to go with him.

She reached out her hand to him. He seized it between his hands, as if she was going to fall.

He stood up while keeping her hand in one of his. He started to walk her toward the door through which they both had come.

The floor felt now to her as if it were made of Jello.

"Jello was what the sisters made, Wolf, when the flu came through the dorm," she said. "Raspberry Jello."

"You don't want Jello, do you, Rabbit?"

"No," she said, "I don't feel like eating. I am so dizzy. I have a bad head-ache. My whole body hurts and I'm so hungry. No, I don't feel like eating."

"That is what depression feels like. You probably know that already. We'll go sit a while," he said. "It'll be okay."

She didn't answer. He walked her in a direction away from home.

-19-

She was handing Wolf the covered glass dish with the lasagna in it – reaching it out to him in her right hand. Meeting his eye, thinking he had it, she let go. But he did not have it. The dish went crashing to the floor, shattering, throwing the food and glass shards every which way, splattering the good brown dress and matching jacket from Giovanni with red sauce, ruining it.

She woke up suddenly at the crash.

Ruined, she thought.

"I'm sorry to get you up," Wolf said. "I am going to need you to come down to read over and sign something soon."

She looked around and realized she was in the bed in her room at Wolf's house. Wolf was sitting on the edge of her bed with Hunter standing close at his side. Wolf handed her a glass of water.

"Drink more water," he said. "I'll go make coffee. Come down soon. They'll be here soon."

She looked at the clock and could see it was just after ten in the morning. She wasn't wearing the brown dress or the matching jacket. They were hung up in the closet. She was still wearing what she had worn to work the day before: khaki slacks and her blue button-down shirt. Now they were wrinkled and sweaty. But no tomato stains.

Now it was all coming back to her. She sat up and peeked over to the desk to see if The Jerk's letter was still there. Gone. Wolf must have it downstairs. He had taken The Jerk's hand out of her room.

Her head throbbed, the daylight coming through the crack in the curtains jabbing at the back of her eye sockets. She had drunk far too much last night, and now she remembered throwing up not long after they'd come back to the house. Wolf had helped her clean up her face and then given her water with lemon squeezed into it, to try to get her to drink it all down.

He'd said to her, "That's *it*! This household has thrown up *enough* lately and we are not throwing up *anymore*!"

And then, when she found herself crying like she was a spring rain, he had laid down with her and held on to her and told her to try to go to sleep. It was over, he said, and the rest of it would be over soon, too. It was over.

Did she dream that at some point they had gotten up and gone to the gym?

She got up slowly out of the bed now, went to the bathroom, closed the door, and emptied her bladder. She took two aspirin out of Wolf's medicine cabinet, held them in her hand, and stared at herself in the mirror for a moment. A hangover this bad sure did make her look older. If The Jerk could see her now, he'd recoil in horror.

The idea made her feel good.

She popped the aspirin into her mouth, cupped her hand to fill with cold water, and took several sips in a row.

The night before was beginning to cohere. From the spot under the arrivals and departures board at 30th Street Station, after she gave him back his gun by giving him her backpack, Wolf had walked her over to a French place he obviously knew from years past. The maître d' had greeted him like an old friend, asking why his wife was not with him.

And then the maître d' had looked at Maddy and pulled in his breath and said nothing more. She thought she must look quite awful to silence him that way.

He showed them to a table in the back, near the kitchen door. Wolf asked the waiter to bring bread and butter right away and when it came, Wolf tore off a chunk of the small crusty loaf and smeared it thickly with the soft butter and gave it to Maddy, telling her to eat.

Then he quickly ordered for them wine and food, and he did it with so little joy, so little thought, she felt lousy-upon-sad for having taken away his pleasure.

"I'm sorry," she said.

He did not answer by asking her what she was sorry about but answered instead, "Don't be so stupid, will you?"

She found his uncharacteristic rudeness towards her very satisfying.

Then he just started asking her all about The Jerk, handing her more buttered bread, refilling her wine. How old was she when he started touching her? Kissing her? And did he have intercourse with her?

She just answered his questions over bread and some sort of limp salad and tepid onion soup. She told him of how The Jerk preferred it, fucking her fast, missionary position, to get into her and out of her as fast as he could. How the first time it had hurt so, and after that it hurt less physically, but each time her sense of confusion felt a little greater.

Still, it was better than nothing, right? Better than the nothingness.

She told him she still didn't like the missionary position.

This is an odd first date, she thought to herself about three fast glasses in. And then she caught herself at the idea and laughed without explanation.

He soon ordered another bottle and grumbled to her that the food here wasn't as good as it used to be.

"Maybe you're just a better cook now," she said to him. "Maybe you just have higher standards. I have higher standards now."

She remembered now some more of what she had told him – how The Jerk smelled of cigarettes and cheap aftershave, how he used to take her down to his basement on the pretense of using the weights to fuck her, how she had she felt this strange, baffling tension of not wanting to go and knowing it was a way out, a way out of her parents' black vortex of Catholicism. How she had to stay because it was the only way to go.

"I don't understand how he could have done it to another girl," she had told Wolf, as he had cut up her meat and mumbled that it was overcooked.

"You think you were special?" Wolf asked with a degree of sarcasm that she didn't know he had in him.

"No," she said, "and yes. I mean, I thought he would have had to stop after me, because – because – "

She could hear her voice starting to slur from the wine. Yet more alcohol seemed like a good idea at the time. It had numbed so nicely her fingertips and blunted so well the shock of the letter.

"The priest who ran my school told me – he told me after my parents died – he was going to tell the police. About The Jerk."

"Eat," Wolf said, loading her fork with the stringy meat and a little of the limp asparagus.

"Does it mean what he did to me wasn't – that they didn't – "

"Rabbit!" Wolf said impatiently. "Eat!"

She took the forkful into her mouth, put the utensil down with a clinking of silver against china, and chewed. She knew he was right, that it was over-cooked. But at the moment she was having to focus enough on the effort of chewing that she had no real thoughts about the taste.

"*Of course* what he did to you was illegal," said Wolf, drinking down his own glass of wine. "And immoral. Don't be ridiculous."

Why was he seemingly so angry at her?

"So, why...I mean, Wolf, why didn't they...?"

"Someone didn't do what he should have done," said Wolf, scraping more food from her plate onto her fork and handing her the fork.

She asked him, why didn't they do what they were supposed to do?

He said there were plenty of reasons this happened. Someone knew somebody. Or someone didn't want a scandal.

"It's often the case," he explained with great effort, as if she did not quite understand English, "sometimes, if one thing comes to light, then a lot else does, too – a lot else comes to light – and then – then there is a much bigger mess. And then all the people who have dirty hands – "

He stopped speaking.

"I think," she said, as the waiter came over and opened another bottle of the same wine, "I think, Wolf, they don't like the idea of a girl calling out the patriarchy."

She reached down into her left pocket, pulled out the wad of cash she had stolen from his wallet, and tucked it under the edge of Wolf's plate.

The waiter looked at her with a cocked head, pulled the cork, and handed it to Wolf.

Wolf simply put the cork on the table, not bothering to look at it or smell it.

"I think, Wolf, they think that if a girl calls out the patriarchy and succeeds, then the whole system is at risk, and it might all come tumbling, tumbling down."

She paused.

"Down," she said again, for no particular reason.

The waiter poured wine into each of their glasses and set the new bottle on the table, a napkin tied around its neck. He had tied the napkin so tight, Maddy tugged at her shirt collar with her fingertips in thoughtless sympathy for the bottle.

"You're not wrong," Wolf said.

She thought for a moment she should tell him about *Wilhelm* and the patriarchy, but she couldn't formulate a thought clearly enough to convey it. Wilhelm and the grants. Wilhelm and the patients. Wilhelm and the bodies. The smell on the intruder's hands. She should tell him.

"Did you see him again, after your parents died?" he asked.

How did Wolf know about her parents dying because of The Jerk?

Oh, that's right: She had told him, over the limp salads and bread, about that day – the day her father found out and went to kill The Jerk. How Maddy wouldn't get in the car, because she didn't want to deal with it. How the next time she was with her family, it was at the funeral home. How the place smelled moldy – how it smelled of old, moldy flowers and damp linens.

"Did you see him again after your parents died?" he asked again.

She shook her head.

He did not reply, so she said more.

"Silence from him until now," she told Wolf. "I mean, he might have tried when I was in the convent to reach me. But if he did, the sisters didn't let word through. The sisters formed a black and white wall for me. A black and white wall, hung with rosaries."

He nodded.

"And being in the convent for two years with the sisters," he asked, "that *never* gave you the feeling of faith?"

The way he asked made it sound as if she still had a chance to salvage something for him. But she almost guffawed at him.

"Christ, no, Wolf," she said. "Why the fuck would being with the sisters make me think their way was *the right* way? All these smart women being blindly obedient! A waste of feminine intelligence."

He didn't answer.

"Where is Hunter?" she asked.

"I locked him in the house," Wolf said. "When you took off, I didn't want to have to manage a dog while I was trying to find you. Maybe that was irrational. He might have helped."

"I still feel bad taking Bobby's dog when he lost his father."

Wolf did not respond. He just buttered another piece of bread for her.

With the morning light pushing in, she was brushing her teeth in the bathroom now to get rid of the residual taste of vomited onions and the acidic aspirin tablets, thinking about all this, remembering little parts of what came after – walking back home from the restaurant, her moving slower and slower as the alcohol leaked from her stomach into her blood out to all the extremities, making her anatomy and physiology all slower and slower. Alcohol: a fine preservative.

Finally, he had picked her up, reaching down under her armpits with his hands and pulling her onto him as if she were a big child, lifting her arms over his shoulders, pulling her legs around his waist, letting her head flop down on him, falling asleep for the last few blocks. But not good sleep – that awful sleep that comes with drunkenness. Sour, uncertain, cobblestone sleep.

Once in the house, he had put her down on the couch and pulled off her shoes, taken Hunter out to let him pee, fed the dog, and then carted Maddy up the stairs. She had told him she thought she had to throw up from drinking too much, and he had taken her quickly to the toilet.

After he had cleaned up her face, he had sent her to her room. He had closed the bathroom door for a minute to pee and then gone and gotten her water with lemon in it.

Coming into her room, he had found that she had not laid down as he had expected but had instead gone to get her suitcase out of the closet to start packing. Her big suitcase laid on the bed, zipped open. Hunter was standing looking from one of them to the other, trying to ascertain what he was supposed to do.

"What are you doing?" Wolf had asked.

"I will have to go," she had explained, opening the top drawer of the dresser and looking in it, seeing her socks neatly tucked together in pairs. She had felt so unsteady. She knew she should shove these in her shoes to save room in the suitcase, the way she always did. But that seemed a lot of work just now – figuring out which socks would fit into which shoes.

He had put the water glass down on her night table and come over to the dresser, next to her. He had closed the drawer. Then he had gone over to the bed, zipped up her suitcase, and put it back in the closet.

"But Wolf!"

"You don't have to go, Rabbit," he had said. "You stay here and finish your work until it's time to go back to Indiana."

"But I can't go back to Indiana."

"Why not?"

"Because he ruins everything," she had explained, starting to cry.

That, she now remembered, was when she had reached the point of the kind of self-pity that drowns anyone within twenty feet.

He ruins everything. He ruins everything.

Wolf had pulled her to himself, moving them both to the bed, lying down with her on top of the covers. She had been crying and shaking and saying over and over again, "He ruins everything."

But Wolf didn't do that annoying thing some people do, of telling you to stop crying, of telling you everything is going to be okay when it's obviously not. He had just stayed so quiet.

And she had felt so uncontrollably loud.

. . .

She reached the kitchen table just as the two officers arrived at the back door. This time it was a woman officer she had not met before plus the fellow who had been here last time, after the intruder – the gruff and somewhat snotty cop who had observed to Wolf aloud that Maddy was describing "the wrong guy." As if she had been intentionally unhelpful by being attacked by someone other than the guy they'd been looking for.

Wolf let the two of them in and asked them to remind him how they took their coffee. The woman said black or with a little milk, if he had some. Officer Snotty said in a voice too loud and too demanding that he wanted his with four sugars. The woman gave Hunter a proper greeting, but Officer Snotty just ignored the dog.

"Where is it, Wolf?" asked the woman.

Wolf nodded toward the counter. Maddy could see that was where the letter sat, back in its envelope. The woman picked up the corner of the envelope with a pair of tweezers she pulled out of her pocket, holding it in the air for a moment as if it were a dead worm. Officer Snotty produced a plastic bag and held it open for her. She dropped the letter in its envelope into the bag. Then she put the tweezers back in her pocket, took the bag from him, and sealed it.

"Well, here we are again," said Snotty. "Here we are again, taking another statement from Ms. Shanks, in your kitchen, Wolf. Same scene, different day, all over again."

Wolf shot him an angry glance.

What, Maddy wondered – did Snotty think Maddy was just making shit up to get Wolf's attention? That seemed to be the implication.

Wolf gave the two of them their coffees, then set down a third cup of coffee for Maddy, topping it off with a half-inch of milk. He reached up to the top of the refrigerator and took down a couple of sheets of paper, laying them on the table in front of Maddy. He handed her a pen.

She could see he had written out a statement for her, about The Jerk.

"Correct it and sign it," he said.

Yes, she could see what he had done – written down what she had told him last night about her relationship with The Jerk. Just a simple factual history. No emotion, no psychological analysis of the kind she was inclined to do. No intellectualizing. Just descriptive prose – dry, historical prose, even when it got to the part about her family all dying. All told in the first person as if she had written it down, even though she had never told the story quite like this, in the neat presentation of a seemingly cool-headed historian.

She read it twice. Then she corrected a couple of small things and inserted a few additional details between the lines he had written, keeping the tone he had chosen, as if she were editing a colleague's draft research paper and needed to not disturb the author's voice. When she was just about finished, she looked up to see them all watching her.

"Wolf, please, Wolf. I don't want to deal with this," she said quietly to him, as if the other two could not hear her. "Please, Wolf, I don't want to deal with him. I want to go on with my plans. I don't want to deal with him and be derailed."

"You won't have to," Wolf answered. "I think – well, we think there will be a statute of limitations problem for you, to be honest. We just need your statement with the letter, to stop him now. This will help us do that."

"Okay," she said.

She smoothed the page out with her hand and signed it: *Madeleine Shanks*.

"Let us do our work, and you do yours," he said.

"Okay," she said.

"Work on your *own* work."

"Okay!" she said sharply. "It's your problem now. He's your problem now. Hunter, come here!"

Hunter came over to Maddy and she held onto his collar with one hand and smoothed the fur on his back and over and over with her other hand.

The woman officer asked Wolf if she could use his bathroom, and he pointed her up the stairs.

Everyone remaining in the kitchen grew quiet. In Maddy's mind, dealing with the question of Wilhelm was somehow coming to be about her part of having to take care of Katie, and she was physically starting to squirm at the discomfort of this confused thought. Officer Snotty was putting more sugar in his coffee, his spoon going clink, clink. Maddy tried to refocus, but all she could do was wonder how she was going to tell Wolf that, for her work, she needed to go to New York, to the library, to look up Schlesinger 1888. He wasn't going to like her going to New York, especially not without Hunter, but she couldn't take the dog on Amtrak, and going to New York to see Schlesinger 1888 was her little part of the Katie problem. Not The Jerk problem, but the Katie problem. That was Maddy's part, dealing with Wilhelm.

Wasn't it?

She paused her thoughts for a minute to try to understand the logic here. Then she suddenly remembered – last night – a new variation on the nightmare about Margaret Lovisa. The twisted metal growing out of Maddy's abdomen – that was there, still, always, as usual – but now the person in the jar was not Maggie Lovisa, but Katie.

But how could Maddy know that girl was Katie when she had never met Katie?

Now Wolf was talking to Snotty about scheduling. It was dawning on Maddy that Wolf was speaking about what his colleagues should do while he was gone for the next couple of days. Wolf was going to be gone for a few days? Maybe that was for the best. She could be her disorganized self alone. He would not fuss over her. She could do what she wanted.

She got up now and walked over to get the phone. She picked up the receiver in her hand and started to dial Indiana.

Wolf came and took it from her, putting it back in the charging cradle.

"I just want to call Liz," she said, reaching to pick it up again.

"No," he said, stopping her again.

What did he mean, "no"? Why couldn't she tell Liz what had happened?

The woman showed back up from the bathroom and Wolf resumed talking to Snotty and now also her about what they should be doing while he was away.

Maddy moved again to grab the phone.

"No," he said to her again, this time more aggressively. "You can't call Liz right now."

What was he talking about? Was she going to be required all over again to keep this all to herself, merely hoping someone would do something this time? Were the Philadelphia cops going to just be another black-and-white wall, with guns for rosaries, vaguely protective of her but useless otherwise?

"Why not?" she asked Wolf. "Why can't I call Liz?"

"She's going to be here soon," Wolf said to Maddy. "She should be in the cab from the airport now."

"Who is?" Maddy asked.

"*Liz*," he answered. "I called her last night. Asked her to come immediately. She's on her way here."

Maddy looked at him sharply, trying to scrutinize his face. Was he telling the truth?

The doorbell rang and she ran to the front door of the house with Hunter following her. Opening the door, she found the postman. He handed her a large and heavy box with her name printed neatly on the label. Wolf came and shut the door and took it rapidly away from her. Scrutinizing the return address, he calmed down. He laid the box on the coffee table.

"For you, from the National Institutes of Health," he said, sighing in relief. "It's just work. Nothing more. Just work."

She went over to the table to look. The response to her Freedom of Information Act request – Wilhelm's grant reports.

"I thought maybe it was trouble," Wolf explained, squeezing his eyes closed for a moment in an uncharacteristic gesture and then opening them to the sound of the doorbell ringing again.

He went over and opened the door.

"Are you Wolf?" asked Liz, standing on the step second from the top.

He nodded, took her outreached hand in his, and pulled her up the steps and in. Maddy thought it looked as if Wolf were pulling Liz onto a boat. He closed the door behind her.

With Wolf standing next to her, Liz adjusted the overstuffed bright yellow messenger bag slung over her shoulder and looked around the room. She found a man and a woman standing quite still near the base of the stairs across the room. And here, here near the couch was her best friend, standing rather like she had frozen in time, looking at her. Why was she so still, and whose dog was this next to her?

"Mad Girl," said Liz, lifting the strap of the bag over her head and putting it on the floor. "You okay?"

"I feel so stupid, Lizard," Maddy answered quietly.

"Yeah," said Liz.

'I feel so stupid. And dead. And ugly. And used."

"Give me a fucking break. You're not *stupid*," said Liz. "We'll both get cleaned up and we'll go to the museum together today, to work. And then you'll remember that you're not *stupid*. You're getting a Ph.D. You're on a full ride. They don't give stupid people full rides."

"But I'm so tired."

"We're both so tired," Liz replied. "But we both need to work today. You've got dissertation work. I have a paper that needs to be submitted. Work doesn't stop just because we're tired, Mad."

Maddy didn't answer.

"As for feeling dead, you're not that either, Mad One. I brought my running shoes. We can go running after we work today. Dead people don't run."

Still, Maddy did not respond.

"And you feel *ugly*? We'll find some thrift stores and both get something new to wear. I need something new anyway, so Margie doesn't get tired of looking at me."

She could tell that Maddy was working now simply on not crying.

"And used? You feel *used*?" Liz asked. "Fuck, Maddy, you *have* been used! We have *all* been used."

Liz let out a short laugh. But it was clearly not a laugh of joy. No one else in the room joined her in laughing.

"We have *all* been used, Mad. But, you know, we are not used up. Not you, and not me. Not yet anyway."

Maddy looked closer at Liz's face. She had forgotten how Liz's very short haircut accentuated her strong cheekbones. She had forgotten how clear Liz's green eyes could look.

She had forgotten what it was like to feel so grateful for long-familiar flesh.

-20-

"Don't think you should go with him," Maddy said in a quiet voice. A moment later she added, "I don't think so."

Liz sat up in the bed a little to look over at Maddy, to make sure she was just talking in her sleep. It was around three in the morning, and Philadelphia seemed so quiet from this second floor of John Wolf's house, as it had the night before. It felt almost like Liz and Maddy could be back in Bloomington where one might hear a passing flock of sorority sisters, or maybe a beer delivery truck, but nothing much else at this hour.

Seeing Maddy's eyes closed, Liz laid herself back down.

I don't think you should go with him.

Who was Maddy talking to, and who was the "him"? Perhaps she was dreaming of telling Katie not to go with The Jerk? Or some patient not to go with Dr. Wilhelm?

It was impossible to guess about Maddy's fantastical dreams. Liz wondered if she herself had dreams similar in quality and quantity to Maddy and just didn't remember them because she slept more soundly than Maddy. Well, she slept more soundly than Maddy except when sleeping *with* Maddy.

This was the second night of crappy sleep for Liz, listening to Maddy talk her way through the night awake and asleep. After this, Liz would go home, back to the woman with whom she wanted to share a bed, and she would be able to catch up on lost sleep. She could stand this – one more night of wondering what was going on beneath the surface of her stressed-out friend's mumbled words.

Maddy twitched and frowned.

"Everything is okay, Mad Girl," Liz said quietly, unsure whether Maddy could hear her. "Phoenix Dumpling?" she added in a cheerful whisper in the hopes of leading Maddy's subconscious down a more enjoyable path, toward Professor Butterfly.

But maybe she shouldn't try adding words to the stewing – maybe it would backfire and leave Maddy dreaming of something crazy, of Colin ending up on her dissertation committee, as a monarch, or on a trapeze made of noodles, or some such. Maddy's mind did love to turn words into objects, objects into persons, persons into messengers of her suspicions, of her longings.

No, Liz probably should not whisper suggestions to Maddy's simmering brain. On the other hand, whatever Maddy dreamed, it would probably be entertaining to hear about over breakfast, the last meal they'd have together on this trip before they would need to say farewell at 30th Street Station. Liz would hop on the local train to the airport, and Maddy would take Amtrak up to New York for the day. And Maddy could usually remember her dreams if Liz asked her within a half hour of waking.

"Are you *sure*?" Maddy asked in a clearer voice, startling Liz into a feeling that Maddy could read her thoughts.

But no, Maddy was still asleep, presumably talking to someone other than Liz.

In a way, it was good that The Jerk had written that creepy letter and sent it here to Maddy. Now the police might finally do something about him.

(Why hadn't Liz previously pushed Maddy to turn him in to the police, Liz wondered to herself uncomfortably? Why had Liz just assumed whatever could be done about The Jerk had long ago been done?)

The distress that the letter had set off in Maddy was unwelcome, but she seemed to have recovered her balance in the last couple of days. And the letter had caused Wolf to ask Liz to get right on a plane to come help Maddy, so thanks to the letter, the two had managed to have two solid days alone together here, working and wandering around the city, and they were both better off for it. And it hadn't cost Liz much of anything other than time and some favors of people covering for her in Bloomington. Wolf had paid her back for the flights and even the cab from the airport, and before he'd left to go see his family up in Massachusetts, he had told Maddy and Liz to eat whatever they wanted, so the trip here had cost Liz almost zero, which had freed Maddy up from any guilty feelings and turned her down-right happy for a few minutes at a time.

Maddy had started digging through his freezer and considering their options as soon as Wolf had left. She had been like a kid opening presents under the tree. Hunter seemed to be picking up on her improved mood as he stood at her side and wagged his tail at her exclamations.

"Coq au vin, Liz! And minestrone! Not like stupid dorm minestrone – the good stuff, cooked with a rind of parmesan. We'll have to buy some good crusty bread to go with it and use the Amish butter."

In a way, it had been a bit like a paid vacation for the two of them even if they'd had to work for chunks of both days. Liz had told Maddy as she was rifling through the freezer that they really *had* to work while Liz was here – that Liz had to get a paper revised in the next forty-eight hours. That was true, but it was also true that Liz knew that getting Maddy right back to working would help keep Maddy from obsessing into the darkness. As it was, as happy as Maddy seemed to be with Liz, it felt as if Maddy might still be circling the edge.

"Did Wolf really go north to go see his family up in Massachusetts all of a sudden? Or was he going to Long Island to deal with The Jerk and he didn't want to tell me that?" Maddy had asked Liz again, a few minutes before she had fallen asleep.

"Listen, you shithead," Liz had replied. "*I don't know and you don't know.* I've told you that a million times now. You can ask him when he comes back."

"I don't want to ask him, though, Liz," said Maddy, as she repositioned her pillow. "I don't want to deal with it. I'll just deal with Wilhelm. I'll deal with Wilhelm, and Wolf will deal with The Jerk. Division of labor."

At that, Maddy reached over and grasped Liz's wrist for a moment.

"Speaking of divisions of labor, thank you again for coming, Lizard. It was so kind of you."

"Oh, do shut up, Sister Mary Madeline," said Liz. "You sound like a fuck-ing Midwestern nun."

"Go fuck yourself," Maddy laughed.

"That's better," said Liz. "Shut up! Go to sleep. We have to be up early for your train and my plane. And you promised to make me Wolf's good coffee and to let me drink it in silence before we go."

Liz thought about the note Maddy had already prepared to leave for Wolf, in case he returned from his trip before Maddy got back from New York.

Wolf, I am going to New York just for the day, for research, to go to the New York Public Library for a text I need to look at that I can't get another way. Don't worry – I am not going to Long Island or anything. Bobby has Hunter for the day. My plan is to be on the train that gets back at 7:25 p.m. If I don't make that train for some reason, I'll call and leave you a message. We ate all the coq au vin, so that's gone, and most of the venison chili, too. Also some other things. Liz said it was excellent. Hope your trip was good. See you later. – Maddy

Maddy had insisted that Liz add a little written testimony at the end so that Wolf would believe Maddy that she wasn't going to New York to see The Jerk, so that Wolf wouldn't worry and freak out. But Liz wasn't sure how she felt about Maddy implying to Wolf that the "research" of the trip was dissertation related. Liz knew why Maddy was going to New York – to see Jimmy Heathcote to talk to him about Wilhelm and to try to examine Schlesinger 1888 for herself at the New York Public.

Liz took the pen from Maddy and added:

Maddy wants me to tell you she's really going to NYC to go to NYPL because she's looking into something about specimen acquisition. That is true. And I know she's telling the truth because her nose didn't turn red like it does when she bluffs in poker. (You should let her play next game because you can easily earn back some food money from her.) And she's right about the food – excellent, thanks. Thanks for having me and for paying for the trip. – Liz

After that, they had had a short argument about whether they should mess up the stack of sheets Wolf had left in the living room for Liz to use to sleep on the couch. Maddy had said they should unfold, wrinkle up, and refold the sheets to make it look like Liz had used them, and Liz had said fuck that, that it wasn't any business of Wolf's whether they shared a bed sometimes. But Maddy had answered that there wasn't any point in causing him consternation, and this way maybe he would invite Liz back. To which Liz had responded that Maddy should just hurry up her work and come home already and get out of this sexually repressed house.

"Try the other one," Maddy said now, still asleep.

Liz wondered what the other one was. A door? A pastry?

Having two days and two nights with Maddy had been as much what *Liz* needed as Maddy, even if the sudden trip had temporarily disrupted just about everything at home. At least, for once, after Wolf's call asking Liz to hurry up and get on a plane to Philadelphia, Margie had seemed to realize what Liz needed from Margie wasn't an expression of jealousy but a little understanding as she tried to help out Maddy.

Of course, Margie might feel less understanding if she knew that Liz had taken Maddy out to a lesbian bar she had heard was worth checking out in Philly. And Margie might feel downright upset if she knew that Liz and Maddy had been sharing Maddy's bed, something Margie didn't know the two friends did when one or both of them had had a rough time.

Liz thought back to how it had started, two years ago, when she had been on a bus that had been hit by a truck. Liz had been thrown across the bus, coming down on the edge of a seat, somehow hitting a pole in the process. An older woman who had been sitting next to her had been much more badly hurt – there was a lot of blood and chaos in the aftermath. Liz ended up with a broken wrist and a black eye, and Maddy had come to meet her at the hospital, fetching Liz's car so she could drive Liz back home.

Liz was so grateful for Maddy's fussing over getting her home and comfortable that she didn't chastise Maddy for her fucking annoying habit of turning on the blinker way too soon. Liz realized on the short drive home from Bloomington Hospital that Maddy probably didn't exactly enjoy rushing to a hospital after hearing about an accident.

Maddy had listened so carefully to all the discharge instructions from the ER nurse, and she had brought Liz back home and made her food and spent the night with her and one additional night after, to make sure Liz was okay, all because the nurse had told Maddy about the side effects of the pain meds and worried Maddy unnecessarily. Liz's pet rat Broc had gotten so stressed about the splint and the odd-smelling bandaging on Liz's wrist, Maddy had had to calm him down with egg noodles and lettuce and a game of chase-the-finger. They'd fallen asleep talking about what Broc must be making of it all and woken up to find Broc and his brother Oli sleeping in the bed with them because Maddy had forgotten to put them back in the cage.

And then there was the time when Liz's mother was getting the breast biopsy, when Liz came over to Maddy's in a tangle of worry and Maddy had ended telling her to just sleep over so they could talk and not worry about getting Liz home after that. And then there was the time when the two of them had been walking home late from Bullwinkle's and a couple of creeps looking like they had crawled out of the sticks accosted them and wouldn't leave them alone, calling them "dykes," and they had both been rattled, and they slept together at Liz's house. And the time when Maddy discovered her Visa debit card information had been stolen and she got so stressed out about money worries. All those times they had decided to sleep next to each other because it just made sense to be like rats.

But then, all those times were before Margie had moved in with Liz.

When Wolf had stacked the neatly folded sheets and blankets on the couch and showed Liz how best to block the street light from coming in the curtains in the living room at night, Liz didn't bother to tell him she was sure Maddy would want Liz to sleep next to her. The extra blankets were helpful, though, since Maddy and Liz had long ago learned they slept better next to each other if they each had their own sheet and blanket. Maddy was a bedding-hog in her sleep and Liz was a light sleeper who would be awakened by Maddy pulling on a sheet as she turned. Liz wondered if Wolf had managed to get any sleep when he had had to spend the night with Maddy, after the letter came.

He had been taking good care of Maddy – that was clear. And for that, Liz was grateful. Maddy had gotten a ton done on her dissertation, and Wolf had even fattened her up a few pounds. The new weight looked good on Maddy. Maddy had told Liz she had had to go and buy some new bras because the old ones weren't fitting right, and Liz could tell that her cup size had gone up a notch even before Maddy said anything – Maddy had a more mature female shape now, something more likely to attract men who were into *mature* women. That was good. Liz was grateful, too, that Wolf was romantically and sexually unavailable – that Maddy couldn't get entangled with Wolf, a guy too old for her, and Catholic, and long distance, and not portable.

But Maddy did talk about him a lot. About his cooking, his worldview, his taste in music, his work, their late-night philosophical and theological conversations. At some level, Liz thought, Maddy must be so relieved that Wolf had found out about The Jerk. He would no longer have to wonder about her initial irrational fright about going into his basement to do laundry, and he would now understand why Maddy had elected to go to a convent for two years. He would believe her now that she had not done it because she had any faith in her, any interest in being Catholic. She had done it to gain her freedom, not to be held captive.

Why didn't Maddy just tell Wolf her suspicions about Dr. Wilhelm? Liz had told Maddy twice she thought Maddy ought to tell Wolf, to see what he thought about what Maddy had found – the anachronistic collection of bodies in Wilhelm's lab, the pattern in his publications of at first bragging

224

about the collection and more recently dropping the subject, the way so many of those in his collection appeared to have died from heart problems even though there didn't seem to be a clear anatomic or physiological reason for that pattern – his references back to Schlesinger 1888 as if one researcher mentioning heart-related deaths in two dwarf brothers in the late-nineteenth century was adequate to explaining the pattern of sudden death in Dr. Wilhelm's patient population, with no further pondering. Why did Dr. Wilhelm have no paper dedicated to that specific issue – the supposed pattern of cardiac-related deaths – when logically he should have had *several* on it by now? And why, more recently, was there a total lack of cause of death cited when Dr. Wilhelm mentioned in his publications using biological material from a new specimen?

And then Nick DesJardins' sudden death.

Maddy had shown Liz the timelines she had sketched out using different color highlighting for different issues with abbreviations tracking specific patients. The specimens available to Wilhelm increased over time, but Liz reminded Maddy that was to be expected simply by virtue of the fact that some patients would die every year, and Dr. Wilhelm's patient population was growing by virtue of his reputation. So of course the absolute number of deaths would go up.

But the mention of cardiac problems as the cause of death had gone steadily and then suddenly dropped around 1999 – about four years ago. Now Maddy had his grant reports to the NIH thanks to the Freedom of Information Act request, and she was going through them and filling in the details where she could, of where every body had come from. Whose it had been, when they died, how they died, and what he did with the information gleaned. At one point, Maddy handed Liz a page from the stack of grant reports, with Maddy having underlined and put an asterisk next to one passage:

Our research team has the largest clinical population and largest teratological and pathological specimen collection in this field of growth and metabolism studies, and thus we are uniquely able to carry out key studies in this area.

"That same line shows up, year after year, in his reports, Liz. It must have been a convincing argument."

"Four decades of continuous NIH funding is damned impressive," said Liz, "and there are people who would kill for it."

Liz meant it as a joke, but Maddy didn't laugh. Maddy just put her head back down and kept reading.

More alarmingly, Maddy seemed to be finding clear evidence that Dr. Wilhelm had reported different causes of death for certain patients in the published record versus his grant reports. Why would that be?

Maddy told Liz later, when they went out for a run with Hunter, that Maddy would talk to Wolf about it when she had enough to make a reasonable case – a reasonable case that there had been too many convenient deaths of people whose bodies were particularly good postmortem research material – if she ever had enough to make such an argument to Wolf. But until she had it, she wasn't going to talk to him about it.

"I'm not going to risk my entire career by suggesting that someone of his prominence is a killer, Liz," Maddy had explained as they stopped for a moment so Liz could re-tie the drawstring of her running pants.

"If you just tell Wolf, it won't get out – no one will know but him," Liz had answered. "If he finds something, if he agrees with you, then it goes forward."

They started the run back up with Maddy loosely holding Hunter's leash.

"But Wolf told me, Liz, that people who become friends with cops have a habit of starting to think they see crime everywhere, like they are little deputies. I'm not going to make an ass of myself. Especially not when Officer Snotty seems to think that I'm just looking for police attention. Wolf can deal with The Jerk right now. And I'll make up for Katie, I'll make it up to Katie, with my own work dealing with Wilhelm."

Maddy had tried to explain to Liz three times why Maddy thought what had happened to Katie with The Jerk meant Maddy had to not drop the ball on Dr. Wilhelm. Maddy had tried once as Maddy showed Liz the museum herb garden, once over breakfast, and once at the record store where they were looking for an album to gift to Wolf as a thanks for bringing Liz to Philly.

But each time, Maddy's reasoning hadn't quite made sense to Liz. She understood Maddy had some kind of thick guilt over Katie. But the implied idea that there was a certain amount of justice to be dealt in the world and everybody should take a chunk of it to work on – that dealing with Dr. Wilhelm meant Maddy was at some metaphysical level dealing with The Jerk – this was batshit. It was like something out of one of Maddy's fantastical dreams, where neurons crossed and created narratives that made no sense.

Liz could understand Maddy's fear – that she could be seen as an attention-seeking conspiracy theorist by bringing forward her Wilhelm hypothesis. That wasn't an unreasonable fear. Liz certainly didn't like to produce an extraordinary claim without extraordinary proof – no more than the next self-protecting scholar. But the sooner Maddy got this side-tracking issue out of the way, the sooner she would be back to finishing her dissertation. And the less likely she would put herself at risk – professional and personal.

Rolling over to her left side in the bed, Liz tried adjusting her shoulders and her hips to relax her muscles. She was looking forward to being back home by tomorrow in the early afternoon, back home to Pumpkin and Spice, back home to Margie. It now seemed clear to Liz that at least part of Wolf's plan had been for Liz to come and fix Maddy's head while he was away so that he didn't have to come back to spaghetti-head Maddy.

And Liz had made some progress in that regard – getting Maddy to rest a little and run a little and sleep a little, getting food into her without letting her drink, to steer her off the darker path. Liz was surprised she had managed at the bar last night to keep Maddy sticking with ginger ale, but maybe Maddy's hangover from the night of the letter had been bad enough that Maddy didn't want a drink for a few days.

Maddy hadn't asked Liz why she would drag her out to a bar and then tell her not to drink – Maddy knew Liz's aim at going out together wasn't the possibility of drink but the company of a lot of women, the idea of going to a place where Maddy could dance freely, even erotically if she felt like it, without male trouble, without concern. It was the right choice even if it did always feel a little weird to come to a lesbian bar with her hopelessly straight best friend.

She had taught Maddy years ago that there wasn't any point, if a woman at a bar hit on Maddy, in Maddy protesting that she was straight.

"Either they won't believe you or they'll take it as a challenge," said Liz. "So, just say you're presently unavailable."

At the Philadelphia bar, Liz had wandered off for a moment and come back to hear Maddy telling a woman, "I'm terribly flattered by your interest, but at the moment I have a raging case of gonorrhea! Gotta deal with that first."

Maddy said it with such a bright smile, Liz had to wonder what the other woman made of it.

The dancing, the escape, had obviously done Maddy good. And Liz had gotten to wear to the bar the shirt she'd found at the second thrift store they'd wandered into. Well, Maddy had found it – "Liz, this is absolutely perfect for you!" Liz thought at first Maddy was nutty to be suggesting a Western-style cowgirl shirt, with shiny snaps and red piping, but once Liz tried it on, she realized Maddy was right.

Maddy had a weird ability to push Liz into things Liz would have felt wrong but that then seemed so right. Like using an old-fashioned wall calendar to deal with planning for the big deadlines at the lab. Or picking out a flowery and sentimental card for her mother on the birthday right after the biopsy. (Maddy had been right that it had been a moment for shedding all Liz's usual ironic posturing.)

Had Maddy always been the way she was – without the need or ability for the kinds of social conventions that made most people stick to what was "expected" of one – or had that come after her life had been turned upside down when she was fifteen? Liz had the sense maybe Maddy had always been this way – unpredictable, unfettered by norms, prone to get into trouble. This probably wasn't so much a post-Jerk personality as the one that had gotten her into the situation with The Jerk in the first place.

Not that she was blaming Maddy.

Liz wondered what Jimmy Heathcote was going to turn out to be like when Maddy met him later today in New York on the Lower East Side. Maddy had found out about him – about Heathcote's suspicions about Wilhelm – rather by accident. Maddy and Liz had gone to lunch, leaving all their work in Maddy's office at the museum, and when they had come back, Shirley had been there looking through what Maddy had left – several stacks from the FOIA response, stacks of Dr. Wilhelm's grant reports.

Maddy had stopped in the doorway, startled.

Shirley had looked up at her and said, "You haven't been talking to Jimmy Heathcote, have you?"

Shirley had stared at Maddy, and Maddy had stared back at her. The dog had looked from one face to the other, trying – like Liz – to understand what was going on between their looks. When to fill the conversational gap, Liz had asked who Jimmy Heathcote was, Shirley would not say. Shirley just left – not angrily, but quietly.

"Who is Jimmy Heathcote?" Liz had asked Maddy, closing the door after Shirley.

"I don't know," Maddy had answered. "We have to go back to Wolf's place so I can call Bess McFarlane and ask her. She'll tell me."

They had worked about an hour more in the hopes Shirley wouldn't find it too weird that they were leaving. They had stopped by Shirley's office on the way out, with Liz telling Shirley it was good to meet her, and Shirley returning the same sentiment, with a pleasant enough smile.

"You're not going to ask Liz to sign a donation form?" Maddy had asked, trying to lighten Shirley's mood. "She worships science, like us."

228

But it was a line that fell flat.

Liz had thought to herself that it was odd Maddy had been talking about Liz donating money to the museum – why would Maddy or Shirley think that Liz, a graduate student, had any money to give?

They'd gone back to Wolf's place and Maddy had called Bess, and then Maddy had called Jimmy Heathcote, setting up a time to meet with him in New York the next day. From listening to Maddy's end of the call, Liz could tell what Jimmy had told Maddy – that he had also thought there were too many suspicious sudden deaths in Dr. Wilhelm's patient population, and that it wasn't a coincidence that they were all in cases where the patient had promised her or his body to Dr. Wilhelm and where the body was considered interesting. Jimmy had told Maddy that he had been specifically disinvited to the annual meeting as a result of his ideas.

When Maddy had hung up with him, she and Liz had just stared at each other a while.

"A good scholar remembers the null hypothesis," Liz had said. "You have to consider that enough evidence might show that you are completely wrong – that there is *nothing to see here.*"

"The whole world, save at most a couple of us, would believe that," Maddy had answered. "So I don't think I myself have to put a lot of energy into considering the null hypothesis."

"That is a very sloppy way of thinking, Madeleine Shanks."

Maddy had stood up and gone over to stick a finger into the dirt of the slightly wilted basil plant on Wolf's kitchen windowsill, to see if it needed water.

"Have you ever known me to be a sloppy thinker, Elizabeth Coopersmith?"

-21-

Liz's visit had left Maddy sorely missing the lovely bubble of the campus in Bloomington, so it was hardly a surprise to Maddy that she had spent chunks of the morning finding herself mentally back there. The creek-of-a-river that formed the spine of the central part of the university grounds, with the tall brown oaks lining it like vertebrae; the limestone buildings with their deep-sill casement windows and heavy parapets; the feeling that every ununiformed passer-by over thirty was thinking about something merely and magnificently academic.

Oh, it felt good to be momentarily back home, with Liz and Pumpkin at most a mile away from her, no matter where she wandered. Only here, in this Bloomington space – in this small, plaster-walled university seminar room with its walnut molding and fluorescent lighting – here now was this raucous argument breaking out, about Maddy misusing research funds.

"So, let me get this straight," said Charles, the classmate who was always trying his best to undermine Maddy. "You accuse Dr. Wilhelm of this and that, but *you yourself* misused your NEH research monies to pay for trips having nothing to do with your proposed research – taking, for example, a costly daytrip to New York to go talk to a dwarf about his conspiratorial suspicions?"

"A *person with dwarfism*," Maddy corrected him in her head. "I mean, *a little person*. And the issue of Dr. Wilhelm and his collection of bodies may not have been in my dissertation proposal or my NEH grant proposal *per se*, but it is still related to the history of specimen acquisition. So, it's *related* to what I said I was working on for my dissertation. Back off."

"Now, Maddy, that's a real stretch. I must agree with Charles, I must say," chimed in Professor Carlyle, Maddy's dissertation director, blowing his mole-pocked nose in his old cotton handkerchief and putting it back in his pants pocket before straightening his bifocals to see her more clearly. "You know, Maddy, as I've told you before, studying anything in the last fifty years means you are doing *journalism*, not history. You're here to get a Ph.D. in *History*."

"Quite right," said Giovanni without looking up. He was doodling something in his notebook and his hair was doing that thing that looked so casual and so designed all at once. "Misappropriation of funds for personal interests, my dear Maddy – tsk tsk! Quite inappropriate."

"Oh, come off it, Giovanni," Maddy answered him, throwing her hands up in the air as she mentally stood before this panel of men. "You know perfectly well the reason you went to the meeting in Cambridge four months ago wasn't to *hear the papers*. It was to *hook up*. With me. And you used your research funds for that trip. So don't go pulling your holier-than-thou crap on me, Professor Mastromonaco."

Giovanni dropped his notebook and pen on the table in shock and made a two-hand gesture to indicate he thought that she should shut up. She figured the gesture was Italian, but she understood the translation.

"What's that?" asked Dr. Carlyle, tilting forward his head to look right through the top part of his glasses, first at Maddy and then at Giovanni. "What's all this? Have the two of you been – have you been – "

Maddy's brain was trying to figure out what wording the stately Professor Carlyle would use to ask if she and Giovanni had been fucking. *Seeing each other* was the best guess. It didn't quite capture the carnality, but it was probably the most Old Man Carlyle could muster.

"Phoenix Dumpling?" asked Colin with a smirk, holding up the fancy black-lacquered chopsticks Maddy had bought for him at the Philadelphia thrift store while shopping with Liz. Maddy had wrapped them up with a note for Colin and asked Liz to send them to him through campus mail when she got back to Bloomington from Philly.

"Not *now*, Colin," Maddy groaned, although the thought of Colin alone sounded pretty great. She could use the short distraction.

Maddy shook her head to dispel this scene. She looked up from her southbound trudge along the dirty sidewalk of Broadway to see the Flatiron Building before her. Manhattan had a liveliness and a layer of filth that just made Philly feel so miniature, like the city of a model train set.

She adjusted her backpack, again having the sense it was just too light to feel normal without her computer. She had left it back at Wolf's place knowing she might be walking into not the safest part of New York. The last thing she needed was to have her backpack stolen with her computer in it. But was the stack of clean towels in Wolf's bathroom the best place to have hidden her laptop? It seemed unlikely that, if someone broke in, they would look there for anything valuable. But what if Wolf came home in a state that for some reason required three towels, and he pulled on them without carefully taking them off the stack one at a time, and her laptop went crashing to the floor?

This was an irrational thought, she realized. It was getting harder to stop the irrational thoughts and the imagined mash-up scenes from coming in simply because of being worn out. As if on cue, Maddy yawned and then yawned again.

She had come upon Union Square and was working her way along the edge of it, south and then east. For once, her Amtrak train had come in only fifteen minutes late, which left her early for her appointment with Jimmy Heathcote. So, she figured, she might as well make the two-and-a-half mile walk from New York's Penn Station to his place in Alphabet City. The weather wasn't exactly pleasant – overcast and just barely topping forty degrees – but it wasn't raining or snowing, either.

She imagined for a moment how nice it would be to be back in the Indiana Memorial Union, sitting near the roaring fire in the big limestone fireplace of the first-floor lobby space, sitting at one of the old wooden tables, working through some text...or just to be way up in the stacks of the IU library, way up on the tenth floor, where the history of science books were housed....

What if for some reason the New York Public Library wasn't going to be open later today, after she met Heathcote?

What if she ran into The Jerk while walking in New York City?

What if another 9/11 happened today – how was she going to get back to Philadelphia or find a place to stay?

What if another 9/11 was already in progress and Liz's plane was one of the ones hijacked this morning?

She sighed.

In some ways, the steady invasion of these irrational thoughts – like a single stream of ants coming out of a crack in the sidewalk – presented less of a problem than the thoughts that seemed simultaneously rational and irrational.

There was, for example, the belief that if she told Wolf at this point what she thought had been going on with Wilhelm – including that he had at least one accomplice, namely the man who had broken into Wolf's house, but maybe also Dr. Tate? – that Wolf would nod and say he would take care of it and then he would, in fact, do nothing – he would just tell her to finish her dissertation – and she would go crazy from another experience of No Justice.

And why *was* she here in New York, to talk to Jimmy Heathcote about Dr. Wilhelm and to look at Schlesinger 1888 and not in Philly tying up the loose ends of her dissertation research so she could go home?

"Phoenix Dumpling?" Colin suddenly asked her again. He said it as if he thought it might in fact be the answer to her question of why she was prolonging her time away from Indiana.

Maddy had to wonder if he was on to something – was she doing this investigation and extending her stay in Philadelphia because of wanting to stay with Wolf – because of a sexual attraction to Wolf? The way his arms looked, just after a run; the way his hands looked when he handed her pages of her manuscript or a plate of food. Listening to herself at the record stores talk to Liz about Wolf had made it so obvious, her attraction to him. When Liz had commented on how the new weight looked good on Maddy, how it had given her a pleasantly mature shape, Maddy had blurted out, "Who would have thought it would take a celibate Catholic man to make me a woman?!" And Liz had just cleared her throat in awkwardness.

Maddy could not deny to herself that she was hoping that tonight he would meet her on the 30th Street Station platform when her train came in and be ready to talk with her. She hadn't seen or heard from him since he had left, just after Liz arrived. She kept picturing him on the platform waiting for her.

But what would they even talk about? She didn't want to hear about The Jerk if Long Island was where he had really been. And she couldn't press him about his supposed visit to his family in case that was a lie he had politely told her to free her from thinking about The Jerk and the need for some member of the police to finally deal with him. And she couldn't yet tell Wolf about Wilhelm and her trip today to New York, especially if she found out *more* but not *enough* about Wilhelm. And there was no way she was going to find out *enough* on this one trip.

Back in Bloomington, seated on the plaid-covered couch in his small wood-framed house, Colin pulled Maddy by the hand, out of this thought, down onto his lap. She didn't resist. She put her right arm around his neck and looked at him with a knowing smile. He moved his knees apart in such a way as to cause hers, too, to fall open a little. The clever and determined maneuver to open her legs made her wet.

He took in his right hand the chopsticks she had sent him through campus mail and gently grabbed the tip of her nose, tugging lightly as if her nose were a pile of wasabi and he wanted to take just a little bit. Then he brushed the hair away from her left ear and did the same with her earlobe. She let out a shaky sexual sigh. While they both looked down to watch his hand, he unbuttoned the top two buttons of her shirt. Now he very carefully slid the shirt down her shoulder, exposing her shoulder, and then he lowered her bra strap, too. He reached around and unclasped her bra through the back of the shirt, and it gave, falling away from her breast.

"*That's* what I want," he said, quietly. "The nicest dumpling – and a little larger portion size than I remember?"

He carefully repositioned the chopsticks in his hand, like a child playing Operation, took hold of her nipple, and tugged on it while he looked in her eyes.

"Jesus, Colin," she mumbled. "Listen, listen, listen. Colin. I've had a very complicated visit to Philadelphia – it hasn't been easy – so if you could please – "

"I'll be extra nice," he said. "And you can tell me what you'd like to have."

And she imagined soon opening her legs to him, with him using those chopsticks to tease and tug on her labia.

"Jesus, watch where you're going, lady!" a man carrying a large box yelled at her, as he moved past her on the sidewalk.

Maddy mumbled "so sorry" and immediately felt stupid for sounding like an apologetic Midwesterner.

She turned left on 10th Street, heading east.

. . .

"Can I help *you*?" the man sweeping the front of the barroom asked with a tone of skepticism as Maddy walked in.

234

She figured he probably didn't see a lot of young women with backpacks walking in at this establishment at this hour of the morning.

"I'm here to see Jimmy Heathcote," Maddy answered, taking in the size of this fellow. He had to be six-and-a-half feet tall and weighing close to three hundred and fifty pounds. It was one of those moments where she didn't quite feel the same species as the human before her, being of such a different size.

"You want to see Jimmy Heathcote? *I am* Jimmy Heathcote!" he answered.

Then he laughed at the look on Maddy's face.

"Just kidding."

He turned to the back of the barroom and bellowed.

"Jimmy! Girl here to see you!"

From the back trudged forward a red-haired man, maybe forty years old, maybe four feet tall, with all the telltale signs of achondroplasia, including the chin and the nose. What was it about the condition that led to those facial structures, Maddy wondered? She ought to know by now, at least from reading Dr. Wilhelm's work. But the lessons on bone development wasn't why she had been reading it.

"Maddy Shanks," she said, reaching her hand out.

He shook it without reply, motioning her to a booth on the side of the room.

"What can I get you?" he asked.

"A coffee, if it's not too much trouble," said Maddy.

"No trouble," he answered, wandering off.

She sat down on the booth bench, took off her jacket, and tucked it next to her. She opened her backpack and took out her notepad. She had purposely brought a fresh one, figuring that it would signal to Jimmy that she was taking him seriously and that it also wouldn't have any of her notes that might predispose him to think she already believed this or that.

She looked around the bar. It felt like one of those places that existed specifically to service the people who needed alcohol like medication three times a day. The pictures on the wall looked cheaply printed and long outdated, the frames covered in dust. The front windows were covered in smoky-purple translucent plastic laminate, the kind of window covering designed to make it hard to see in. Or maybe it was designed to make it feel as if it were always night – as if it were late enough to be drinking? Everything from the booth bench to the tabletop felt a little sticky.

Jimmy delivered Maddy a cup of coffee. On the side he had put two small containers of creamer and two packets of sugar. For himself he had gotten a drink that looked like a cola but that Maddy had a feeling had something stronger in it. She could smell rum, and she thought the odor was coming from his tall glass.

"Thanks for taking the time to talk to me. You didn't come to the meeting in Washington?" Maddy started, by way of small talk.

"They wouldn't let me if I tried," he answered, looking in her eyes to see if he could read her reaction. "They don't like me coming around anymore, with my suspicions about Dr. Wilhelm."

"Who told you that you couldn't come?"

"Shirley Anseed called me," Jimmy replied. "Said she'd been asked to call me. I don't got email – I don't got a computer. They give me a small room upstairs here."

He took a sip of his drink, and then a longer one.

"Don't matter anyway. If they won't give me the travel help to come, the travel money, no way I can come, and they said they won't no more. You know, that was the thing every year I – you know, the meeting?"

He didn't finish the thought. She wasn't sure what to say. She knew what he meant – that the annual gathering had been personally important, as something to look forward to every year.

"What you said on the phone," he said, "you wanted to talk to me about what I think?"

Maddy nodded.

"You sent by Dr. Wilhelm, to talk me out of it, to convince me I'm wrong, or whatever?"

"No!" answered Maddy, putting her coffee cup down too firmly on the saucer. "On the contrary. I've frankly been wondering myself – there're just – signs. There are signs I don't like."

"And how did you find out about me?" Jimmy asked.

Just then the big guy turned up the music system loudly, and the speakers started blaring head-banger rock.

"Can you shut it OFF, Frank?" Jimmy yelled.

Frank turned it down, and yelled back at Jimmy, "You're supposed to be working!"

"Give me ten fucking minutes!" Jimmy yelled back.

He took another long drink.

"I found out about you by accident," Maddy explained. "Shirley found me at the museum looking through Dr. Wilhelm's grant reports. When she saw me doing that, she asked me if I had been talking to Jimmy Heathcote. She wouldn't say who that was. So, I called Bess McFarlane, and I asked her who Jimmy Heathcote was."

"What'd Bess say?"

"She said that you had been coming to the meetings for years, but she had the feeling you had been pushed out of the group because of talking about how you thought too many people who had promised their bodies to Dr. Wilhelm had died – that a lot of them had died suddenly, in Philadelphia."

He didn't answer, so Maddy continued.

"Bess said she was kind of worried about you."

Jimmy harrumphed as if he had no patience for Bess's worry. And yet, Maddy thought the sound came with some degree of gratitude that Bess was concerned about him. Were his eyes damper than they had been a minute before?

"Bess is the mama to everybody," said Jimmy.

"Is your own mother alive?" Maddy asked, unsure where her question came from.

"I don't know," said Jimmy. "When I was born this way, she and my dad gave me up – gave me up to an institution. My mother and my father, they were society people, up in Darien. They didn't want no midget kid."

Maddy wasn't sure what to say. She had learned a long time ago not to reassure people when they were speaking an ugly truth. She hated it when people tried to reassure her about the ugly truth of having her parents and her sister die. And she had learned over the years that *not* squashing ugly truths with shallow platitudes meant people told you more. And then you found out more.

Sure enough, in the face of Maddy's silence, Jimmy continued:

"I went to go find my parents, years ago. My mother answered the door – I think it was her – and she just started screaming at me, 'You can't be here! You can't be here!'"

He took another drink.

"So, I left."

"Well, that sucks royally," Maddy said. "My parents thought I was a lot of trouble, but they at least kept me. Until they died when I was fifteen."

"You got something wrong with you?"

She wanted to answer *he* had nothing wrong with *him*. But she knew he would think she was pouring saccharine on his festering wounds.

She just shook her head.

"How'd they die, your parents?"

"Car crash. With my sister."

"I'm sorry for your loss," he said.

She felt a weird burst of happiness from being with another New Yorker for just a moment. *I'm sorry for your loss* – what the stranger in New York says at that moment! *That's how we phrase it here,* she thought, *like the way we say "the city" when we mean Manhattan.*

Almost as if he could read her mind, he asked her where she was from.

"I grew up on the Island," she said, and Jimmy nodded. "But I think of myself as being from New York."

He got up, went behind the bar, and brought the coffee pot back to refill Maddy's cup. He took the pot back to the bar along with his own glass and came back with his glass full again. She thought she detected a little unsteadiness in his gait.

"So, what you want to know?" he asked Maddy.

"I'm an historian," she said, "so I think about these things in terms of dates and places. Could you sketch out for me the ones you're wondering about?"

"Yeah, that's how I think about it, too. People and places and the dates. What other way?"

Jimmy pulled a wad of napkins out of the metal napkin holder and took Maddy's pen from her hand. He started writing down for her what he knew. He filled up the first napkin:

Roberto Montenaro, died in Philly hospital while there to see Dr. Wilhelm, 1990.

Casandra May Winiper, died in same hospital, 1991.

Maggie Lovisa, died in Philadelphia on a park bench the day before she was to see Dr. Wilhelm, 1997.

He handed the first napkin to Maddy and started on the second.

"Ordinarily," he said, "I don't write them down. If I remember them, if I remember them all, then they can't be lost."

It sounded almost superstitious. He filled up the second napkin:

"Name something like Tongay Waytoka?" Jimmy said aloud, as he wrote that down.

That was a boy from Zimbabwe, he said; a dwarf teenager who was also an albino. Died around 1990 in a hotel while in Philadelphia to see Dr. Wilhelm.

Baby Joseph LaCasse, died the day after being seen by Wilhelm, 1985?

238

He handed Maddy the napkin and she read it.

"A baby?" Maddy asked.

Jimmy nodded.

"He said to me once, when I told him about my family, that my life was an example of why the conditions should be prevented."

"But you know," Maddy said, watching Jimmy scribble down more names on a third napkin, "of course with all these conditions, with their co-morbidities, some people are just going to happen to die."

"You think it's such a coincidence that they sign over their bodies to him and then they die – and that the ones of us with the most so-called 'interesting' conditions are the ones who die when they get near him?"

(Maddy remembered now what Dr. Wilhelm had said, when she mentioned Bess's condition – osteogenesis imperfecta: "I have one.")

"I ain't interesting," Jimmy added. "Glad I ain't interesting to him! I'm just a plain old achon."

"Did you know that Nick DesJardins died at the meeting in D.C.?" Maddy asked.

Jimmy's mouth fell open.

"*Jesus.* Dr. Day-Jay."

The way he said it – "doctor day-jay" – made it sound almost like a rapper's name. Maddy wondered if Nick knew that was what Jimmy called him.

"Jesus," Jimmy said again. "Dr. Day-Jay – he was always so nice to me. He used to call me sometimes and ask me how I was doing and talk to me about my parents and what they did. How they rejected me. And now Wilhelm and him – Jesus. He always fucking trusted Wilhelm. He thought I was being totally stupid."

"But listen!" said Maddy. "Nick had signed his body over to someone else – to the Cleveland Clinic. Dr. Wilhelm won't get Nick's body – in fact, Dr. Wilhelm's competitors have got it and they'll have it."

"You *sure*?" asked Jimmy. When Maddy didn't answer, he pressed: "How do you know it went to Cleveland?"

"Dr. Wilhelm said that," Maddy said, suddenly feeling a little stupid.

"If I was you, I'd check," said Jimmy. "Nobody ever fucking checks anything he says. They just fucking take his word for everything."

He pulled out another napkin and wrote down two more names, dates, and what he knew.

"How is Bess?" he asked, handing Maddy the napkin.

"She seems good. She has got herself the Cadillac of chairs," Maddy answered, giving a small smile. "And she's damned proud of those two kids."

"God love her," said Jimmy, leaning back and looking sentimental. "There was a time, you know, when I thought she and I might – "

He said nothing more. She waited. About twenty seconds went by.

"I don't know, Jimmy, isn't she's kind of short for you?" Maddy observed with a shrug of her shoulders, and Jimmy let out a sudden burst of laughter and held up his hand to high-five Maddy.

"Sort of slutty, too, don't you think, Jimmy?"

At that, the two broke up laughing hard for a moment.

"Can I get you something to eat?" he asked her. "Everything here is plain shitty, but the place next door makes a good egg and cheese on bagel. It's okay-good on the onion bagel."

"Let me buy us both one of those," said Maddy. "I owe you."

She almost added that she could charge it to her research travel budget. But then she thought better of mentioning a research budget to Jimmy.

. . .

Maddy took a big breath as she ascended the grand marble stairs of the New York Public Library's main branch. It had taken a long while to get through security – a tour bus had come just before she arrived, disgorging a flock of tourists who drifted from taking their photos with the lions to wandering inside. She walked steadily up to the second floor and turned to head through the room of computer terminals into the great Rose Reading Room.

As soon as she arrived at the room, as if reflexively pausing at the doorway of a church to dunk her fingertips in the holy water, she stopped and looked up at the reading room's ceiling – the magnificently restored ceiling, no longer hung with plastic and scaffolding, the painting of the blue sky with the orange and pink clouds of the Hudson School. She felt suddenly the silly spiritual rush of being in a great cathedral of books. Dr. Wilhelm's library ceiling might be deeper in referential meaning, but it had nothing on this one.

The afternoon light was streaming in through the tall, plain-glass windows, coming off the trees of Bryant Park, and her nose could just pick up the scent of expensive paper and the leather-and-glue of quality bindings.

She sat down for a moment at one of the long tables, took off her backpack, and pulled out her pad of note paper. She had tucked Jimmy's scribbled napkins into the back of the pad between the last sheet and the cardboard backing. Now she flipped the pages of the pad over the top so she could look carefully at the napkins. He had filled up almost a half-dozen with what he knew and suspected. She would have to check this information carefully against her own notes and timelines when she got home. But she could already see that some of what Jimmy indicated matched in genders and dates several deaths that she had marked as possibilities in her own timeline. Several of these people had supposedly died of heart problems. All seemed to have been autopsied by Dr. Wilhelm, at least in terms of the representations of the causes of death named in his grant reports and his publications. How handy for him that he could be the one to say what they supposedly died of....and his claims didn't always match.

Over the bagels, Jimmy had asked her why she had ever thought that what Dr. Wilhelm said what they died of was actually what they had died of. She had been *so stupid* in assuming Wilhelm's representations should ever be taken as accurate. *Of course* it might be the case that he was simply making the deaths look natural in his own reporting. She would need to get the death certificates if she could. In most of those cases, someone else should have signed the death certificate – someone else should have tried to determine cause of death – right?

Maddy pulled her hair brush out of the front pocket of her backpack, took her hair out of the ponytail clip, combed it, and fastened it back in. It was time to go ask for Schlesinger 1888. She packed the notepad carefully back in her backpack and went up to the clerk's window to explain what exactly she was looking for.

"Have a seat," the worker told her, brusquely. "It's going to take a while to get that one."

She sat down not far from the clerk's window and thought about this text.

From the point of view of a researcher in the history of medicine, it didn't make a lot of sense that such a document would be here, at this particular library. Looking in the online records while she was visiting Booker in Bethesda, this was the *only* copy she and Booker had been able to locate. Why would an obscure pamphlet on the subject of the death of two brothers with dwarfism have ended up in the New York Public?

Sure: maybe it was just part of a big collection that a doctor had left to this library. Maybe it had been acquired in an unusual cache from some bookseller in Europe. But it was the kind of thing she would have expected to be at the National Library of Medicine, or the Wellcome Library history-of-medicine collection in London, or more likely a medical-historical library in some German-speaking land, given its origin. Not here. This wasn't going to be a place the average doctor or historian came to look at a relatively obscure medical text.

And why would Schlesinger have published this material in a *pamphlet* and not a standard journal article? It was supposedly published just before he died, based on the date – it seemed to be perhaps the last thing he had published. By then, Schlesinger had had a long record of journal publications and books. Putting it in a *pamphlet* – that felt so *eighteenth*-century. Out of its time. In fact, it would have been more trouble for Schlesinger to publish it in a pamphlet than a journal. A journal article simply would have required him to send the manuscript to the journal editor and, with his reputation and the good story, the editor would surely have published it. A pamphlet would have required Schlesinger to commission a printer and to go through the trouble of managing the publication and distribution.

Dr. Wilhelm had certainly appealed repeatedly over the years to Schlesinger 1888 as proof that people with growth deficiencies were known to die of heart problems. It seemed an explanation for the pattern supposedly associated with patients in his clinic. But it was hard not to notice, as Jimmy had done, the correlation between the deaths and those who had particularly unusual bodies or who had promised their bodies to Dr. Wilhelm.

This all smelled to her like Schlesinger 1888 constituted a fake. A fake designed to minimize any surprise at the pattern of the deaths among his clinic patients. To make it look like the deaths in his clinic population were part of a long historical pattern, not something special to his patients.

But if Dr. Wilhelm had faked this text, how could it be that there was a second original in the New York Public, a copy that must have come by a different route than the one in his own collection? Making two fakes might have been almost as hard as making one. Maybe he had had both made at once?

More likely this was the right question to ask:

Wilhelm's original had supposedly been lost in the accidental fire at his library a couple of years ago – but *was* the one housed here a different "original" than the one Wilhelm had had? Or was this the same copy as the one that had been in Wilhelm's collection?

She was going to try to find that out. Maddy knew that Dr. Wilhelm had given various members of the little people community photocopies of his own "original" of Schlesinger 1888 over the years. Nick had said he had a photocopy of Wilhelm's original and Maddy knew that Bess had one, too.

242

Maddy had asked Bess to send her a copy of her copy, to Wolf's house. Meanwhile, she had purposefully brought a disposable camera with her here, so that she could photograph this one. In a few days' time, this would allow her to compare her photos of this New York Public copy to the photo-copy of Wilhelm's "original" coming from Bess.

She couldn't be sure the pamphlet here at New York Public would show any special features that would mark it as the same or different from the one Wilhelm had copied from his own collection to give to Bess and the others. But nineteenth century paper, particularly paper for pamphlets, was reliably crumbly. If the shape of the crumbled edges of this one matched the shape of the crumbled edges shown in the copy that Bess had...well, that would seem to suggest this was, in fact, the same single "original." And that would be significant. More than significant, given Wilhelm's claim about a fire having destroyed his copy.

The clerk called Maddy over and handed her an acid-free folder with the pamphlet inside.

"Be careful," he warned. "It's marked fragile."

She wondered why on earth they would give a random patron without gloves a fragile old document. But then there wasn't a lot of rhyme or reason to the big public libraries.

And that's why, she thought to herself, *Wilhelm would put it here and not in a more logical library. Easy to slip into the collection here.*

She knew exactly how she would do it, if she wanted to insert a faked text into a collection like this. She would order a stack of books on subjects related to the subject of the fake. Then, when returning the books, she would casually turn over the pamphlet and say that she had found the pamphlet inside one of the books. She would tell the clerk that the pamphlet needed to be individual-ly catalogued. And then she'd keep an eye out for it showing up in the online index, to see that it showed up.

You'd have to count on them doing their job, and not setting it aside or sending it off to some other collection without leaving a trace. But they probably would, as you hoped. They wouldn't have any other easy way to deal with the stray dog of a text than to catalogue it and add it to the collection.

Maddy sat down and carefully pulled the six-page pamphlet out of the folder. Sure enough, the paper looked and felt to be late nineteenth century. It had that characteristic grey to it – the color of the boiled potato dump-lings they sometimes served at the convent.

Of course, it would not have been very difficult for Wilhelm or whoever faked it for him to get blank paper from the right period to use. Maddy sometimes came across sheets of very old paper just like this. Booksellers and researchers would find such paper in the archives of researchers or bound in at the end of long published volumes. These blank old pages would be perfect for creating fakes.

Wilhelm would have had to make sure the printing also looked nineteenth-century. But if he couldn't figure out how to do it himself, there were surely printers, especially in Europe, who could pull this off for a fee. Paid enough, a printer probably wouldn't ask a lot of questions.

And of course it had to be a pamphlet. Dr. Wilhelm could not fake a journal article. It would have been too easy for anyone to look and see, in bound library copies of the journal, that the article didn't really exist. And anyone like Maddy could see that the journal indexes like the Index Catalogue were missing the supposed journal article. That would have made no sense – someone would have discovered by now a journal article to be a fake.

But a medical *pamphlet* – the absence of any sign of it in the big indexes would be easier to explain. Not every index was going to pick up every pamphlet. And all Wilhelm had had to do was to keep citing it now and then, to get others in his field to cite it, too, so that a sort of record of it was created in the modern medical literature, suggesting it really did exist. In the medical specialties, when it came to talking about old historical texts, they all just copied each other's citations, not following the rule of looking at the text yourself. They all just cited it as if they had seen it. And if they *did* want to see the original to read it for themselves before citing it, they would have just asked Dr. Wilhelm, and he would have happily supplied them a photocopy.

Nobody was going to do what she was about to do – compare this one to the supposed other copy.

Now she looked more closely at the text. She knew already what the contents would say, based on what Dr. Wilhelm had reported about the text in his own publications. But she read through it carefully anyway, translating it in her head from German on the fly, delicately turning the pages. Here was the story of one brother, then another, both dying of heart failure, almost exactly two years apart. Here was Schlesinger postulating on the connections between growth deformities, heart development, and cardiac stress.

Maddy reached into her backpack and pulled out the disposable camera. She wasn't sure if she was allowed to take photographs of the texts here, so she quickly set up the camera in her lap and then leaned over the text holding the camera near her chest, snapping several photos, turning the pages, and snapping more. As she had hoped, the text had several marks on it that ought to make it distinctive enough – including places where the paper had crumbled on the edges, a stain of some sort on the third page, and a smudging of a couple of lines of print on the fifth page.

She hoped the camera was doing its job. There would be no way to tell until she had the film developed.

Now she sat down, slipping the camera back into her bag. She was done so quickly, she didn't quite know what to do with herself. So, she decided to sit with it just a little longer to think about it.

Are you from Dr. Wilhelm's library? she asked the pamphlet in her head. *And are you going to stay here now, or are you going to disappear somehow before I can show you came from Philadelphia for the purpose of looking like you were a second original? Will you reappear somewhere else, looking like a third?*

She thought about this last possibility for a minute. Then she pulled an index card and a blue ballpoint pen out of her bag. She used the pen to scribble in one spot over and over again on the index card, until the spot – about the size of a grape – was dense with ink. Now she rolled her right index finger back and forth across the ink spot, lifted her finger, apologized to Schlesinger in her head (as if saying a prayer to the dead), and stuck her inked finger in the center of the fourth page.

There it was. Her fingerprint marring the text, smack dab in the middle of a section on the death of the second brother. If Wilhelm tried to now move this item to a third location, he would be forced to carry with it her own body's mark.

She put the pamphlet back in the folder, licked her finger, and wiped it off on her jeans. She went back up to the desk and handed back the folder.

"The thing is," she said to the clerk, "I need to know the acquisition record on this text."

"Sure," said the clerk without looking up.

He used his keyboard to enter into his computer the code from the folder. He scanned the screen to make sure he had the right one, printed it off, and handed it to Maddy.

She thanked him and took a few steps away to let the next person come up. She looked at the acquisition record. Her heart picked up ten beats a minute.

There it was – *provenance unknown*.

The first record of its being in the collection was just a couple of years ago. Right around the time of the supposed fire in Dr. Wilhelm's library.

He had surely done exactly what she had imagined she would have done. He had become worried someone was on to him, and he needed to try to make this text look more real than he had bothered to until then.

So, he had claimed it had been destroyed, and he had relocated it here, to make it look like there had been at least two copies in the world, one independent from him.

He had brought Schlesinger 1888 to New York, New York – the place everyone goes to start life over, to become more than they are – only eventually to be found out, if they became a little too famous.

. . .

Maddy stood in the aisle in the line of people waiting to get off the train at Philadelphia as the train shimmied, shifting across a switch from one track to the next. The bottle of wine she had started drinking at Penn Station in New York and finished not long into New Jersey was wearing off. The full realization of the call she had made to Shirley, while she had been waiting in New York City for her train back to Philly, was sinking in.

She should not have called Shirley, especially not having drunk two glasses of the wine on an almost empty stomach. But the day – Jesus, *the day* – Jimmy and Schlesinger, and then seeing in Penn Station a man who for a startling moment looked so much like The Jerk – and then scanning the crowd as she did, in a panic, to see if she could find Wolf –

Once she calmed down a little, she had looked at the clock, seen it was five minutes to five, went to the pay phone, and used her phone card to dial long-distance, to Shirley's desk.

"Shirley," she said, "it's Maddy."

"Where are you, Maddy?" Shirley asked, in a voice that sounded worried, though perhaps not for Maddy. "Where have you been today?"

"I'm in Penn Station, in New York. I went to see Jimmy Heathcote." Shirley did not answer.

"Shirley, who got Nick's body? Who got Nick DesJardins' body?"

"Dr. Wilhelm did. I learned that today. He has it."

Maddy said nothing. Shirley continued:

"He got it after the autopsy in D.C. Turns out Dr. Wilhelm showed the medical examiner the donation form, so he got it, because Nick hadn't yet formally signed with Cleveland."

Maddy did not answer. Shirley made the clinics sound like competing sports organizations. And Nick himself had quipped to Maddy that Shirley was the exclusive recruiter for Dr. Wilhelm's team.

"Maddy, what did Jimmy tell you?"

Maddy thought about what to say. Just then, the station dispatcher announced the arrival of her train, saying it would be boarding on track 12. She should hang up.

But it felt rather as if the receiver of the payphone was glued to her hand and her ear.

"What did Jimmy tell you, Maddy?" Shirley asked again.

"He keeps it all in his head, Shirley. All the names and the dates and places. For him, it's an oral history."

The announcer had called the track number again.

"I think he can't possibly be right, Maddy," Shirley had said, almost too quietly for Maddy to hear.

...

The train lurched and stopped, as Maddy and all the people in the line to disembark fell forward a step.

The conductor called again "Philadelphia! Thirtieth Street, Philadelphia!"

He opened the door and the line started to move.

Maddy followed the people in front of her, looking down to make sure she put her foot down correctly on the metal steps. A few feet clear of the train on the platform, she looked up. There was Wolf, already standing next to her, with Hunter at his side. She felt Wolf's gaze wash over her face, and she suddenly felt as if she should have pulled herself together better on the train – fixed her hair, put some powder on her nose.

He reached out to take her backpack and put it over his shoulder. She bent over to greet Hunter, who gave her nose the lick of a friend. Maddy found herself suddenly afraid Wolf might speak of The Jerk, so she stood up and hastened to speak first.

"Wolf, Liz and I ate practically everything, so what did you make?" she asked, as if they had been talking about dinner for some time.

"I told you I went to New England, to see my family, Rabbit," he said, as they made their way up the stairs to the station lobby. "So, I made a lobster bisque."

"Wolf, you know that's not the best use of lobster," she said.

"Why don't you try it before you conclude that?"

She winced inside, wondering if he found her insufferable. She hadn't even brought him anything from New York – not so much as a real bagel – and now she was doubting what he'd made her for dinner. What the hell was wrong with her? She was insufferable. She had realized about a year earlier that after people got to know her for a while, they were likely to find out she was this way. Maddy tried to avoid being around anyone in particular too much or for too long for that very reason – because eventually they'd find her just such an asshole. Not that she cared that much what people thought of her, she told herself. She was who she was and she had long ago learned that endlessly seeking the approval of others came at too high a cost.

Yet with Wolf...

They came up into the lobby, finding themselves right under the giant arrivals and departures board, where they had been just four days before when she had been lost, and he had taken to kneeling, to ask her to let him help. The two of them paused and looked up as if there was something they needed to see. The dog waited patiently. The listing for her train was just starting to rotate away.

She wished now so much that she could not be an asshole. He had made lobster bisque for her. He had taken the trouble to meet her at her train, *and* he had made her something to eat for dinner, something different, no doubt something at least very good, if not excellent! Why had she responded by telling him he had misused the lobster?

As if he could sense what she was thinking, he reached over and took her hand in his. He shifted his fingers around to intersperse her fingers with his, locking his fingers around her knuckles to the back of her hand. The way he was holding it, she thought, felt like he intended to keep her hand clasped to his for a long time. Perhaps until they reached his house?

Would he see her ink-stained index finger when they sat down to eat and ask her why it was blue?

She thought back a few hours, to her visit to the American Museum of Natural History. Finding herself with two empty hours in New York – between returning Schlesinger 1888 in its folder to the clerk and the departure time for her train back to Philly – finding herself standing near the library service window drowning in the disorientation and the clarity of the acquisition record – *provenance unknown* – she had felt pulled to her old friend, the whale. Two hours, she figured, would give her enough time.

From the library, she took the subway up to the natural history museum stop, on the west side of the park, and she went straight from the entry way to lie again under the blue whale on the cold parquet floor in the dark quiet of the Hall of Ocean Life. *Of course*, she thought to herself as she made a beeline for the whale, *the museum was all the same*, exactly as it had been when she had come again and again growing up – all the same but for a new exhibit here or there. Her great blue whale wasn't going anywhere.

She had walked into the Hall of Ocean Life and came face to face with it immediately. The sight felt so restorative, it seemed almost as if, if she wanted, she could just go find her sister lingering in the gem and mineral room, as she always did.

She had descended the stairs to get underneath the whale, and laid down, putting her backpack under her head, her feet on the floor with knees pointing up at the beast. Hung majestically from the ceiling as if swimming right through the hall, stretching almost a hundred feet long, the beautiful foam model of her fellow mammal still felt as if it existed specifically in order to be the magical antidote to that feeling of The Jerk leaning over her. His letter of a few days ago had brought back to her in small waves that stinging sensation of pollution, as if he could induce a bloom of jellyfish in her uterus. But this big, magnificent thing, this fine huge mammal, it would wash her clean of him with its strong wake, protect her with its dense mass from the world caving in from above.

Lying on the floor, feeling the sea lions of the dioramas looking on, she had taken her index finger, still stained blue from her marking of Schlesinger 1888, and she had held it up as if to touch the whale. One blue mammal connecting to another. The species difference meant nothing. For they had both been born warm-blooded. They had both been born with hair and with brains ready for language and kinship. They had both begun life attached to their mothers and had then been set free. Their bones – all the different bones – they all came down to the original ancestor bones millions of years before, no matter whether now the bones shaped the human, the whale, the rabbit, the wolf. One blue mammal swimming toward another.

Wolf let go her hand to manage the station door, letting Maddy and Hunter go in front of him while he held the door. He adjusted Hunter's leash in his right hand and reached over again with his left to take Maddy's, wrapping his fingers again through hers. It felt to her as if he were pulling her, through the murky waters of the city air.

-22-

She woke up to the sound of Wolf snoring quietly in her bed next to her in the deep end of the night.

Maddy always slept on the right side of a double bed for some reason, but after he had brushed his teeth and put on his sleeping sweatpants and t-shirt, and he had come to her bedroom and given Hunter an order to lay down near the desk, Wolf had motioned to Maddy to move over in the bed, out of her usual spot, toward the side of the bed nearest the closet. She guessed either he wanted to sleep between her and the door or he was just used to being on the right.

She remembered now how he arranged the blankets to tuck his in along his side, to keep Maddy from being under the same blanket as him. She had told him that's what Liz did, to keep Maddy from hogging the blanket all night.

His blanket wasn't tucked so neatly now.

She had been yawning her way through dinner even though his funny take on lobster bisque had caused her to brighten and exclaim that he was culinarily insane – a lobster bisque made with a coconut cream, flavored with saffron and turmeric and dotted with bright red fresh pomegranate seeds, poured over pan-fried rice cakes full of crispy bits of scallion. And with it, a hoppy pale beer. So exactly right.

She kept oohing and ahhing at the flavor. It seemed as if her noises of delight were the reason he had two of the bottles in quick succession, and then a third. He was having trouble not smiling at her inarticulate exclamations about the flavors, and so she tried to cool it, to save him the embarrassment.

Over seconds, he asked about her research trip. She said only that she had learned a lot. She wished it had been time to tell him. But it had not yet been.

Tomorrow morning, she thought to herself, she would drop off the camera at the drug store to have the images from the library processed so that, when Bess's photocopy of Dr. Wilhelm's original of Schlesinger 1888 came in the mail to Maddy at Wolf's house, she could compare the copy Bess had to the photographs Maddy had taken at the library. And she would tell Shirley in the meantime – first thing tomorrow – that Jimmy was just nutty and she had just been humoring him.

And then, every second the museum was open to her, Maddy would work madly to get as much as she could for her dissertation, to grab as much information as she could, like a monk watching the monastery burn, she thought – she would rush to the museum's library and save what she could. It was not really on fire, of course – it was only that she would soon be unable to continue there – something was going to give – and she had to try to save her dissertation.

She had tried to calm herself by reminding herself that she could always change course in her dissertation if she couldn't get the texts she needed. But the odds of having funding to stretch all the way to the end of her degree... too risky. She wondered if she ought to tell Wolf right now about Wilhelm. But she had to get it all lined up, like billiard balls. She had to make sure, in order to be taken seriously, that when she gave it all to the police, they did not think she was merely distracting herself from her dissertation with a fancy flight. She needed them to understand the opposite was true: that she was, in fact, being responsible, not irresponsible.

(Why did she even feel like she had something to prove to them? Was this house just that much like the convent?)

Was delaying the responsible thing to do? Was Wilhelm going to be able, in the meantime, to destroy her budding reputation as a scholar? Eliminate her ability to go to every single anatomical museum and archive? Or would she first be able to prove what it was she and Jimmy knew?

Surely Wilhelm would not make a further move on another patient if Shirley had told him that Maddy was looking at his grant reports. That would make him hesitate. That gave her time. Had Shirley told him?

"What are you thinking so intensely about?" Wolf had asked her at dinner, getting up to serve her thirds.

They were using his lovely, broad-bottomed, dark-blue soup bowls for this dish. Wasn't it always the best food, Maddy thought, when he took out these bowls? Nowadays her mouth salivated like Pavlov's dogs when she saw him pull a pair of these out of the cabinet. He had laid two rice cakes on the bottom of the bowl and spooned out the bisque over it, not so much that you couldn't still see a little of the browned tops of the cakes peeking out from the bisque, like an island coming out from the ocean.

Oh, the taste of the rice cakes soaking in the seasoned coconut cream. The feeling of the pomegranate seeds bursting in her teeth, releasing their sacs of fluid.

"Rabbit, what are you thinking so intensely about?" he asked again.

She replied that she had to work very hard the next few days because she was working on two projects at once.

"Your dissertation and – ?"

"Look, Wolf, sometimes as a scholar you have to just manage two related projects because the timing is right in terms of the research you can do. That's the case here. I'm trying to get two things done at once while I'm here."

She did not want to tell him that she might have to go soon – leave Philly – because her access to the museum would be cut off. If she said it, he would ask her what was going on. But she could tell that her vague answers were leaving him unsatisfied and confused.

She thought about what it was she could ask him so they could talk about something else – but she just yawned again. He observed to her that it looked as if she would have no trouble sleeping that night. She scrunched up her face and said she wished he was right, but she was afraid she would struggle to sleep.

"I can't explain it, Wolf," she confessed suddenly to him and to herself, "but it feels a little bit now like being back to the first days in the convent? Where will I sleep – where will I be able to sleep? Between the attack and now The Jerk knowing where I am – I mean, I appreciate having Hunter near, but I feel – I feel – I feel dislocated. Am I good enough to be kept?"

He had presented, in response, a rare and complex visage for a human, she thought – a combination of concern and hope and pain and a need to say something that he could not say?

"Wolf, maybe it is because Liz was just here," she added, trying to reassure him that it wasn't something he had done wrong.

She drank down a half-bottle of beer in three fast gulps, feeling the hops light up her palette like sun on a field. Why couldn't it brighten her brain?

"Maybe, Wolf – maybe it is just because of The Jerk showing back up – the letter, I mean – and then you going suddenly away, and Liz coming suddenly, and bunking with Liz like in the dorm of the convent, when Sister Mary Grace was sleeping near me in the first days, to keep an eye on me the first few days – I don't mean Liz is Sister Mary Grace, I mean Hunter is. The way Hunter is keeping an eye on me. He's kind of a quiet nun of a dog. Maybe that's why it feels like the first days in the convent?"

Wolf had nodded in a way that suggested specifically that her remark about bunking with Liz had just confirmed his reading of the stack of sheets they had left undisturbed on the couch.

The feeling in her chest was one of sudden loss. She had felt suddenly overcome by a wish that she could just read his mind and know where he had been the last few days – had he, in fact, gone to see his family up in New England? Or was this lobster purchased in New York or in Philadelphia merely as a ploy to comfort her with that fiction, the fiction she had suggested to him somehow days ago in this kitchen with Officer Snotty looking on – that she could now just forget about The Jerk because Wolf would take care of it all, Katie and The Jerk and all – the fiction spoken when Maddy had told Wolf that she didn't want to have to deal with The Jerk at all ever again?

Had he, in fact, been on Long Island, taking care of it? Had Wolf, in fact, just seen The Jerk? Was her life just going to keep cycling like this? Was The Jerk somehow going to get Wolf killed, too, like her family? Or at least take him away from her again and again?

"Where is the lobster from, Wolf?" she asked plaintively, putting her spoon down and starting to look like she might soon cry a little, exactly like an exhausted child. "You haven't told me – you haven't said where you got this lobster meat."

He pushed back his chair quickly and came to grab her, pulling her up into his arms and holding on to her very tight as she dissembled.

"Fuck. Fuck, Wolf. Even if you told me," she said, pushing words through her strained mouth, "how would I know that you were telling me the truth?"

"You want to discuss epistemology?" he asked, sitting down in his chair and pulling her down on this lap, putting his arms back around her.

"No, I don't fucking want to discuss epistemology!" she said, almost laughing.

"I promised you I would take care of it. I did not lie. And I got lobster. So you know I'm not lying about anything."

He reached around her and grabbed his beer from the table and drank down what was left in the bottle.

"You really want me to tell you what's happening with The Jerk, Rabbit? Or do you just want to know we are dealing with it?"

"The latter," she said. "If you tell me too much, then you will summon the bastard – he will show up tonight."

Wolf pushed her shoulders back a little and looked at her face to see what she meant.

"Show up in your dreams?" he said.

She nodded.

She did not tell him the nightmare she had had, just before the alarm clock had gone off that morning to wake her and Liz, about The Jerk and Wilhelm being the same person. A frogman – a limb cut off, a limb grown back; amphibious, able to hide under the surface of the water, in the reeds, where it could not be seen.

"Pull yourself together," he said, firmly but quietly. "You know you're strong. You have got to pull it together, Rabbit, and admit that this bisque is a *very* good use of lobster of unknown origin, *much* better than you expected, and so you should trust me. You should trust me when I go on to make us turkey later this week."

"But I've told you a thousand times, Wolf! Turkey is the *stupidest* meat – it dries out so fast, like wax dripped on a cold surface – "

"Nah-ah-ah!" he said, waving a finger at her. "Have some faith in me, woman!"

She grabbed his finger and held it, wrapped tight in hers.

"If I promise not to put a move on you Wolf, would you please sleep in the bed next to me tonight?"

She said it as if this was what they had just been talking about – not turkey. She added that she desperately needed sleep, that she had a shitload of work to do the next few days on her dissertation and the related research project, and she could not if she did not sleep. Before he could answer, she told him quickly that Liz had found that if they just didn't share a blanket, then Maddy wouldn't drive her crazy with blanket-hogging all night. So if they just used two blankets, maybe she wouldn't make him crazy all night pulling on the blanket.

And he had said okay as soon as she shut up.

Now he was asleep in her bed, and she awake, and she wondered what to do.

Were he not here, she would likely let her mind wander to the sexual, used her fingers to get herself off, to try to go back to sleep. She had long since learned this was the best way to calm her night mind, to leave consciousness behind again.

But here was Wolf, lying right next to her – here was Wolf, smelling a little of toothpaste, saffron, laundry detergent, and his sweat. She moved a little closer to him to try to pick up more of the sweat. Her motion stirred him, and without opening his eyes he reached out and pulled her towards him, with her facing him. Her face was in his chest.

She wasn't sure what to do. It seemed clear that he was still asleep. There was, at least, a blanket still between most of them, at least from her sternum to her knees. Maybe she should pull herself away, not cause him the consternation of waking up holding her like this. Although, for all she knew, the same thing had already happened the night of The Jerk's letter – she could barely remember what had happened that night.

She was slightly twisted, her knees out of alignment from her ankles and hips, and it was starting to get uncomfortable. His grabbing and pulling her in like that had so startled her, she hadn't thought to shift herself to a good position before he stopped moving. And now, she realized, she wasn't going to be able to hold this pose much longer. *Was* he asleep?

"Do you want to talk epistemology now?" he asked very quietly, as if not to wake Hunter, but she let out a laugh too loud.

The dog stirred and then went quiet again.

"What are you thinking about, Rabbit?"

"Everything, I suppose," she answered.

"Yes," he said, "night thoughts – night, the time when it seems that all can be known."

"And that all will forever remain *unknown*," she answered.

"Yes."

He was right – the night was when it seemed that all could be known. It must have been what drove the astronomers of the Scientific Revolution – Tycho and Kepler and Galileo. It was night, not day, that brought on Enlightenment.

They said nothing for a moment, and she finally turned away from him to her left side, to relieve the cramping starting to happen in her right hip. Instead of pulling away from her, he surprised her: he let her finish adjusting herself and then wrapped his arm again around her, pulling them closer together in a gentle motion, his front against her back. She could feel his heat through the blanket. She focused on the sensation for a moment, feeling as if it were the sun on her back.

"Are death certificates public documents, Wolf? Even old ones? And new ones? All of them?"

"I suppose so," he said, yawning. "We never have trouble getting them, of course, for law enforcement investigations, so I can't say I've ever tried outside of my official capacity. But yes, I think they are public. If there is one you want, you should be able to get it."

Get *it,* singular, she thought – he must be presuming there was just one she wanted.

He yawned again.

"What else would you like to know, Rabbit?"

"Why does saffron cost so much?"

"It is such a tiny part of the crocus bloom, and it's so much trouble to get it from the flower to the cook. So, the cost is high."

"Right," she said, "the stamen of the crocus."

"No, not the stamen," he answered. "The stigma."

"What are you talking about? Crocuses have stigma?"

He let out a little laugh at her question.

"I would have thought you'd know this, Dr. Anatomy," he said. "The female part of the flower that receives the pollen – the female receptacle – it is called *the stigma.* The stigma is female."

"The female is stigma! Fucking patriarchy," she said, hoping that would make him laugh, and it did. "Anyway, I don't do plants, I do animals."

"Well, now you know: saffron is of the stigma, not stamen. Let *me* ask *you* something," he said. "What is your favorite commercial packaging for saffron?"

"Well, I don't think I've ever bought it, but in terms of what I see at stores, I think I like it best when it comes in one of those tiny little glass vials, as if it is a special medicine. That's so much better than the little paper envelopes, which look just so much like what moist towelettes come in. The envelope-style packaging takes away from what I think must be the joy of the formal ritual of using saffron. The tiny little glass vials in the bigger glass herb jar are the best, don't you think?"

"Absolutely," he said. "Now you are making sense."

They said nothing for a while, but she had the feeling, with his nose being near the top of her head, that he was breathing her in.

If only he were not so hung up on such a foolish notion of sex. By the time she would take off her pajamas he would have an erection if he didn't have one already, and she could just climb aboard and relieve them both.

And yet, for a reason she could not articulate to herself, this spooning with him was strangely satisfying, in the most pleasantly carnal way. Perhaps if Adam and Eve had had this – a warm bed with two blankets, a dark-night conversation about the packaging of saffron – then all the trouble of being human might have been averted. "Knowledge" could have come to mean more than a euphemism for that feeling right before an orgasm.

"Wolf, how do you know when you *know enough* about something to draw a conclusion?"

"Do you mean how does *one* know when *one* knows enough, or how do *I*, John Wolf, know when *I* know enough?"

"How do you, John Wolf, know when you know enough to draw a conclusion – about a crime? For example?"

"I know that I know enough," he said, "when I know I can say what I know out loud in a calm and steady voice, in complete sentences."

She did not answer.

There was, for a moment, the sound of a single plane flying overhead.

"How do *you* know when *you* know enough, Madeleine Shanks?" Wolf asked.

"I don't normally think of myself as intellectually immature, Wolf," she answered. "But today, on my way home from New York, I realized I don't know the answer to that. That was why I was asking you."

The sound of the plane faded out.

"But then," he said, "then shall I know even as also I am known."

"Corinthians, 1-13," she replied as if taking a test, and she could feel him nod.

He let out a long and sleepy sigh.

She dragged a net through her brain and caught the contextual verses, still there, still in her memory. She spoke them aloud as if reading from the book at mass:

"For now we shall see through a glass, darkly; but then face to face. Now I know in part, but then shall I know even as also I am known. And now abideth faith, hope, charity, these three; but the greatest of these is charity."

257

"Sometimes translated as 'love,'" he answered. "Sometimes it is translated as faith, hope, and love."

She smiled in the dark, understanding in this moment why it could be that *charity* and *love* would be understood the same concept. *Charity-lobster, provenance unknown.*

"I think that Saint Paul was wrong on this one," he told her, in a very sleepy voice. "I think that, of faith, hope, and charity – or of faith, hope, and love – one is *not* the greatest. One of those three is not the greatest of the three. They are all the same."

"They are all the same?" she asked. "You mean they are all of the same level of importance, or that they are all the same thing? Faith, hope, and love?"

"The same thing, Rabbit. Faith, hope, and love – they are all one and the same thing." He brushed her hair off her neck. "Think on that for us, and I will go back to sleep for both of us."

He was soon lightly snoring again. She, too, started to fall back to sleep. But there – just on the other side of her eyelids – there was Maggie Lovisa. She was still in her jar, but now she was dressed in the black-and-white habit of the West Virginian sisters, reading to Maddy from the hymnal:

For now we shall see through a glass, darkly; but then face to face. Now I know in part, but then shall I know even as also I am known.

Maddy woke like a cork surfacing from waters deep.

-23-

Four days later, Wolf came in his back door at the end of his workday to find Father Tad sitting at the kitchen table reading from his prayer book. Hunter could soon be heard coming from the living room to greet Wolf, the tags on the dog's collar jingling lightly.

"Good evening, John," said the priest, closing the volume and looking up.

"Hello, Father," Wolf answered, furrowing his brow and petting Hunter on the head. He turned and put his keys and wallet on the counter along with the few items that had come in the mail. (He no longer had to remind himself not to put his gun there.)

"Maddy must have let you in, Father?" Wolf asked.

"Yes, John," replied Father Tad, holding one finger up to his lips. "Shhh. She wasn't feeling well. She's asleep on the couch. She asked me to come and walk her home from the museum this afternoon," he explained in a quiet voice.

The priest stood up, walked over to the refrigerator, opened it, and pulled out a butcher-wrapped package. He handed the package to Wolf and closed the fridge door.

"Maddy said we had to stop and get some groceries because she had told you she would get the food on the way home. I told her that I could walk her and Hunter home and then go get whatever you needed. But she said I would get the wrong kind of chicken – that you are 'particular' about your chicken."

Wolf nodded, still looking confused.

"This seems like unnecessarily expensive chicken," said the priest. "She also said we had to get the ingredients for 'green goddess' dressing. That didn't sound like your kind of thing to me – green goddess dressing."

"No, she is right," Wolf said. "I found a recipe in a cooking magazine she gave me. It's very good with roast chicken and vegetables. It has fresh herbs. It's creamy."

Wolf wondered why it sounded like he was apologizing for the sin of a condiment.

He opened the brown butcher paper and looked at the fresh chicken, poking it a little through the cellophane wrapper on the inside. It looked just right. Hunter was below him, his nose in the air picking up the scent of the raw bird meat.

"John," Father Tad asked, "why is she still here?"

When it was clear Wolf wasn't going to answer, the priest reminded him confession was available the next day. Wolf tried not to look annoyed. But his body language conveyed the truth – that he was not interested in apologizing for particular types of chicken or creamy salad dressing or for any other charity toward Maddy. He put the meat back in the refrigerator and checked to make sure Maddy had gotten some buttermilk. She had.

"Father, why didn't Maddy call me to get her home, instead of you?"

"She told me she didn't want to bother you at work," answered Father Tad. "It was no trouble for me, John – I did have to skip a meeting this afternoon to go get her, but it was not a gathering I wanted to attend. The bingo ladies are having a dispute, and they wanted me to mediate it. Only they don't really want me to mediate it – they want me to take sides."

The priest went back to the table and picked up his prayer book. He did not sit back down.

"Will you be staying for dinner, Father?" Wolf asked, walking over to the kitchen doorway and leaning into the living room. He could see Maddy on the couch under a blanket, not moving.

"I would like to stay, John, but I'm afraid I should get back. Mrs. Rojewski is expecting me for supper at the rectory, and she will be miffed if I cancel now."

"Maddy asked you to stay here at the house, until I got home?"

The priest nodded as he put on his jacket. Wolf saw him out the back

260

door, locked it, got himself a tall glass of tap water, and drank it down slowly. He told Hunter with a nod of his head and a verbal command to go back to Maddy, and the dog followed his order. Wolf looked through the mail. There was a letter addressed to Maddy from a Bess McFarlane, from an address in North Carolina. He wondered if it was, in fact, a letter from The Jerk, sent under a fake address. But the postmark did read North Carolina. He resisted the urge to open it.

Then he noticed the answering machine blinking with a new message and pushed the button to play it back.

"It's Jimmy again," said the unfamiliar man's voice. "Listen, if you're serious about looking into it all, call me." There was a pause. "I hope you're not fucking with me."

Same basic message as yesterday, only a little more urgent sounding.

Wolf had asked around at work today to see if anyone knew of a Jimmy who might be trying to reach him. But no one did. Even though it was the second call of its type to his machine, it still felt like a wrong-number dial to him. The only Jimmy he knew had a relatively high-pitched voice. This man didn't.

He drew and drank a half-glass more of tap water, went into the living room where Hunter was lying by the coffee table, and sat down on the edge of the couch, right next to Maddy's hip. He put his hand on her forehead. Her temperature seemed normal – she wasn't hot or cold, not sweaty or clammy. He pulled her hand out from under the blanket and felt her pulse. Normal.

She was stirring at his touch.

"What's going on, Rabbit?" he asked, putting his hand on her cheek. His hand was still cold from the outdoors, and he hoped it would wake her enough to get an answer. "Father said you weren't feeling well."

She opened her eyes and squinted a little, looking at him.

"I passed out at the museum," she said, closing her eyes again as if her lids were too heavy to stay up. "Twice, I guess. I thought I'd better come home."

"That's not good," he said. "I mean, it's good you came home. But not good you passed out."

He thought back to the morning and remembered that Maddy had eaten a good breakfast – he had been getting up early to make her big breakfasts since her trip to New York, after Liz's visit and his own trip north. Maddy certainly hadn't complained of this new big-breakfast morning routine. She had been finishing off plates as large as the one he had made her the first time she arrived at his house, that night in the rain.

And he knew she had taken a sandwich of leftover roast turkey for lunch that day – so it could not have been that she had passed out from hunger. Yet neither did she seem to be vividly ill.

"Hey, Rabbit, why do you think you passed out?" he asked, putting his hand on her forehead again.

"Dr. Wilhelm," she said. "He said I had a seizure, and I should go to the hospital with him."

She seemed still half asleep – so groggy. A small drip of drool hung at the corner of her mouth.

"A seizure?" said Wolf. "Then you *should* have gone to the hospital, Rabbit."

"They kill people at the hospital, Wolf," said Maddy, still without opening her eyes.

Now she took her hands up to her head and rubbed her face like she was trying to wake herself up. But it did not seem to work. She put her hands back down next to her sides.

"Is Hunter here?" she asked, with her eyes closed.

"Yes, he's here," answered Wolf.

"You staying too?" she asked.

"I'm not going anywhere. Why don't you sleep longer," he said, tucking the blanket around her torso, "and I'll make the chicken and all, and wake you up when it's ready?"

She did not answer. She seemed to have already fallen back asleep.

He took her pulse one more time. His touch added to the dream she was having, of being under water, in the weedy pool of an estuary in the midst of an incoming tide, her trying to look up to see him as he reached down from above to fish about for her wrist. She was trying to open her eyes in the muddy water.

...

She finally placed the feeling: Nocturnal Adoration. That strange and wonderful moment of standing out on the driveway of her childhood home on Long Island, the neighborhood so completely silent, and looking up at the stars in the black of the night. Her father would come out of the house soon, to let her into the car, to go over to their church, to enact the bizarre Roman Catholic ritual of the little all-night-long prayer brigade that volunteered to adore the exposed communion wafer, displayed so carefully on the altar as if it really were the Body of Christ, with call-and-response prayers. Every hour through the night manned by a different little group charged with the shift work.

Her father liked to sign up for the three a.m. to four a.m. shift for some reason. And, unlike her mother and sister, Maddy liked to go. She liked to go for just this moment – the moment before and after church of standing on the driveway, in the silence, adoring the stars. Adoring the structure of the universe. She could feel in her skin and her nerves the erotic thrill of *the idea*. But what idea?

The idea, she figured now, that she could see the true structure of the universe – see it not because she was brilliant, or godly, just because she had fully accepted her humanity.

How funny to have this same sense of wonder, of erotic thrill, in an ordinary Philadelphia bar. Above her was not the universe of stars, but cheap, faux-stained-glass, ceiling light fixtures. Around her was not the open night air, but the overheated, beer-soaked atmosphere of this place. And instead of silence, there was Bobby singing a song a few feet from the table, strumming on his guitar and gazing at her, his mic a little too loud.

Nevertheless, in the dreamy buzz that she figured must be the after-effect of whatever Dr. Wilhelm had slipped into her sandwich or her soda to make it look like she had had a seizure – perhaps some drug capable of giving her an actual seizure – she knew, in fact, she was experiencing the same thing – *the idea* of the universe. The relinquishing of herself to the awesome beauty of the truth.

She must have had a look of amazement on her face, to have Bobby looking at her that way, singing as if to her. He must have misunderstood utterly why she was looking this way, with him thinking she was so deeply moved by him and his music, not realizing that her wonder came from what she could see now in her mind's eye: the steady mapping out of the data points of Wilhelm's acquisition of the bodies, as if tracing the constellation Sagittarius, the centaur archer. The arrow being drawn back on the bow.... (Her father would come soon to unlock the car.)

Yes, this buzz, this post-drug buzz – that and the photocopy from Bess. It was all Maddy needed to know for sure. Now she knew for sure that Wilhelm had killed patients for their bodies. And that he must have by now definitely figured, given the actions he was taking against her, that she knew what he had done.

And somehow in this moment, because of the dog *Canis Major*, she knew, too, that what she felt in her for Wolf was love. Which meant she was capable of love after all. How funny! Who cared that it might all not lead to anything? Who cared that she might not ever be able to figure out exactly how Wilhelm had done it all, or to prove what Wilhelm had done? Who cared that Wolf might not feel the same, or that it could never lead to anything more than this extraordinary expansive sensation, or that it might be gone tomorrow? Here it was.

How beautiful – how absolutely exquisite – was the structure of the universe when beheld by a person abandoned to her full humanity.

Hunter stirred a little and flopped over to lay his head on her feet. She reached down under the bar table and scratched him behind the ear, and he lifted his head a little in acknowledgment. The way that dog looked at her, with deep affection, was exactly how she felt about him. Indeed, she thought now, it was the realization of her quick and primal expanding love for Hunter that had made her realize what she was feeling with Wolf.

Sitting next to her, Wolf reached his right hand to Maddy's face and pulled her lower eyelid down a little to look at her pupil. She said nothing. There was no point in telling him that she was dopey and stupid and labile because of whatever Dr. Wilhelm had slipped in her turkey sandwich or her drink. That little attempt by Wilhelm wasn't the thing that mattered. The thing that mattered was that through this attempt to get her to the hospital, Wilhelm had completely destroyed the null hypothesis.

She would tell Wolf soon, after she figured out *just a little more*.

He had seen her (yawning over the plate of chicken) open the envelope from Bess that he handed her, her eyes growing wide on seeing the photocopy contained there. There it all was: the same jagged edges; the old stain on the third page; the smudged lines of print on the fifth page. Everything but her own fingerprint. There was all the proof it was that the "original" of Schlesinger 1888 at the New York Public was in fact the same "original" that had been in Wilhelm's own library before the supposed fire.

To be sure that she was not remembering the New York Public version incorrectly, she left the dinner table suddenly, ran upstairs, and retrieved from her desk the photographs she had had printed at the drug store from the disposable camera. When she came back down to the table, Wolf had the photocopy and envelope from Bess in his hands. He was obviously trying to understand why this photocopy of a nineteenth-century text would have her so agitated – why someone would have mailed her this from

North Carolina. She grabbed the photocopy pages from him and compared them to the photographs. There was the absolute proof: the crumbled edges matched. It all matched.

There was but one reason Wilhelm would have moved this text from his collection in Philadelphia to the library in New York: to make it look like the backstory he had been telling was real. Nobody else was ever going to check the New York Public version against the remaining photocopies of the Wilhelm library version. Nobody but an historian was going to think about the provenance.

Nobody checks anything he says, said Jimmy.

She almost told Wolf. She almost held up the index finger of her right hand, to tell him what she had done with that finger at the New York Public. But no, this was not the moment – she needed to clean up her argument first.

She put her finger back down in her lap. She needed to rouse herself fully out of this stupor and put it all into a clearer, more elegant presentation than what she had composed so far. Something Wolf could immediately appreciate, the way he had her dissertation. Something Officer Snotty could not doubt.

She knew that, as with Wolf's ongoing nightly reading of her expanding dissertation manuscript, he was going to *question* parts of what she said about Wilhelm – ask her if this or that claim was the *only possible* explanation, ask her if she could trace how this body got from here to there. So, she would have to be careful, before giving this to him to hold in his hands, to make it as strong as it could possibly be.

Honestly – she acknowledged to herself now – she also wanted this glorious moment alone with her findings, the moment of revelatory bliss that comes *before* the world sees what you've found – the Edenic moment in which you know you've birthed something new, something meaningful, something unlike anything else. To hold the babe in her arms before life's inevitable questions and challenges.

Yes, she realized now – with the warmth of Hunter turning her ankle so hot it felt almost sweaty – it was *just like* the lines from Revelations – the lines they would read at Nocturnal Adoration, the passage that always sounded like it was written by the homeless schizophrenic who would hang out near Mario's, where her mother got the Saturday pizza –

And there appeared a great wonder in heaven; a woman clothed with the sun, and the moon under her feet, and upon her head a crown of twelve stars. And she being with child, travailing in birth, and pained to be delivered. And there appeared another wonder in heaven; and behold a great red dragon, having seven heads and ten horns, and seven crowns upon his head. And his tail drew the third part of the stars of heaven, and did cast them to the earth; and the dragon stood before the woman which was ready to be delivered, for to devour her child as soon as it was born.

She wanted to hold the whole new work, what would be her perfectly revised study of Wilhelm, before they devoured it. Before Officer Snotty and the policewoman and Wes and Manny and Neller and Wolf pulled out their forks and knives to see if they could swallow it.

Tomorrow she would wake fully out of this drugged fog and call Jimmy and tell him he was right. She would tell him that her work in the last few days since she had met him in New York had borne out their suspicions. That there was a clear pattern of patients with particularly interesting conditions dying either under Wilhelm's care at the hospital or when he was in close proximity. That three of the families that she had reached in the last couple of days had death certificates that showed causes of death inconsistent with what Wilhelm had reported on the cases in his own grant report and publications. There was only one reason he would be lying about the causes of death. She was sure when she got more of the death certificates, she would find more.

Someone behind her suddenly reached an open bottle of beer over her shoulder, as if to hand it to her. She tilted her head back to see it was Wes. He still had his coat on. Before Maddy could react, Wolf reached over and took the beer and put it on the table in front of himself.

"Not tonight," he said to Wes, without further explanation.

Maddy looked at Wolf and caught his gaze.

"Have you ever realized," she asked Wolf, "how *beautiful* the universe is when you see the whole thing?"

"What the hell are you *on*, woman?" Wolf asked, again pulling down the skin below her eye.

-24-

As she walked to the museum the next morning, Hunter by her side, Maddy realized she had forgotten how annoying money in her shoe could be. The twenty-dollar bill she had stuck in her right dress boot between her sock and the inner sole was starting to chafe at her foot's arch. And she could hear Liz's voice in her head saying, *Seriously, Mad Girl — like twenty fucking dollars is going to save you?*

But it was just an old habit, sticking some money in her shoe when she was going to be in a risky place. Her mother had made Maddy and her sister do this when they went into the city alone, each put a twenty in a shoe, so that if they got mugged, they'd have some money. "Mad money" she called it, and Maddy always wondered about the meaning of "mad" in this phrasing.

When she had first arrived in Philadelphia, she never would have thought that the museum was going to become a place that made her feel the need of mad money. The streets on the way there or on the way back, maybe. But not the museum itself.

Now she took the opportunity of a sudden widening in the sidewalk in front of a men's clothing shop to pull herself and Hunter out of the pedestrian flow, to pause. She crouched down to talk to the dog.

"Listen, Hunter," she said.

He stared into her eyes very intently. He held his head quite still, but his back half remained a little jittery. She could tell he was feeling, as she was, the wake of the commuters passing by.

"I need you to stay near me all the time today – do you understand?"

His ears moved forward a little and he licked his lips on the left side.

"Hunter, I need you to make sure you *understand* you have to *protect* me. The last thing I want is for Wolf to find out what I've written on my arm. If I get hurt, he's going to find out. And then he's going to be *really angry* with me for not talking to him sooner."

As if Hunter could read, she pulled up her sleeve and showed the dog what she had penned that morning on her left forearm, just above her wrist, in large letters, in blue permanent marker: *Emergency contact Det. John Wolf,* along with his phone number at the station.

"Be a good protector," she said giving Hunter a kiss on the top of his head, feeling his ears part a little to accept her kiss. "Be a good dog."

She stood up and started them back on the walk to the museum. The feel of Hunter's gait on the leash recalled to her the awkward moment last night when they were walking back from the bar from Bobby's show. Wolf had said something about Wes and then something about Bobby, but Maddy did not respond to either remark. The remarks seemed to her to be tossed-off and odd apologies from Wolf, and she had been busy wondering about whether drugs given to someone in the last moments of life might survive fluid preservation in a jar or somehow persist within a skeletal specimen.

Then Wolf had looked over at Maddy walking Hunter and had said to her in what seemed to Maddy a too-formal tone, "I am quite glad that Robert gives you good company."

Maddy had looked at him briefly and had almost said "you mean Hunter," but had decided it best to bring no attention to the slip. But soon she could tell by the way Wolf cleared his throat that he had realized that he had just called the dog by Bobby's father's name.

Finally, ten steps later, she had realized what she should say, and she said it: "He's a real *dog*, Wolf!"

And Wolf let out a snort-laugh.

"Thank you, Rabbit."

She had handed him the leash. She had thought about telling him that she wished he would sleep with her tonight as he had the night she had come home from New York a few days before. But she had so appreciated everything he had said to her that night, about her strength, she didn't want him to think her weak. And she had spent much of last night thinking about what they were going to do if he slept in her bed again and, in their sleep, something happened that Wolf would quickly regret.

Plus, part of Wolf's purpose in taking Hunter from Bobby had obviously been to help Maddy sleep *without* Wolf. And Maddy had managed to convince Hunter in the middle of the night to ignore his training to stay off the furniture and come up on the bed and sleep next to her, where she could put her arm over him. She could sleep with Hunter that way again tonight.

She wondered if Wolf had seen her sleeping like that – with Hunter in the bed – and if that was why he had slipped on the walk home and called Hunter "Robert."

A block short of the museum, they passed another dog on a leash, and Hunter gave the other dog a sniff and then looked up at Maddy.

"Good boy," she said, feeling like he was looking for reassurance that he had his loyalty right.

Her plan today was to ask Shirley out to lunch – to eat out in public, where nobody could put anything in her food or drink easily – and to try to figure out what Shirley knew and didn't know. Today, she thought, she needed to work on that part of the Wilhelm research. It seemed to Maddy an important part of the puzzle and she had been swinging back and forth, in her midnight musings, between thinking that Shirley was just a dupe to the idea that Shirley was in on the whole thing – that, in fact, Shirley had been the intruder, the attacker. But she realized the latter idea made no sense; the intruder had clearly had a male build and was skinnier than Shirley. He also moved much faster than she figured Shirley could. And he moved like a male – something about the sexed motion of the human pelvis?

Hunter trotted up the front steps of the museum in front of her, knowing where they were going. She followed behind him, saying only a quick hello to the person at the front desk and heading down the stairs to the room she had been using as her office. Just coming into the doorway of her little space, she could see Shirley there, packing Maddy's things into a file box.

"Shirley?" said Maddy, stopping just inside the door. "What's up? What are you doing?"

Shirley turned and Maddy tried to read her face. Uncharacteristically, she was wearing all black. Her lips were pursed, and she was breathing audibly through her nose.

"You need to go, Maddy," said Shirley.

Maddy could feel Hunter looking up at her waiting for a clue about what he was supposed to do. He was obviously picking up on the irregularity of the situation and Maddy's sudden tension.

Shirley continued her task of collecting Maddy's books and papers into the box.

Watching her, Maddy felt immediately relieved that she had not left any of her research on Wilhelm here – not since when Liz had been here and Shirley had walked in and seen Maddy had Wilhelm's grant reports. After that, Maddy had been careful to keep that material at Wolf's place.

But Shirley obviously had some reason to be kicking Maddy out.

Hunter let out a whine and Maddy looked down at him. He turned his head as if to point to the hallway. There was Dr. Wilhelm.

"Feeling better than when you lost consciousness yesterday, Miss Shanks?"

Maddy grabbed Hunter by the collar and retreated into the room. She wished she didn't look as alarmed as she was.

"What's going on, Shirley?" Maddy asked again.

"We can't have you here, Maddy," said Shirley, looking not at Maddy but at Dr. Wilhelm who was now standing just inside the doorway. The room felt so crowded with the three of them and the dog. "If you have a problem with a seizure disorder – and a dog for it – *a dog* – well, the liability."

"Yes, the liability," said Dr. Wilhelm, nodding. "The medical society must think about the liability. And if you won't go to the hospital when a reasonable person would, well."

"I see," said Maddy.

Hunter gave a small march in place as if he felt the need to make a movement but was uncertain where to go.

"Sit, Hunter," Maddy said, releasing his collar.

The dog did as commanded, and Maddy moved to help Shirley collect the last of her things into the box.

"I'm sorry, Maddy," said Shirley without looking up.

"Well, I'm not sure how I'm going to get this heavy box back home with my backpack and Hunter, Shirley. Cabdrivers won't like to take a dog, I think."

"I have a grocery cart in my office you can borrow!" Shirley said, with a glimmer of her old helpful self. "Come with me."

She took Maddy by the hand, as if Maddy didn't know where Shirley's office was, pulling Maddy past Dr. Wilhelm and down the hall. Hunter came close behind them.

"Maddy, Maddy, Maddy," said Shirley, as soon as they were in her office and out of earshot of Dr. Wilhelm. She released Maddy's hand and grabbed her folded grocery cart from next to a bookcase and gave it to Maddy. "Listen, I need this back, and you should specifically bring it back to me at seven tonight, here."

"But the museum will be locked up then, Shirley," said Maddy.

Shirley glanced at the doorway.

"Just come then to the side door – I will let you in."

She said it in a near-whisper. Then she added, in a much louder voice, "I'm sorry, Maddy, but you know, liability. And you have enough material to go finish your dissertation in Indiana."

She nodded at Maddy.

"Okay, Shirley," answered Maddy, nodding back. "I'm sorry to have been a burden. I apologize for that."

Holding the handle of the wheeled cart in her right hand, Maddy wrapped her other arm up and around Shirley's back, to give her a fast hug.

Maddy did it not to bestow a gesture of warmth, but to see how Shirley reacted.

Shirley's response – the uncomfortably hard embrace you give to someone who is kin, the kind of hug that feels like a marking – told Maddy what she needed to know.

...

Good thing for the power of prayer, Maddy thought cynically to herself as she waited for Shirley to open the door to her and Hunter. On a normal night, Maddy would have had to explain to Wolf why she was going out with Hunter in the evening for an indeterminate amount of time. But Wolf had told her over breakfast that morning that Father Tad insisted Wolf come for dinner at the rectory so they could then go together to the hospital to visit Wolf's wife and pray together. This meant she would likely be back home before him, and, even if she were a few minutes late coming back from seeing Shirley, she could just say she had been out walking Hunter.

Or she might finally tell him what was going on? She might pull her draft report and her key Wilhelm files out of the upper cabinets in his kitchen, pull them out from where she had just stashed them behind the popcorn popper and the pressure cooker, and finally show him what she had?

When was Shirley going to open this door?

After being sent home by Shirley that morning, Maddy had spent most of the day cleaning Wolf's house. She wasn't sure what else to do, finding herself back home by ten a.m. after being ejected from the museum. There was just so much work she could do on her written Wilhelm thesis, since she had to make changes on the paper copy; there being no printer here, she could not make changes on the computer and then reprint it all before Wolf returned from the hospital.

She wondered if Wolf was going to notice all the tidying-up when he got home. The margin between how he kept house and how clean she could get it was thin, but she thought she'd done a good job cleaning the insides of all the kitchen cabinets and the oven. He might notice that she had dusted and neatened all his books in the living room, too, and had washed the insides of the windows, all except in his bedroom.

She told herself all this cleaning was the least she could do after the money and effort he had put into having her. But she knew she was doing it because she had to do something physical as she formulated and jotted down more of her argument behind her Wilhelm thesis. Something about the odor of the vinegar and water solution she was using on the wooden cabinets – the solution they used to use in the convent on the floors – it felt right for the mental list of questions for Shirley that she found herself composing, questions she would ask Shirley that night back at the museum. And it was the cleaning of the kitchen cabinets that gave Maddy an idea of where to stash the important Wilhelm material while she was gone to the museum tonight. She didn't want to leave all that work out, just in case someone broke in while she and Wolf were both gone. And there was no way Wolf was going to randomly look in those cabinets. She knew that nowadays he made popcorn in a regular pot with a lid – he made fun of people who made popcorn with a dedicated device, the way he made fun of people using a special tool to mince garlic.

She had paused, between emptying and refilling the cleaning bucket and jotting notes on the paper copy, to try to reach Liz by phone a few times. But she got no answer on the first two passes and reached only Margie on the third. By around four o'clock she had also pulled out her suitcase and started to pack, starting with the dressier items she knew she wasn't going to wear again on this trip. She also worked on packing non-essential books and papers into two boxes she could ship back to herself. It made sense to go ahead and start packing her things, she thought. Who could tell how soon after Wolf heard about her exile from the museum and her Wilhelm research that Wolf would say it was time she go?

Liz finally called back around five.

"I'm headed home soon, Lizard, back to Bloomington," Maddy said, trying to say it brightly. "Wrapping up things here."

"Everything okay?" Liz asked. "What happened in New York? I know I should have called you, but everything was so crazy when I got back and – "

"Pretty sure there's something there, Liz. Schlesinger 1888, pretty clear it is a fake – "

Maddy ignored Liz's exclamation.

"— anyway, I'm going to turn it all over to the police and head home."

"Good," said Liz. "That's the right thing. Let someone else attempt repeatability – see if you are right. Let it go. Come finish your diss. Take care of that. You know when you're coming – which train? Want me to pick you up in Indy?"

"Not sure which train yet, but I thought I'd ask Colin to get me in Indy," said Maddy as she pulled out the bag of dog food to give Hunter dinner. "Been a long time since I got laid. We can catch up in the car and get the niceties out of the way on the drive."

"Yeah, I did send Professor Butterfly the chopsticks through campus mail, so presumably he'll remember who you are," Liz replied.

Then there was a pause as they both took in the awkwardness of what Liz had just said.

Liz moved them past the gap by asking how Wolf was. Maddy overrode the instinct to answer that she had come to conclude that he smelled better than any dish she could imagine, and that a recent trip to the gym with him suggested that, while the average person might wish to spend nights on a warm beach lying under Ursa Minor, Maddy would much prefer a night under Wolf's pectoralis major. She hoped Colin's body wasn't going to feel too wrong – too thin, too academic.

Now she rolled her head around her neck and looked at her watch – five after seven. Where was Shirley?

Funny, Maddy thought, how sex had become her default mode for distraction during times of stress. Must be, she thought, some primal instinct, something urging her to the would-be reproductive path in the face of threat? Thank god for reliable IUDs.

Hunter had grown tired of standing next to her outside the side door, so he sat down. Realizing that perhaps Shirley was waiting for Maddy to knock, Maddy did, four times, rather quietly. The door opened and Shirley took the folded grocery cart from Maddy and closed the door rapidly, as soon as Maddy and Hunter were in. Shirley had on just one small light in this big reception room next to the garden, and Maddy could see only glimpses of faces from the great murals on the walls.

"You're late," said Shirley.

"I was standing out there waiting for you to open the damned door."

"Why the hell wouldn't you knock?! Someone might have seen you."

It wasn't like Shirley to yell at Maddy, or anyone.

"I'm sorry, Mad," said Shirley, walking across the room towards the doorway that led to the stairs down to the basement level. "I'm stressed out. Let's go break into the brain-softening medicine in my office. I have some Punt e Mes we can throw over some ice, if whoever used the ice tray last filled it."

Maddy hesitated. Shirley certainly didn't seem to be faking it – and there was that hug that morning –

From the other side of the room, Shirley turned to ask Maddy what she was just standing there for.

"Is Dr. Wilhelm in the building, Shirl?"

"Of course not!" answered Shirley. "Are you *crazy*? I told him this afternoon that I was going away for a few days, to go attend to a sick friend. I don't know what I'm going to do. I thought you could help me figure that out."

"Okay," said Maddy, now following Shirley down to her office, with Hunter at her side. "It's just that yesterday..."

"Yeah," said Shirley, stopping in the small common room with the refrigerator to grab two mugs and fill them with ice, "you assuming the same I am? That he slipped you something? Probably went with some traditional herb, knowing him. A good old-fashioned toxin like belladonna."

"No hallucinations," replied Maddy. "Not belladonna."

Now they were in Shirley's office. Shirley pulled open a filing drawer and retrieved the bottle of sweet vermouth.

"I keep the bottle filed under 'intestinal parasites; traditional treatments for.'"

She poured them each a generous serving over the ice and they sat down on either side of her desk.

"Did I seize?" Maddy asked, giving Hunter an order to lie down. She waited to see Shirley drink before taking a sip herself.

Shirley shook her head no, swallowed, and took another drink.

"You simply passed out – twice. Needless to say, I understood why you didn't want to go to the hospital."

"Did you tell him that I was looking at his grant reports, and that I'd gone to New York?"

"I told him that the day before, Maddy," said Shirley. "I felt I had to tell him – but I should not have. Obviously."

"So, you helped me call Father Tad?"

Shirley nodded. "It wasn't easy to figure out who you were telling me to call, but eventually I got it. I remembered you had said you spent a couple of years in a convent – you know, back when you told me that, I thought you were joking. But then I remembered that you had been in a convent, and I figured you really were asking me to call a guy who is a priest!"

Shirley had drained her cup and poured herself more.

"Sort of sucks without the orange slice. Sweet vermouth is supposed to be served with a nice orange slice, Maddy, if you drink it this way – straight."

"Well," said Maddy, "I'm hungry. Let's order in something that comes with orange slices."

"You're a genius!" said Shirley. Then she added, almost as if talking to herself, "And that's why Dr. Wilhelm slipped you something."

Maddy moved Shirley's phone toward her. Just in case, she wanted to be fully in control of the food.

"How about Szechuan Wok?" Maddy asked. "Got the number?"

Shirley opened her top desk drawer, rifled through the business cards scattered there, and handed Maddy the one for Szechuan Wok. Maddy dialed and was immediately put on hold by the person who answered the phone.

"Whatever the drug was, Shirl," Maddy said, covering the receiver with the palm of her hand, "it felt like the proof. Plus, I sure did get a nice buzz, and a great night's sleep."

She thought back to the night of sleeping with Wolf, once again; he said he was worried about her sleepy, goofy behavior and asked if would be okay with her if he slept next to her again. She only hoped she hadn't done anything awkward in the middle of the night.

"Make sure you order the orange slices on the side, Maddy," Shirley said standing up and bending over to retrieve a copier-paper box, putting it on her desk. "I don't want soy sauce in my vermouth."

"What's in the box?"

Shirley took off the lid. Maddy stood up to look through the contents.

"I found that list on your desk, of the things you still wanted to look at here for your dissertation," Shirley answered. "So, I spent today after you left photocopying all those for you – well, almost all of them. There were a couple I didn't find. I know it's a big box – I can just ship it to you in Indiana, or wherever you want. I didn't want you to – to – "

"Oh my God," said Maddy. "You are just the best."

"Thank you, miss, we try," said the host on the line. "You want take-out or delivery?"

-25-

Shirley handed Hunter another piece of beef. He was hanging close to Shirley, lying next to her leg, because Maddy wouldn't give him any of her share. The three of them were on the floor in the main exhibit hall, Maddy and Shirley leaning up against the cabinets that contained the collection of various items retrieved from bodies after death – bullet fragments, a shark's tooth, and a tiny, inhaled toy car.

It wasn't a big room, but in the quiet of the museum being closed, it felt larger than it ordinarily did. Shirley had turned on just a few of the cabinet lights when Maddy asked if they could eat their dinner in this room. She told Shirley honestly that she regretted spending so much time here with the texts and not enough with the bodies. She could tell, though, that Hunter didn't feel comfortable amidst the smell of so many bodies. He kept squirming and looking to Maddy.

"Do you suppose," Maddy asked, "Dr. Wilhelm is going to make it hard for me to work at all anatomy museums now?"

"Depends what happens next, I suppose," answered Shirley, using her disposable chopsticks to push some of the General Tso's chicken onto her paper plate and handing the container over to Maddy. "You're not the kind of historian doctors like. I told you, they want you to record their glory, like an angelic scribe. Instead, you've decided to pursue the idea that Dr. Wilhelm is – that he is – "

"A serial murderer," said Maddy. "The exact diagnostic term finally came to me after I thought about it, after I talked to Jimmy Heathcote."

Maddy had already told Shirley while they were waiting for the delivery about her conversation with Jimmy in New York, about the Schlesinger 1888 at the public library, and about the death records that didn't match the causes of death named for various patients in Dr. Wilhelm's grant reports. She had also told Shirley what she knew about the circumstances surrounding Nick DesJardins' death.

"I still wonder, Shirley, if Nick's death was my fault – because I told Dr. Wilhelm that Nick was going to leave his body to Cleveland."

"Yes, Maddy, it's your fault," said Shirley, dishing herself more rice. "It's definitely your fault that Dr. Wilhelm murdered somebody."

Maddy could detect the sarcasm in her voice.

"Aren't you scared, Shirley? I mean of him?"

"I know I ought to be more scared than I am," answered Shirley, "particularly given what happened to you yesterday. But I have this notion he wouldn't touch me because – because he thinks I will defend him."

"Will you?"

Shirley didn't answer the question. She was staring up at a cabinet that contained a fetal series showing the development of the human from near conception to full-term, a jarred set of specimens taken from a combination of miscarriages and intentional abortions.

"It's funny, isn't it, Maddy," Shirley said, pointing her chopsticks to that cabinet. "We develop, bit by bit, month after month, and we never know when we will suddenly end. The nice thing about Dr. Wilhelm's approach seems to be that he makes it quick, you know? That's how I'd like to go – quick."

Maddy couldn't tell if she was serious now.

"Shirley," Maddy said, pointing her own chopsticks to a different cabinet, one holding the skeleton of a male giant standing next to the skeleton of a female dwarf, "I've read that that display used to consist of the woman with dwarfism holding, in the open palm of her hand, the skull of the fetus she was pregnant with when she died in childbirth. Why isn't she posed like that anymore, with her fetus's skull held in her hand?"

Shirley let out a snort that made Hunter cock his head at her.

"We got in trouble for it. They said it was insensitive. You know what,

Maddy? When I started working here, we could all luxuriate in the fascination with the abnormal forms of the human body – we could party with the pathological, dress up the teratological, to enjoy the absurdity of the human condition. Now we are only allowed to stare and celebrate the *beautiful* and the *perfect* in our culture – and we must treat all the abnormality as if it is a terrible *tragedy*. I'm no good at that. I can see the pain and the suffering, but I just can't see the tragedy. I think it's all grand."

Seeing Hunter poke his nose at Shirley to ask for more food, Maddy called him over to lie down closer to her. He got up and reluctantly moved to Maddy's side.

"Dr. Wilhelm thinks they're all tragic, of course," said Shirley, "and it should all be prevented. Prevention, sure, I suppose. But there are always going to be the abnormal among us."

Maddy observed aloud that at the dinner at Dr. Wilhelm's house, it had sounded like Shirley had agreed with him and Dr. Tate.

"I am perhaps sometimes too quick, Maddy, to say what I think they want me to say? You are not very good at that."

Maddy nodded and asked Shirley if she could pass her anything. Shirley answered that if there were any pot-stickers left, she'd take one, and Maddy passed her the tin of that dish. Maddy shoveled some rice into her own mouth.

"You know, Maddy, Dr. Wilhelm gave me checks over the years."

Maddy had her mouth full, so all she could utter was, "Huh?"

"He'd write me checks – large checks – like a thousand, or two thousand. Personally. Him to me. They were always around the time someone I had helped with died."

Maddy stopped chewing. She swallowed.

"Helped with?"

"Maggie Lovisa," said Shirley, staring now at the skeleton of the dwarfed woman next to the giant. "I set up the meeting on the park bench, between her and Dr. Wilhelm, the day before she was supposed to visit his clinic. The day she died. And Marco Santelli – I delivered from Dr. Wilhelm to him the drugs that Dr. Wilhelm said he needed to take the day before the special research scans. The day he died."

Maddy did not respond.

"So, you know, there are records, Mad. There are records of him paying me. He said they were gifts. But there are records of what look like him paying me."

"Jesus, Shirley," answered Maddy, putting down her plate on the floor on the side away from Hunter.

"Yeah, and all those years I got all those people to sign all those forms – even you."

Shirley looked down at her chest and used her fingers to fish a rolled piece of paper from her bra. She handed it to Maddy. Maddy unrolled it and saw it was the cadaver donation form Maddy had signed.

"Right after your priest friend came and picked you up yesterday, I found that form and I hid it," Shirley said. "Dr. Wilhelm didn't know I had one signed from you – but I didn't want him to ever find out."

Maddy tore up the form into small pieces and threw them into the empty container that had held the beef. Using her chopsticks, she stirred the bits of paper around in the leftover sauce, to soil them.

"He even has one from Jimmy Heathcote, thanks to me," said Shirley, watching Maddy.

"Well, he's never going to want Jimmy – too ordinary a form. Just plain achondroplasia."

"Agreed," answered Shirley. "Whatever good things you can say about Jimmy Heathcote – and you can say a few – he is blessedly boring for a dwarf."

"So...you're not going to defend Dr. Wilhelm, are you? You're not going to sow doubt to help him?"

"Loyalty is such a funny strong pull, isn't it, Maddy?"

"Yes," said Maddy. "My best friend Liz, who you met, she studies rats. And she says it's just about who we are near – who we are near the most is to whom we become most loyal. That it *feels* psychological, even spiritual, but that loyalty is just about biological proximity. About smelling each other."

Shirley nodded.

"Maybe," Maddy said, attempting a joke, "I should have spent more time in your office."

"But it's not just Dr. Wilhelm, Maddy – it's the whole thing. The society here, the medical society that's employed me for almost thirty years. The scientific establishment – because you know, if you're proven right, Maddy, it's going to create terrible feelings towards medical research among the general public. You're going to be harming medical research."

Maddy didn't answer. She knew that Shirley was right, but she also knew that the idea of protecting Dr. Wilhelm to protect medical research was morally absurd. It was not just because she was raised Catholic, was it? – this feeling of needing highly-specific justice, no matter the collateral damage?

"And yet," continued Shirley, leaning over to put her hands on the floor to push herself up to a standing position, "and yet I have always believed that the best thing to do is to pursue the truth and not worry about the unintended consequences. That, it seems, must be the ultimate loyalty – loyalty to the pursue of the truth – if we are to live in a world that is centered on science, knowledge, light, truth."

She went over to the cabinet that contained the mid-nineteenth-century collection of Native American skulls, one that Maddy knew had become the subject of a repatriation attempt. Maddy stood up and joined her at the case. Hunter sniffed longingly at the plates on the floor, but he did not take any food.

"Some of the people in some of the tribes," Shirley said quietly, "they don't want to know the DNA analyses on the remains they say are their ancestors. They say that is not where their truth resides. But you and I know that the causality found through biology and physics – the material history – is typically far more accurate than the causality claims provided in human myth."

"And you know as well as I do," said Maddy, "that human myth can suppress material history for generations. People push away scientific truth if there's something they want so badly to believe. There are many who will think Dr. Wilhelm a hero, an unquestionable hero. They won't be able to see the evidence."

"And this is where the police can do better than the historian," answered Shirley.

At that, Maddy told Shirley what she had not before – that the man Maddy was staying with in Philly was, in fact, a police detective, and that Hunter was, in fact, a retired police canine.

Shirley turned, looked and Hunter, and laughed.

"That's why he's such a good dog!"

Maddy didn't laugh. She told Shirley that she had laid out all that she knew in a draft report, with annotated appendices in a series of files that she could easily turn over to the police.

"Why haven't you turned it over to the police already?" asked Shirley.

"I wanted to understand it all – to get it all down, first."

"You know what they say, Maddy. There are two kinds of scholarly projects – perfect and done. Maybe it is time you acknowledged that and let this project of yours go out for review."

Shirley ran her fingers over the glass of the case and let out a sigh.

"Would you take me home with you tonight, Maddy, to your policeman friend's house? I don't feel like meeting my end just yet. I may not be perfect, but I think I'm also not done."

Maddy said she would call Wolf and ask him to bring the car. In preparation for heading back to Shirley's office to use the phone, she picked up off the floor the plastic bag from the take-out and gathered up all the trash into the bag. When she had gotten it all, she picked up the empty bottle of vermouth, too, and joined Shirley back at the case of skulls. Hunter came over to stand between the two of them.

"Shirley, I need to ask you about one more thing. That day I didn't come to work, just before I went down to Washington – it was because someone attacked me."

Shirley turned to look at her with a fresh face of concern.

"It was a tall and thin man – I assume it was a man – and his hands smelled like the soap at the hospital. Is there someone in Dr. Wilhelm's group that it might have been? Someone who would go that far to help him?"

"Yes," answered Shirley, taking the trash from Maddy. "Yes. Sergey Goncharov – M.D., endocrinology."

"Why does he come to your mind so quickly?"

"Well, your description, Maddy – tall and thin man, someone who would have been at the hospital," answered Shirley. "But more than that – he told me more than once how grateful he was to Dr. Wilhelm for getting him a green card – that he would be dead back in Russia – that he would do almost anything for Dr. Wilhelm. But he has also seemed so troubled of late. He gave me a gift, a set of nested dolls that he said had belonged to his mother. And he would not say why."

. . .

Wolf picked up the call after just one ring.

"Hi, Wolf," she said.

"Christ Almighty, Rabbit, where have you been?!"

She looked at her watch and realized it was just past nine.

"When I got home, I found the place all cleaned up and your suitcase out and half-packed and you weren't here – "

"I'm sorry, Wolf. I assumed I'd be back before you – I'm sorry. I am wondering if you can pick me and Hunter up at the museum, in the car? And we need to help out my friend Shirley tonight. So, we need the car."

"Rabbit, listen – someone named Bess MacFarlane, the woman who sent you that photocopy in the mail – she cold-called Philadelphia P.D. *about you* and what she says you've been working on about Dr. Wilhelm, and someone figured out she was talking about a person staying at my address, and they called me in, and, well, MacFarlane says.... You know what she says?"

Maddy didn't answer.

"Rabbit!" he yelled angrily.

She thought she had better wash her arm as soon as she could, as best she could. Shirley was packing things into her big handbag but also looking at Maddy. Maddy figured she could hear what Wolf was saying.

"Rabbit, so *this* is the second project you've been working on – about Dr. Wilhelm killing patients?"

"Yes, Wolf. Yes. And that's why we have to help Shirley out. Just come get us. Honk when you are outside. I'll show you what I have when we get home."

-26-

The car rocked a little as Wolf pushed the copier paper box aside to also fit Shirley's suitcase in the trunk. Shirley got in the front passenger seat.

"You sure you have enough room back there, shorty?" Shirley asked, closing her door twice to get it to latch.

"I'm fine," answered Maddy.

Wolf slammed the trunk closed, got back in the car, and buckled his seatbelt.

"I hope I packed the right things," said Shirley. "I assume we're going to have to spend some time with the police tomorrow, and I don't know what one wears to such a thing. I went for a pantsuit set with a scarf that I think says 'I am not crazy, and I am innocent, so don't arrest me.'"

She let out a sigh.

Wolf started the car, pulled out, and headed towards his house.

"Why *did* you wear all black to work today, Shirley?" Maddy asked. "It's not like you to dress so morbidly."

"It's just what seemed right, knowing I was going to have to kick you out this morning, after what happened yesterday."

"What happened yesterday?" asked Wolf.

"Maddy didn't tell you? Dr. Wilhelm slipped her some drug — well, that's

284

what we both assume. She passed out, twice. After just the first time, he tried to get her to go to the hospital – that's what made each of us think he was definitely behind it. No normal doctor tells you to go to the hospital because you merely passed out, especially when you're a healthy young person. Maddy had me call a priest-friend of hers instead. I thought at first she was delirious, asking for a priest. But then I figured out she was serious, and she just wanted him to get her home – not that she wanted the last rites! Her priest-friend came and got her and Hunter."

Wolf did not reply. Maddy started to wonder if she was going to head back to Indiana with Wolf furious with her. Maybe that would be a good thing.

Shirley cleared her throat at the silence and then kept talking:

"Getting one's clothing right for a particular context is *so* important. Did you know, Maddy, that in China, brides traditionally wear red – there, red is the color of happiness, of good luck, good fortune! White is a color for mourning. But here, of course, white is the color of the virgin bride, and red, the color of the slut."

"You ever been married, Shirl?"

"No, Maddy, no," Shirley answered, reaching back between the seats to give Hunter a series of pats on his head. "Not easy for a tall girl to find a fella. And what is love anyway but acquired conjoined twinning?"

"Acute-onset," answered Maddy. "The worst kind. But at least it is typically transient."

"That's certainly been my experience, Mad. But I haven't read the literature. I prefer the scientific literature."

She and Maddy both let out a short laugh at Shirley's joke.

Just inside Wolf's house, Maddy put down on the floor the box of materials Shirley had collected for her dissertation, pulled a kitchen chair over to near the stove, stood up on it, and opened the upper cabinets. She took down the popcorn popper and the pressure cooker, resting them on the counter, and pulled out her files of research on Wilhelm. Then she put the appliances back in the cabinets, closed them up, and put the chair back at the table. She looked over the folders briefly to make sure they were in a logical order, with her draft report on top, and handed them to Wolf as a stack.

He had been just standing there watching her, with Shirley's suitcase in his hand. He put down the suitcase to take the folders. Maddy took off her coat and hung it on the hook near the back door.

"Come on, Shirley, I'll show you my room and we can change the sheets for you together."

"I don't feel right taking your bed, Mad," said Shirley. "You can just give me the couch."

"You won't fit comfortably lying down on the couch, silly," said Maddy. "Come on."

When they came back down, they found Wolf sitting at the table reading Maddy's report, occasionally looking in an appendix folder to look at the documentation she had assembled. Hunter lay on the floor next to him.

Without checking to see if he wanted it, Maddy got him a bottle of beer, opened it, and put it on the table about eight inches from his hand. He reached forward, took it, and drank a few sips without looking up.

"You want some dessert?" Maddy asked Shirley. "I could make you an egg custard."

"Sure," said Shirley, "if it's not too much trouble."

Maddy got out two bowls, a whisk, and the pots for the double boiler. On the counter she set up what she needed in terms of the ingredients. She turned on the heat under the water pot and started to whisk two eggs in the base of the double boiler.

She wondered if she shouldn't be making quite so much noise with the whisk banging against the pot as Wolf was trying to read.

Shirley leaned over the stove to see what Maddy was doing. The egg was foaming and starting to thicken.

"Maddy," Wolf said without looking up, "after that, you go take your bath."

Maddy didn't answer. She wondered what Shirley must think of such a command.

...

"I guess it's called permanent marker for a reason, Hunter," Maddy said to the dog lying on the bathmat as she tried to scrub her arm clean with her fingernails. Adding more soap was just going to be futile, and it was going to make the bath water too soapy. She gave up and leaned back in the tub.

It had occurred to her by now why Wolf had sent her off to the bath: so that he could talk to Shirley alone. What did he want to tell Shirley, or ask her, without Maddy there? Maybe he had seen something fundamentally wrong with Maddy's reasoning or evidence, and he wanted to talk to Shirley about how to tell Maddy? Maybe he wanted to figure out if Shirley was as innocent as she appeared? Maybe he was trying to ascertain from Shirley how quickly they needed to act to avoid Dr. Wilhelm destroying evidence or harming somebody else? Maybe he had asked Shirley to call Dr. Wilhelm to make him think nothing special was going on?

Or maybe he just wanted to know if Shirley was okay and needed anything – any reassurance, any help understanding what was going to happen.

What *was* going to happen?

Wolf had confirmed that they were going to end up with the police much of the next day. Maddy was glad that Shirley would likely be with her. The two of them could crack their inside jokes about anatomy and physiology, and it would give them both some relief from the stress. Maybe the day would be interesting.

Yes, maybe, as with the third and fourth and fifth weeks at the convent – when the initial terror and disorientation had subsided and a certain sense of safety had set in – there would be the fascination of watching a group of people all in the same profession interact, as each inevitably distinguished herself or himself by words and acts, with the steady revelation of character. Yes, maybe it would be *interesting*. That was always better than boring.

Maddy added some hot water to the bath, to warm herself up. She wondered how long Shirley was going to stay with them. She wondered if this meant there was no chance that before she went back to Indiana, Wolf and she would spend one more night in her bed together, the blankets' edges shoved carefully between them at the start.

Of course, now, with the revelation of what she had been doing with the subject of Wilhelm's specimen acquisition, perhaps Wolf's whole view of her had changed. She would now necessarily be Wolf's professional subject.

She wondered to herself if this were the real reason she had put off telling him.

...

Maddy made sure Shirley had everything she might need – towels and extra blankets and a glass for water – before she said goodnight to Shirley and took herself in her pajamas downstairs to the living room. She sorted out the bedding she had brought for herself from upstairs and made up the couch as a bed, with a bottom and a top sheet, and then added two blankets on top. She got in between the sheets and tucked the bedding around her to try to get a little warmer and gave Hunter an order to lie down on the floor next to her. The small lamp by the edge of the couch was still on, but she figured Wolf would turn it off if she fell asleep.

Soon he came in from the kitchen, the stack of folders in his hands, a pencil held between his teeth. He sat down in the armchair near the couch and took the pencil out of his mouth.

"Okay if I sit here, Rabbit?"

"Of course," she answered.

She rolled over on her side toward him. Looking up at him from this position, she realized this was the dog's-eye view of life.

Just then, Hunter let out a long fart.

"That's not my fault," Maddy said as the stink filled the air. "Shirley gave him some of the Chinese food we had for dinner – I told her she shouldn't."

"It's okay. Can I ask you something? What set you down this – this research path?"

Maddy turned to stare up at the ceiling. She noticed a dust web hanging from the light fixture, draping a few inches down. She was surprised Wolf hadn't seen it, but then he didn't much turn on the ceiling light here. She hadn't seen it before either.

"Something must have set you off, Rabbit?"

"He showed me his specimens at his lab," said Maddy, "and then I had a bad dream about one of the women in his collection. She was having a cup of tea, in the jar, talking to me... And then I started looking."

"Okay," said Wolf. "If they ask you that tomorrow, don't mention the bad dream. Just say something didn't seem right."

She wondered if he was worried she would embarrass him. The report itself was probably going to be embarrassing just by its very nature. But then Wolf, like her, didn't generally care what other people thought.

"What can I say, Wolf? I am just generally open to unusual possibilities."

She said it not as if she were proud of it, but as if it were a problem.

"Sometimes being open to unusual possibilities is very much to my advantage," she added. "But sometimes other people use my openness to take advantage of me."

She started chewing on her lower lip.

"But sometimes, Rabbit," he said, "that you are open to possibilities is both to your advantage and to the advantage of those around you."

She stopped biting her lip and relaxed her face.

"So, what do you think of my draft?"

"You use too many adverbs," Wolf replied.

"Yeah," she said. "I always try to fix that before submission. I wasn't planning to submit it to you just yet."

"When *were* you?"

She couldn't tell what his tone was – merely curious or still angry?

"I don't know," she said. "It – well, it's been complicated."

He didn't answer.

Feeling a little too warm, she draped her left arm down off the couch, and trailed her fingers along Hunter's back. Wolf got up, came over, and sat down on the couch next to her, pushing Hunter aside a little with his feet. She realized he had now seen the writing on her arm. He took her wrist in his hand and pushed back her sleeve, and read aloud what she had written there, including his name and phone number.

"That's your idea of how to stay safe?" he asked, pulling her sleeve back down. "Christ."

"I had Hunter, too," she answered defensively, pulling her arm to her chest. She didn't mention the twenty dollars in her shoe.

He moved back to the armchair and sat down.

"Your report is good, Rabbit. Well composed. I appreciate that you even entertain the weaknesses in your argument, head on."

He said it like he was grading her work.

"I mean," he added, "it's completely bizarre. I don't mean your reading of Wilhelm's actions is unbelievable to me. Like you, Rabbit, I don't have any illusions about human beings and of what they are capable. But it's bizarre to read a report that is written like this – as if it is for a class. No offense. It's not how people normally present suspicions to us. I'm not sure what – what the others – my colleagues – are going to make of it."

"Then you'll have to help me figure out what to wear," she said, glumly.

"It doesn't matter what you *wear*," he answered in an exasperated tone.

It was clear he immediately regretted much of what he had just said, as he mumbled something meant to sound friendlier.

Hunter let out another fart.

"Damn it, Hunter," said Wolf, "go to the kitchen."

He pointed and the dog got up and obeyed the command.

"You know, Rabbit, when I got you the dog, Hunter was meant to keep you *safer*."

"Right, Wolf, I know."

"So instead, you think you can use him to take *more* risk?"

She didn't answer. She was starting to feel overwhelmed by his criticisms.

She wasn't sure what she expected would happen when she would finally show him her report on Wilhelm, but it wasn't all this. She had expected something more like his reaction to her dissertation – interest, scholarly debate, and then a little unembarrassing praise. She had hoped for that.

"Well, you will now take it over," she said in a quiet voice. "And when you're done asking me questions, then I have to go back to Indiana."

"What?" he asked. "I can't hear you."

"I have to go back to Indiana," she said louder.

"Yes," he said.

She rolled over the other way, toward the back of the couch. She wanted to ask him if they could go to the gym now, but she knew they couldn't just leave Shirley home alone. Shirley would be fine alone with Hunter, of course, but if she woke up and they weren't there, that would be rude.

She could hear him leafing through the pages of her report again. After a few minutes, she heard him put it down and crack his neck.

"Rabbit," he asked in a gentler voice, "why did you spend today cleaning?"

"I don't know," she said. "I guess because I have been a lot of trouble."

For a moment, there was silence in the house. Maddy could hear the refrigerator condenser turn on.

"No, *I* have been a lot of trouble," Wolf finally answered. "To you."

She rolled over and looked at him. He was leaning forward, his elbows on his knees.

"What the fuck do you mean, Wolf?" she asked. "How the fuck can you say that *you* been a lot of trouble to *me*?"

"Pushing you," he said. "Pushing you to work so hard to finish your degree – although I know you push yourself. Pushing you to eat. I mean, I know you like to eat, but…Well, making you go out to Bobby's concerts. Making you take Hunter. Calling your best friend to come without even asking you."

"You certainly have a fucked-up understanding of what trouble looks like," she answered him, finding it impossible not to smile a little. "Were I to stay longer, I could show you some more what trouble *actually* looks like."

He bent over and untied his shoes. He kicked them off under the coffee table, turned off the light, and climbed onto the couch, getting behind her. As he spooned in behind her, she adjusted the blankets so he could have some. Now he had his arms around her, his head on the pillow, with her head on his bicep. She loved having her nose this close to his armpit.

"You're definitely the most troubling houseguest I've ever had, Matthew Shanks," he said.

She pulled his forearm to her chest and took a deep breath of him. But just as she could hold that lovely Wolf-soaked gallon of air no longer, he whipped his arm away and bounded over her.

"Maddy," he said with clear alarm in his voice.

She feared he was about to tell her they couldn't keep doing this – he had used her ordinarily name instead the name he had given to her – but instead he headed for the kitchen and told her to come with him.

"What, Wolf?" she asked, following him. Hunter stood up as they came into the kitchen.

"One of your folders – Jimmy Heathcote – I just realized – it hadn't occurred to me the messages might be for you. No one but Liz ever calls for you here."

He hit playback on the answering machine.

It's Jimmy again. Listen, if you're serious about looking into it all, call me. I hope you're not fucking with me.

"Yes. That's Jimmy Heathcote," said Maddy, her mouth feeling suddenly dry. "How many messages has he left?"

"Just two," said Wolf.

She stared at him thinking what Wolf was presumably also thinking – that Jimmy would have assumed she was getting the messages and not calling him back for some reason.

"Well, it's too late now," said Wolf.

"What the fuck do you mean, it's too late now?"

Hunter was looking from her face to his face and back again, trying to ascertain what he was supposed to be doing in this moment.

"I just mean it's almost midnight, Rabbit, that's all."

"Oh, Jesus, Wolf," she said, pressing her left palm against her breastbone to try to stop her heart from banging around. "I thought you meant – that I had again – that – Nick – and Katie – and"

"Stop," he said. He pulled her hands together into his. "Stop. You have to stop thinking you are somehow responsible for everyone you cross paths with, that you're responsible for everything they do, for everything that happens to them."

"If I don't think about that, then I might make a fatal mistake again!" she yelled at him. "Don't ask me to be fucking *naïve*, Wolf!"

"Be quiet!" he said, in a loud whisper. "Shirley is probably trying to sleep."

He motioned to Maddy to sit down and ordered Hunter to lie down. Hunter obeyed. Wolf pulled two tumblers down from the upper cabinet to the left of the sink, put them on the counter, opened his bottle of Jameson's, and poured them each a glass. He told Maddy again to sit down. This time she did.

He sat down across from her. She expected him to say something, but he said nothing. She sipped the whiskey down slowly, feeling the fire fall down her throat. He drank his just as pensively.

"What?" she finally asked.

"Your research on Wilhelm – the report, specifically – you took it up intensely after Washington, after Nick died?"

"Yes," she answered.

"But it is also about Katie and The Jerk, isn't it. About not letting a terrible person go unchecked in his ways. About not failing to take care of other people, not put your own needs first."

She did not reply. So, he continued:

"What you said just now – about trying not to make *another* fatal mistake – Rabbit, would you please tell me why your family died?"

"Car crash," she said, wondering what he was getting at. "You know that."

"No," he said, getting up to get the bottle and pouring them each a little more. He put the bottle on the table this time. "Tell me why. Why they really lost their lives."

"Car crash," she said again.

He sighed.

"You know why my wife is going to die, Rabbit?" he asked. "Because I was a shitty enough husband that she cheated on me with my best friend. So, they were in a car together that got hit by a crane. It was my fault, because they wouldn't have been in the car together if I had been a better husband. So I am responsible for it."

"That's a completely bullshit construction of culpability, Wolf, and you know it. You can't be responsible for the crane."

He drank back the rest of his glass. She did the same.

"Why did your family lose their lives?" he asked again, after a moment.

"Car crash," she answered.

"Why do you think the car crashed?" he asked.

"Because," Maddy answered, "because – you're asking me to state the obvious – I was in a relationship with The Jerk. They died because of my decisions."

"That's a completely bullshit idea, Rabbit, and you know it."

"Not really, Wolf. If I hadn't been in a relationship with him – if I had done something about The Jerk – if I had not been wanting something from him, some kind of, well, love, I suppose – then my father would not have angrily bundled everybody into the car to go kill him. My father wouldn't have crashed the car with all of them in it. So any logical person would see I am responsible."

"Right," he said quietly. "Like my wife's death is my fault."

"What is your point?"

"My point is that you can't be morally responsible for something you had absolutely no intention of causing. Your family. Katie. Nick. You can be responsible for a sin that might *lead* to a disaster, but you can't be responsible for the *disaster* – and in the case of The Jerk, Rabbit, you can't seriously come to some kind of facile conclusion that *you* were responsible. You were still practically a *child*."

"My father had a very expansive notion of sin," Maddy replied, putting her chin up in the air a little, as if she were naming a point of family pride. "My father told me that if I thought of a sin – if I so much *dreamed* of a sin – it was the same as consciously committing the sin. So, of course, the failure to anticipate that disaster might result from one's action or inaction – it must simply be an accessory fault."

"Your father was a terrible theologian," said Wolf, getting up and getting them each a glass of tap water. "How could God possibly hold you responsible for something you had no real control over, like a dream?"

She did not respond.

"So, your father held you responsible for The Jerk, too?"

"Of course," she said. "And he wasn't wrong, at some level."

She took several gulps of water. She was wondering now if part of the reason her dreams stayed with her so much longer than dreams seemed to stay with other people was her illogical sense of culpability for what happened in her dreams – culpable not even just what she did in her dreams but for what other people did in her dreams?

"Besides, Rabbit," he said, a good minute into the intervening silence, "why do you care about sin and God?"

"An atheist has to have *some* kind of moral framework, Wolf, to know what to do in the world. An historian ought to be able to think about the morality of action, inaction, and she ought to be able to think about consequences."

"There's a reason we use the phrase '*unintended* consequences,' Rabbit. You act as if there is no such thing as *unintended* consequences to our actions."

"The good historian ought to know the *possible* consequences. And take those into account in what she is doing. Or not doing."

"And were you a historian – a good historian – *at thirteen?* Or even at *fifteen?*"

His voice conveyed a bitterness that reminded her of the night at the restaurant when she told him all about The Jerk. She loved drinking that bitterness from his lips.

He stood up, pushed in his chair, and walked into the living room, turning on the light near the stereo. She and Hunter followed him in to find him looking for a particular record. Maddy gently told Hunter to go lie down in the kitchen while she kept watching Wolf searching. When he found it, he put it on, dialing the volume to the lowest audible setting.

She recognized the tune immediately. Liz had played this record several times during her visit.

"You know it?" he asked.

She nodded.

"*Si Tu Vois Ma Mére*," she said. "If You See My Mother," she added, translating the French title to English.

"*Si tu vois ta mére*," he replied. "If you see your mother..."

"No," she said, thinking he had misunderstood the name of the song. "*Si tu vois ma mére*. If you see *my* mother."

"Madeleine, Madeleine Shanks, *si tu vois ta mére*," he said, "if you saw your mother again, what would she say? Would she say *you* caused it? Would she blame you, Madeleine?"

Now Maddy's lower lip started to tremble. Her eyes blinked rapidly. The combination of the thought of seeing her mother again someday and the song – a song of sentimentality –

She gasped, and hearing her wet gasp, he pulled her to him, to dance.

"It might occur to you someday, Rabbit," he said very quietly, as if telling her a secret, "that if every death that can be traced back in some way to something you did or didn't do, then you are responsible for every single death since the moment you were born. Is *that* what you think original sin looks like? Is *that* what you think your mother did when she let you go to breathe the air of the earth – that she cursed you so fucking hard?"

"It's complete bullshit, Wolf," she answered quietly, now looking up into his face, "and you know it."

He was holding her in a kind of waltz pose, a hand around her back, her left hand raised in his right hand. He moved her slightly side to side with the music, as if they were in a crowded dancehall, too crowded to move more than a couple of inches at a time.

"If you think what you did or did not do makes you responsible for a death you never intended," he said, "then perhaps what you need to realize is that you think yourself far more powerful than you are."

She closed her eyes and leaned her head against his chest. She could just pick up his heartbeat.

"Instead of this arrogance, this idea that you are so powerful, consider instead humility, Rabbit."

"Humility as a route to absolution?" she asked. "Wolf, are you saying humility can be a route to absolution?"

"Yes, Rabbit," he said. "Yes. Not feigned ignorance. *Actual humility.* Humility is one way to get to absolution."

"Legitimate absolution?"

"Legitimate absolution."

He pulled his left hand away from her lower back and placed it on the back of her head in order to keep her exactly where she was.

"Allow yourself humility," he said. "Please."

The top of her head felt suddenly like a drop of rain had fallen on it. One more fell.

-27-

Had Wolf found that last kiss as awkward as she had?

There had been no time for anything more than a hasty goodbye when they said their farewells in the aisle of the train. They had each gone for a cheek but had gone in the same direction and ended up banging their noses, sort of kissing on the lips. Ugh.

They should have taken the opportunity of the time they had standing around on the platform to say a proper goodbye. She should have guessed that when the train arrived – when it came time for him to help her hustle her suitcase, her overstuffed backpack, the shopping bag of food, and Hunter onto the train – Wolf was going to have to get on and off the train fast.

As they had been standing around waiting for the train, there had been a blind woman on the platform feeling the face of a man she was leaving. Why hadn't Maddy done that, she wondered now? Why hadn't she closed her eyes and felt Wolf's face? Sure, he would have told her she was being silly, but he probably would have put up with it. And it might have led to the best dreams during what was bound to be shitty sleep on this long ride back to Indiana. She could have dreamed whatever her subconscious mind would do with the proprioception of his face.

Instead on the platform they had had a conversation he was bound to conclude amounted to evidence of her fundamental weirdness. He had been trying in the time left to show her a few self-defense moves – how to pivot and kick out an opponent's knee from the side; how to punch someone in the nose, hard; how to grasp her keys in her palm so one key would protrude from between her fingers, to make it available to jab at someone's eye. And she had responded by telling him that while everything he was teaching her in this five-minute course made sense, she preferred to disarm people with her charm.

"Yeah, Rabbit," Wolf had answered, "you know, being *completely unpredictable* is not quite the same as being disarmingly charming."

He emitted a little smiling laugh after his admonition.

"I suppose your best defense is your speed," he said, more thoughtfully. "Use that."

"And I can jump," she replied.

"You can definitely jump."

Hunter had his nose up in the air and Maddy thought he looked a little distressed, as if he was picking up too many scents at once. She patted him on his head to try to reassure him.

"Well, then, what have we learned, John Wolf?" she asked, still patting Hunter, sounding as if she were administering a post-course assessment. She asked the same thing again quickly – "What have we learned?" – not sure why her brain kept throwing up this thing to say.

She felt so completely out of sorts, having spent the previous day telling the police all she knew, having had her dissertation research taken away, having to say goodbye to Wolf. Everything felt smashed and uncertain.

"What have we learned from what?" he asked.

"The whole damned thing," she answered.

"I think you have learned how to make an egg custard and how to properly treat a chicken cutlet," Wolf said. "And I have learned how it is you can put so much food away and not get fat."

She asked him with genuine curiosity how that was.

"Because *when* you finally fall asleep, Rabbit, I mean *really* fall asleep," he answered, "you stop talking, and you stop moving, and you turn into a little furnace."

"What?"

"You did it last night. You have before, too. You put off enormous amounts of heat when you finally hit deep sleep. So, I think that's where all the calories are going. Well, that and your brain otherwise working overtime."

She silently wondered if her extreme vasodilation woke him up. She hoped not. If it did, that would mean that when she was sleeping *poorly*, she was keeping him awake with unconscious chatter and movement, and when she was sleeping *well*, she was keeping him awake with waves of too much heat.

"So, what else have we learned?" she asked.

(And now she remembered; this was what Sister Thomas Aquinas had asked Maddy repeatedly in the sisters' car, on the way from the convent to Georgetown, the first time she and Sister Mary Patrick were taking Maddy there.)

Just then the stationmaster had announced the arrival of The Cardinal, bound for Chicago by way of D.C., Charlottesville, Charleston, Cincinnati, and Indianapolis.

"We have also learned," Wolf had sighed, "that occasionally Amtrak can be on time."

When the train's dirty blue engine came into her line of sight, Maddy suddenly thought herself an idiot for not having taken Wolf up on his offer to drive her back to Indiana even if it would have meant having to put up with Father Tad as an unwanted chaperone in the backseat.

But lord, how awkward that would have been. Why hadn't Wolf just told Father Tad no, that he'd drive Maddy back alone, thank you very much?

At least in Indiana, Maddy was going to have Hunter to curl up with. Now, on the train, Hunter was sleeping on the floor at her feet, but at home she could talk him into coming up into her bed, and she could wrap her arm around him and feel his breathing. She had told Wolf she didn't want or need the dog in Indiana, but he must have seen that she didn't fight him hard. And she knew it was going to make Wolf feel better for Maddy to have Hunter.

She kicked off her shoes and rubbed Hunter's side with one of her feet. He lifted his head and looked up at her for a moment as if to see if she needed something, and then closed his eyes and laid his head down again. They had run him hard that day, to wear him out for the long trip.

Maddy stretched her arms and legs, enjoying having so much space to herself. She had as always paid only for a coach-class seat, but Wolf had accidentally scored her a free upgrade. He had insisted they get to 30th Street Station early so he could show his badge to the Amtrak staff and explain that Maddy had to take "this police dog" to Indiana. The station staff had radioed ahead, and when the train arrived, a conductor waved her and Wolf and Hunter up to business class, where the conductor said they had an empty set of seats Maddy could take, with enough room for Hunter to lie comfortably on the floor.

Wolf had made noises implying to the Amtrak staff that he needed Maddy to get this dog from him to some other officer in Indianapolis. Maddy felt a little silly having the conductor think she and Hunter were somehow on official business. But it was so nice, for a change, to sit in the more expensive car. The rows of seats had more space between them, the people were quieter, and the car was delightfully free of children. And she would have sworn Hunter seemed so happy when, right after they entered the station, Wolf had put on a little blue vest that identified him as a working law enforcement dog. All in all, this ruse to get him on the train with her had worked out just fine.

She wondered what Wolf was going to tell her dissertation director on the phone tomorrow. Wolf had offered to call Professor Carlyle, to try to explain what was going on, tell him why Maddy might seem a bit exhausted and stressed, and to explain the dog. And to tell him that Maddy was probably going to be a bit at sixes and sevens because she wasn't going to have all of her dissertation research with her for what might be a few weeks. The investigators had asked to see it and to take parts of it. Now she felt she should not have said yes to that. It wasn't relevant to what they were working on, and God only knew if they were going to be careful with it and give it back to her in the same orderly condition that she had given it to them. It was probably just sitting near someone's desk in a heap of boxes, being ignored. They had even taken the box of fresh photocopied material Shirley had given just her, as if that would be of any use to them.

Wolf did say that if they didn't give it all back soon, he would make copies of all the material for her and send her what they had. But could he?

Was this whole thing going to fuck up her degree? She knew that, if she had to, she could take another year – the department would find her some form of funding, like teaching, because she had gotten the NEH fellowship for this year – but she also knew that the less time she took, the better she would look to search committees. And there were some good jobs opening up for next year that she needed to apply for now, while they were open. Professor Carlyle had been forwarding the notices. The application deadlines were coming up.

She took a deep breath, and then another, to calm herself. There was that Amtrak disinfectant smell. The smell that had reminded her of the attacker's hands when he came at her in her bedroom.

She had told the investigators about the hospital-soap smell only briefly in case they thought that something like a scent was too subjective to pay any mind. In talking with the investigators, Maddy had reminded herself repeatedly of what Wolf had said – that the way he knew he really knew something was that he was able to make the argument calmly, in complete sentences. If they were going to take her seriously, she needed to do that, appealing to facts as objective as possible. Not spending too much time explaining smells or historical contexts.

Wolf had certainly seemed happy with her performance. The way he looked at her at the gym afterwards – after they went home and, at her request, changed quickly to go straight to the mats and the bars – well, he looked more relaxed than she had expected. Maybe that was partly because the police were apparently now keeping an eye on Wilhelm, so Wolf was less concerned than he might have been before?

But then he had told her they hadn't been able yet to locate Sergey Goncharov, the doctor Shirley thought had probably been intentionally helping Wilhelm, the man who had probably broken into Wolf's house to come at Maddy. And that felt unsettling.

An officer did manage to get some photographs of Sergey and show them to Maddy and Wolf, so they would know what he looked like. The photographs were mostly of his face, but there was one where he was standing in a group with Dr. Wilhelm, and sure enough, his build seemed about like what Maddy and Wolf thought had been the intruder's.

Maddy was glad Colin would be picking her up in Indianapolis at the end of this train ride tomorrow night. She didn't feel like talking to Liz right off the train, as Liz was bound to push on all the stress points. Liz would grab Maddy by the wrist and give her stiff coffee and drag her verbally through the fields of the unknowns and the risks of what Maddy was facing. Maddy was sure Liz was going to quickly pull out of Maddy the whole story of Shirley and Maddy having had to spend so much time telling the police what they knew. And then Liz was probably going to poke at Maddy's relationship with Wolf.

By contrast, Colin would presumably have his usual low-key demeanor and be focused on getting laid. He would thoughtlessly order delivery from Phoenix Dumpling, eat a late dinner with her, ask her how her work was going, maybe update her on his butterfly grants, tell her again they couldn't have a steady relationship because of his work, and then help her out.

He probably had no idea how useful this could be at a time like this. She hoped she wouldn't do something stupid like be overly grateful.

Colin had seemed unfazed by her warning him on the phone that she had a well-behaved dog coming with her and that she had had a rather exhausting time in Philadelphia.

"That's how serious research trips are, babe," he said, in a tone that felt a little condescending. As if *she* had not made many research trips before. As if *he* had any experience waiting for a search warrant to drop.

Wolf hadn't been able to answer Maddy's questions about how much of all this would be traceable to her. He thought she was worried about Wilhelm knowing. But she told him that wasn't it – Wilhelm had already figured out she had been researching his grants and talking to his patients, not least because Shirley had told him. That was obviously why he had slipped her something, to try to get her to the hospital.

"I'm not worried about my life, I'm worried about my career, Wolf. Presumably after he's charged – presuming he's charged – it's going to get out that I had a part in it. I think it's going to get out even if he isn't charged. They're going to search his lab and his home – that is all going to get out. And people will find out I'm behind that, given all the people who knew I was doing the research – people like Jimmy Heathcote, and Bess McFarlane, both of whom will talk about it. Well, Wolf, a lot of the jobs I might apply for are either in medical schools or involve joint appointments with medical schools. How many medical schools are going to want to hire an historian who accused a member of the National Academy of Sciences with serial murder? Even if it turns out he's convicted, which you already said could be a long time from now?"

Wolf had had no answer. He had opened his mouth twice, as if to say something, but then each time just closed it.

Too bad she didn't have a sleeper on this train. She would happily curl up with Hunter and try to conk out. It was going to be challenging to get herself in a good sleeping position in this seating arrangement.

She reached into the shopping bag of food on the seat next to her and pulled out the thermos of split pea soup Wolf had given her. She had initially protested that the big steel thermos was going to take up too much room, but he had told her that on a trip this long, she was going to want something truly hot to eat, and he wasn't wrong. He had given her some buttered rye crackers to go with it, and a cut-up lemon, packed in a little twist of plastic wrap, to squeeze into the soup in case it needed a little more sour. She pulled out the pint mason jar of pinot noir he said would go well with almost everything in the bag, including the soup, the hummus, and the salami. The wine, he said, should in fact taste good with everything, everything except the peanut butter sandwiches and the macaroons.

She opened the tray table for her seat, covered it in the faded dishtowel Wolf had given her, and laid out the little dinner. As Delaware went by outside the window, she ate one thermos-lid's worth of the soup and about half of the crackers and drank a little of the wine. Then she put all that away and pulled out something else Wolf had given her for the trip: his copy of Calvin Trillin's *Alice, Let's Eat: Further Adventures of a Happy Eater*. He said she could give it back, along with his thermos, when she saw him again.

"And when will that be?" she had asked.

"I expect it all depends on what happens in the next few days," he had answered. "We'll see what happens with the search warrants."

"Can I call you late at night from Indiana?" she had asked. "If I can't sleep?"

"Of course, Rabbit. There's not going to be anyone next to me that you'll be waking up."

He probably didn't say it to contrast their ways. But that had been the effect.

How strange her little place in Bloomington was going to feel. The other apartments in the divided-up old house she lived in near campus would be occupied as usual with people moving about, but her own part of the house would surely feel as if it had been unoccupied for months. The heat would be turned down. The fridge would be near-empty. Her palm tree was presumably still over at Liz's.

Perhaps in the next couple of days Maddy should throw a small party at her little flat, invite some of the grad students in her program, to warm the feel back up. She could tell the undergrads in the unit next door to stop by, the three nice guys who had the front part of the old house. They were going to love Hunter, and she was sure they wouldn't tell the landlord about him. She was counting on them helping out with the dog now and then.

Yes, with Hunter to keep her from feeling physically isolated, if she just turned on all the lights when she got home and put on some familiar music, it would probably all feel normal pretty quickly. And she could call Wolf. And at the end of the call, he would tell her to eat something, or go running, or to go to sleep. He would remind her of the Liturgy of the Hours.

. . .

302

The porch light came on and Margie opened the door.

"Maddy!" Margie exclaimed, throwing her arms around her returning friend.

Not letting go Hunter's leash, Maddy gave Margie a firm embrace in return. She enjoyed the feeling she had missed, of the tip of her nose poking into Margie's mess of curly hair as she gave her a hug. As always, Margie smelled of sandalwood incense and root beer.

Liz appeared right behind Margie.

"What are you doing here?" Liz asked. "I thought we wouldn't see you until tomorrow, because of Professor Butterfly?"

"Happy to see you, too, friend!" Maddy said sarcastically, giving Liz a hug. "I need to ask a favor."

Margie had bent down to give Hunter a proper greeting.

"You must be Hunter!"

Margie was rubbing his jowls with her knuckles and talking to him in baby talk, and he was wagging his tail. Maddy had taken off his vest on the ride from Indianapolis, so he would know he wasn't on duty.

"I need you to take Hunter tonight," Maddy explained to Liz. "He keeps staring at me and Professor Butterfly" – Maddy gestured with her head at Colin parked in his pick-up truck at the curb – "and we feel like he's going to be judging us all night. He's fed and he's walked and all – can you just take him and I'll get him in the morning?"

"Of course we can!" said Margie, standing back up and taking the leash from Maddy. "Come for breakfast, Mad – I'll make your favorite waffles, with the sunflower seeds and the apple slices."

"Jeez, Mad," said Liz, as if Margie had not spoken, "what's this big dog going to do to Pumpkin and Spice?"

"Just keep the rats in the cage," Maddy answered. "He's a good dog – he's trained not to attack unless given an order. Pumpkin and Spice will be fine."

Liz leaned over and gave Hunter a pat on his head. He pushed his head up against her leg in a gesture of affectionate familiarity.

"Poor creature," said Liz, now scratching him behind his ears, "having no steady family, being handed off from person to person, never knowing where he's going to sleep."

"Yeah, listen, I can tell you from personal experience that that kind of life is not so bad if you are good at making friends," Maddy replied. "Friends who help you out."

Margie cleared her throat and then told Liz to stop being silly.

"One night with Hunter isn't going to kill us, Liz – and you had nothing but nice things to say about him after your visit to Philadelphia. Pumpkin and Spice will be fine if we keep them in the cage."

Margie led Hunter into the house, talking more baby-talk to him.

"Okay, Mad," said Liz, looking over Maddy's shoulder to Colin's truck. "But if this were for any reason other than a night of meaningless sex, I would say no."

"I get that," said Maddy. "And I appreciate it."

"How are things – I mean, in Philly?"

"Things are fucking complicated. I will tell you tomorrow."

"Come over in the morning for your dog and your palm tree and your waffles, and we can catch up."

"Fuck you, too," said Maddy, blowing a kiss at Liz before turning to leave. After two steps, she turned back, just as Liz started to close the door.

"Wait, Liz, do me one more favor? Call Wolf and tell him I'm fine and Hunter is fine, and tell him I am asleep, and I will call him tomorrow?"

Liz nodded and closed the door.

. . .

"There is simply no way for you to give me the sex I need right now," Maddy told Colin as she bent over his coffee table to pick up a pot-sticker with her thumb and index finger. She dunked it in the sauce, popped it in her mouth, and sat down next to Colin on his couch.

She was wearing only his bathrobe, her hair wet from the shower she had taken while he'd gone to get the food. As she leaned forward to take a plate from the coffee table, he also leaned forward, to try to peak into the robe.

"No way to give you the sex you need?" he answered, laughing at her. "Come on, girl, at least give me a chance!"

"Oh, it's not you, Colin," she explained, her mouth a little full from the pot-sticker. She chewed and swallowed. "God, I missed those things. They have just the right amount of garlic. And the mirin in the sauce is just right. Anyway, Colin, it's not any deficiency on your part. I just need – after Philly – the sex I need – "

She leaned forward to move some of the ginger chicken from the take-out container to her plate, and he leaned forward to look into the robe again.

"What makes you think I can't deliver, Maddy?"

"For one thing," she said, "I haven't gotten laid since I saw you last. So, you have to make up for all that time."

"That *is* a long stretch," he replied, holding the container of rice over her plate so she could take some of that. She did.

"How about you, Colin? Have you gotten laid since last I saw you?" She sat back against the couch to eat the chicken and rice.

"A gentleman doesn't tell," he smiled at her.

"A cad who wants to get laid doesn't tell," she replied.

"You do have a quick wit, m'lady."

He picked up the tin of beef-with-broccoli and used his chopsticks to push some out onto his plate. Looking at him do this, she thought about how, soon, she'd be tasting soy-sauce-soaked scallion in the back of his mouth. They both ate without saying a word for a while.

"Well, you say, Maddy, I can't satisfy you tonight because you're just so horny from going so long without, but I think you ought to let me *try*."

"It's not just the length of time," she said. "A lot happened in Philly and..."

She was trying to figure out how one explains in a perfunctory manner that one discovered a series of murders – explains in a way that lets the conversation just move on. This was going to be a bit like learning how to explain that her whole family was gone. It had taken her a few years to learn how to do that. Maybe that experience would make this task easier.

"You need to forget Philly for a bit? Regroup?"

She nodded and he handed her the beef-with-broccoli tin. She spilled some out onto her plate.

"And to be perfectly honest, Colin, I met someone I think I would like to lay, and for complicated reasons, that's just never going to happen."

"Well," Colin answered, "you're welcome to think about him or her while you lay me, if you do me the courtesy of not using his or her name – plausible deniability and all that."

"Kind of you to offer," she said with a laugh.

He leaned towards her, brushed away her wet hair from her shoulder, and kissed her briefly on the neck.

"I'll just take you from behind, Maddy, so my face doesn't get in the way of your imaginings. I know you prefer it anyway."

"Anything but missionary," she answered, like she was reminding him of her taste in ice cream flavors. "Kiss me there again?"

He did, a little slower. It felt good, but it didn't quite do to her physiologically what she had been thinking it might.

"I *thought* I was going to get laid in Philly one night, at least – with some-one visiting from Indiana. But that didn't work out. He's someone I had been seeing sometimes, but he is now on my dissertation committee, so."

Colin pulled his face away from her neck.

"Well done!" he cried. "Now you just have to sleep with, what, three more members of your committee? And then you can turn in complete shit and they'll still have to give you your degree!"

"Shut up," she answered, laughing. "He wasn't supposed to even be facul-ty here. It was an accident."

They ate in silence for a little while longer.

"And, well, some other shit happened in Philly, and I'd like to forget for a little while."

"I might be able to give you the kind of sex that makes you forget every-thing for a little while."

"I need a kind of sex that makes me forget my own *name*," she sighed.

"That's asking a lot," he replied, "but I'm willing to try."

When she didn't answer, he got up to get them more water to drink.

"Colin," she asked when he returned and sat back down next to her, "how do monarch butterflies have sex?"

"The male tackles the female in the air, takes her down, and then he spends up to the next fifteen hours or so pinning her while he transfers his semen."

"Does he at least tell her some good stories during all those hours? Ask her about her work? Let her nap? Get her off?"

"Humans are so weird," he said, sitting back down next to her.

She put her plate down on the coffee table, put her feet up against the table and pushed it away about a foot. The motion made the robe fall open just enough that he could see the line of her thigh all the way up to where he could see just a touch of her pubic hair. She took his plate and put it on the coffee table, slid herself down to the floor, undid his pants, and pulled his cock into her mouth.

"Christ!" he said, as the feeling of her mouth hit him.

He put his hands on her head. But the feeling of his hands on her head re-minded her suddenly too much of Wolf's hand on her head as they had danced in his living room.

She reached up and took Colin's wrists, moving his hands away from her head. She held on to him that way now while she moved her head back and forth.

After a moment, she pulled back.

"How's about you take off your clothes?" she asked.

He did as she asked and laid back on the couch while she mounted him. The feeling of guiding his cock into her vagina felt – well, like the cliché, just like getting back up on her bicycle. (But where had she left her bicycle locked up? Now she was trying to remember.)

"Your hair is dripping on me," he said.

"Why the fuck don't you own a blow dryer?" she asked.

"Why the fuck would I?" he asked. "Anyway, I don't mind you dripping on me – it's hot."

Colin untied the belt of the bathrobe Maddy was wearing, and it fell open. Maddy straightened her body to be sitting upright on him as he laid there. She dropped the bathrobe behind her. He looked at her, taking in the sight of her body from her face to where her pelvis met his.

She rotated her hips to feel him now in this spot, then that spot, then a little deeper.

"Oh, that *does* feel good," she said, meaning it. "Oh, Professor Butterfly, you do feel good."

He was looking her up and down from her chin to her pussy, almost as if he was trying to make sense of her, as if he felt a little wonder.

"Acute-onset conjoined twinning," she said, as if explaining what he was seeing. "Ischiopagus – joined at the pelvis."

"What?"

"Nothing," she said. She was starting to breathe harder.

She leaned over and put her hands on his shoulders. He did have lovely shoulders – muscular like the haunches of a mature hawk.

"Maddy, I think I forgot how absolutely marvelous you look and feel," he said. "How fucking sexy."

She did not bother to tell Colin she had gained a few pounds in good places, thanks to Wolf's cooking and his taking her to the gym. But she thought about it. And then she started thinking to herself that it was strange to be thinking about Wolf at this moment, given that this – this lovely carnal act, this physiologically satisfying feeling – was unknown to that relationship, and always would be.

But there she was, staring off into the air, feeling Colin's cock pressing against the wall of her vagina, picturing Wolf leaning against his kitchen counter, drinking beer from the bottle, smiling at something she had said. She was smiling, too.

She leaned over to French-kiss Colin, searching with her tongue for a scallion in his mouth to orient her to her academic Butterfly. He wrapped his arms around her upper back and kissed her back. He moved his hips lightly to stay with the rhythm she seemed to be enjoying.

There, she thought, there was the mouth that was so specifically Colin's – that slightly-too-muscular, too narrow tongue. The molars that never felt quite clean.

It wasn't the mouth she wanted right now.

She pulled back, sat up, and turned herself to face away from him, straddling his thighs with hers.

"Ah!" he said. "The *female* grabs the *male* in flight! A publishable finding!"

"You're such a dork," she said laughing, looking down to see his erection where it entered her. She had her hands on his knees. He had his right hand on her right hip and his left up where her neck met her shoulder.

Something he did just then – perhaps it was the way he grasped her in a fashion that felt oddly a little too familiar? – poked at her core in a most unpleasant way. It wasn't, she thought, a physical poke.

"What?" he asked, as if he could feel the change in her.

"Nothing," she said.

She was thinking about how unlikely it was that Wolf had tried out different positions with his wife. He and she had presumably accepted the Church's view that the purpose of sex was reproduction. Something at which they had failed.

"Colin? What do you think is the purpose of sex?"

He was now running his hands up and down her back in a fashion that made her think of a boy-child running his toy car up and down a wall.

"Procreation," he answered, with a bit of a gasp. "Obviously. Its evolutionary function."

"So, the female orgasm – merely a byproduct?" she asked.

He reached one hand around to her front and plunged a finger into her pubic hair. His maneuvers were so much clumsier than she had recalled.

"Female orgasm, a byproduct?" he asked. "Not for me. But for nature, yes."

His lost, wandering finger was starting to annoy her. She pulled his hand away and turned herself back around to face him. She affixed his hands on the small of her back and put her own hands back on his shoulders. She started to hump him again.

"I can – " he said.

"Please shut up," she replied.

She closed her eyes and tried to focus on the sensation of the fullness of her vagina. She knew that if she could focus just so, if she could bring her mind to bear on this very intently, then all those unconscious nerves would take over. The magical feedback loop would take over properly. No thinking – no thoughts – nothing clever, nothing knowing.

Absolution through humility, she thought to herself, as if she were telling herself a little inside joke. But all she could see in her mind's eye was the engine of the Amtrak train coming into view the day before.

What have we learned? Sometimes Amtrak can be on time.

Why had Wolf sent her back to Indiana so quickly? Was it that he didn't want to have to worry about her in Philadelphia? That he wanted her gone for the drama of the search warrants and the possible media circus that he said could follow? He knew that Amtrak only ran the Cardinal three days a week, so if he had not put her on the train the day before, it was going to be another couple of days....

She opened her eyes, pulled her hands away from his shoulders and leaned back. She crossed her arms above and behind her head, feeling her own shoulders with her fingertips. She held still and could feel now Colin slowly moving in, out, his hands on her hips. She closed her eyes again, and now she could see so clearly Wolf's face watching the blind woman on the platform feeling the face of her companion, then turning his head to look at Maddy.

Why, oh, why hadn't she felt his face?

She opened her eyes again to see Colin. His own eyes were closed, his visage a portrait of a man close to orgasm – a man holding off. She wondered to herself what Wolf's face looked like at such a moment – was it a variation on the way he yawned, his chin more to one side than the other? Was it like his face looked when he lifted deadweights?

His eyes clenched shut, Colin emitted the small sounds of a man trying to hold on. Now his hands were laid at his sides, his fingertips gripping the couch like an NBA player holds a basketball.

Maddy wondered now if Wolf had known how to make his wife come.

She could picture Wolf's fingertips, specifically the way he held the edge of a tender piece of meat to get a sense of its density and moisture. She could for a split-second picture his fingertips on her own labia that way, held with just the right amount of pressure, rolled gently to light up the glans of her clitoris inside.

How lovely would it be if Wolf could let go everything in his catechism and just touch her that way. How lovely it would be if Wolf would make *that* part of his Liturgy of the Hours, right around five a.m. each day. Light the wick of her clitoris.

But the purpose of sex, Wolf would say, is to create children within the context of the sacrament of marriage.

And what did Colin say? Same as Wolf: that the purpose of sex was to create offspring, albeit, in Colin's view, in the context of species continuity and ultimately evolution.

Fucking patriarchy.

So, what did *she* think was the purpose of sex?

(Colin moaned in a way that made her glad Hunter wasn't here.)

Wait – what *did* she think was the *purpose* of sex?

For the first time, she realized, she did not know.

She did not know.

"How absolutely wonderful," she whispered accidentally.

-28-

Given the lack of any decent sleep on the train, Maddy had been sure she'd be able to sleep anywhere tonight – even a commercial-district sidewalk made of the hardest concrete. But somehow, she had again slept so badly.

Colin had made clear he wasn't thrilled with the idea of her spending the night, so she had told him she'd take the sofa and leave early. But the couch was so uncomfortable, its seat cushions divided in inconvenient spots relative to her frame, the scratchy fabric irritating to her skin. She should have asked him for a sheet.

It didn't help that she'd been trying to sleep in day clothes – jeans and a sweatshirt. She had thought about pulling her pajamas out of her suitcase and wearing those to try to sleep, but she was sure her pj's still had Wolf's scent. She didn't want to overwrite that with Colin's.

She'd spent much of the night thinking about the work she hadn't been doing in the last two months. In Philly, it had been easy to say to herself that she should just focus on her dissertation research and let everything else wait until she got back home. But now that Maddy was back in Bloomington, there was no denying that she had to be working on other things, too: applying for jobs for next year; submitting proposals for conference sessions; working up manuscripts to send to journals.

Well, at least she had these things to do while she waited for the rest of her dissertation work to arrive in boxes in the mail. At least they hadn't seized her computer.

Maddy got up quietly from the couch and folded up the blanket Colin had given her. She pulled her laptop out of her backpack and went into the kitchen where she could plug in to access Colin's internet service. Looking up at the kitchen clock, she could see it was now a little after six in the morning.

She logged onto her university email account and found a message from Professor Carlyle saying he had spoken to Wolf. Would she please come follow-up with him?

And here was a message from Bess McFarlane, also from the day before, asking Maddy if she knew what was going on with Jimmy. Bess said she had not heard from him in days, and she had been trying to reach him.

On reading this, Maddy's stomach churned. Before she left Philadelphia, she, too, had been trying to reach Jimmy. When she had asked Wolf if he thought she should call the bar where Jimmy worked, Wolf had said he'd already called and asked NYPD to check. Had they yet?

Then there was also an email from Liz, from just a few hours before, around midnight.

I called Wolf like you asked. He wants you to call him when you wake up – he said he needs to talk to you. He wanted me to wake you up and put you on the phone, so I had to say you were so dead tired that I didn't want to wake you, because you had gotten no sleep on the train. So, tell him that when you talk to him. I told him he could talk to Hunter if he wanted, and made Hunter speak to prove he was with me, figuring then Wolf would know you really reached here. Anyway, come over whenever – just let yourself in. Turns out Pumpkin is fascinated by Hunter. That rat definitely has a rather dangerous innate curiosity. I should have named him after you, chica.

Maddy closed her computer, unplugged it from the internet connection, and picked up Colin's phone to call Wolf. Then she realized she had better not call him from here. What if he somehow figured out that she wasn't at Liz's? He would be livid if he knew that Maddy was without Hunter.

At this hour of the morning, Bloomington was just a sleepy little college town, and even with the sun not up, there would be no risk at all in walking herself and all her crap the mile or so over to Liz's place. Maddy packed up her backpack and suitcase and quietly let herself out of Colin's house. She headed for Liz's, Wolf's thermos in one hand, the pull-handle of her suitcase in the other. As the suitcase bumped over the sidewalk cracks and the protruding tree roots, Maddy took in a good whiff of the town that had been her home for the last four years. It smelled the way it always did this time of year – a little like wet tree bark, a little like asphalt, a little like people. An early-morning group of three joggers ran by. The sparrows were chattering away.

What a dull and predictable place Bloomington could be after a few years. Like the scenes of a 1940s movie on the classic film channel. The natural and cultural seasonal changes that happened around the year had once felt different to Maddy, even interesting – the exceptional quiet of the library during the frenzy of football Saturdays, the luxury of a long and humid academic summer when campus emptied out and the research spaces all felt sanctified, beginning just after the graduation tulips bloomed near the university gates.

But now, now it all felt so dully predictable. Her role in it all as a studious graduate student just felt predetermined.

Another reason not to consider intentionally putting off her own graduation a year. Much as she would miss being with Liz, it was time to get out of here, hopefully get a job in a real city or at least move to a different college town. Get a post-doc or an assistant professorship. Hopefully the latter. Hopefully tenure-track.

Liz was spending more and more time with Margie anyway. As Maddy reached Liz's house she could see evidence of that. Instead of the repurposed broad-striped tablecloth Liz had been hanging sloppily in the front window as a nighttime window covering, the little rental house now had a proper-looking set of curtains.

Reaching the cement stoop, Maddy looked closer at the curtains through the window. She laughed to herself. There *were* curtains, but they had been made neatly made of the striped tablecloth. Maddy could guess why Margie had done this – no doubt Liz had protested that the tablecloth was perfectly fine as it was, thrown over the curtain rod. No doubt Liz had protested that she liked the print or the color of the tablecloth. And Margie had decided to just use the tablecloth as a compromise, to turn it into proper curtains with an hour or so of sewing.

Putting her key in the door lock, Maddy heard Hunter give out one deep bark. She cringed. She had forgotten that he had been trained to give out a bark when he heard anyone coming in, and now Maddy had probably accidentally woken up Liz and Margie with Hunter's bark.

Dragging her things into the vestibule, Maddy was greeted by Hunter.

"Shh, boy, shh!" she whispered to him, taking off her coat and laying it over her suitcase. "What's this on your collar, Hunter?"

Bending down and feeling it between her fingers, with Hunter holding still for her as if she were picking a tick off him, she could see Margie had knitted him a red and white band to go around his neck right next to his collar. The colors of the university. Margie knew how to welcome a dog to town.

Liz came out of the bedroom stretching and yawning, closing the door behind her.

"Hey," she said to Maddy in a quiet voice. "You have *got* to call Wolf if you haven't by now. He called again around five a.m. again, to see if you were awake. I thought about trying to find you at Colin's but I have no idea where Colin lives or what his phone number is."

Liz handed Maddy the cordless phone from her charger, and Maddy sat down on the couch.

"I'm sorry, Liz, for waking you guys up repeatedly. Did you tell Margie what's going on?"

"No," said Liz. "You know she's a worrier. I just told her Wolf is kind of obsessed with you and that's why he wouldn't stop calling. Then she started worrying about that. So that was stupid of me."

Liz sat down on the couch, very close to Maddy.

"I want to hear what Wolf tells you," explained Liz.

"Okay," said Maddy, "but don't make any noises. And don't be surprised that he calls me 'Rabbit.' I can explain later."

"I can guess."

Maddy dialed the phone and Wolf answered, sounding fully awake.

"Did you get some sleep?" he asked.

"Not much," she said. "Readjustment and all. I didn't realize you had called early this morning – Liz just told me. What's up?"

"Search warrants likely to be executed today. His house and his lab and his office."

"Okay," said Maddy. "Hunter, c'mere."

She slapped her knee gently to get Hunter to come. He came and laid his head between her knees while she petted his head. He looked right into her eyes in the way that made her remember Sister Anjelica saying in a whisper to Maddy that she knew it was against Church dogma, but she felt sure dogs must have souls.

"What are you looking for with the search warrants exactly, Wolf?" Maddy asked.

"Something less circumstantial, obviously."

She didn't answer for a moment. Then she replied:

"Everything in history is circumstantial."

"Well, Rabbit, hopefully we find something today that convinces a jury or a judge to disagree with you about that."

Maddy did not reply this time. After a few seconds, Wolf continued:

"We talked to the medical examiner – I don't mean *we*, I mean the investigating team. I'm not part of the team technically because they know – well, that you were living with me." He cleared his throat. "I mean, they probably think – well, it doesn't matter what they think."

"What did the medical examiner say?" asked Maddy.

"She thinks you're right – that Wilhelm was trying to redirect and distract her during the autopsies of some of his patients. She said that, at the last one, Wilhelm had given her a particularly strange feeling. She's pulling all the records and evidence on them, seeing what they have."

Liz reached over and now also patted Hunter on the head, as if Hunter were a lucky talisman that they each needed to touch.

"Why did they even let him into the autopsies, Wolf? Why did they let him be there for them?"

"You know the answer, Rabbit. He's a specialist in the field. And he was going to end up with the bodies anyway – why should they have suspected anything?"

Again, Maddy did not reply. Since Wolf's comment about trying to find "something less circumstantial," she had been doing a fast double-columned list in her head of facts in her favor versus possible evidence against. It sure seemed like she had enough to prove it, but she could see how some of it might look inconclusive.

And she was thinking about something Shirley had mumbled to her about during a food break on their long first day with the police – that Wilhelm had told Shirley that if Maddy tried to smear his reputation, she'd have a defamation suit on her hands.

"Rabbit," said Wolf, interrupting the silence, "I talked to Professor Carlyle yesterday. I think he understands. He asked me to go over it a few times. He said he just hadn't had to deal with anything like this before and he was trying to make sure he understood it."

"Okay," she said. And then in a more impatient voice she added, "Wolf, to be frank, none of this sounds so urgent that you'd call at five in the morning."

He didn't answer. Liz leaned forward and looked at Maddy, her eyebrows pulled down in a gesture of confusion.

"Wolf, Bess McFarlane sent me an email – she hasn't been able to get ahold of Jimmy. Did anyone from NYPD go check on him yet?"

"I don't know, Rabbit," Wolf said. "I'll follow-up."

"Great," she said sarcastically. "Did they go get Schlesinger from the library?"

"I'll ask that, too," he said.

"Great," she said, in the same cynical tone. "Listen, nothing you've asked or told me hits on something that would be a 5 a.m.-call motivator for you. Because about all this you would say to me, 'There's nothing we can do but wait, Rabbit.' And you would tell me to get more sleep."

"Right. I would say that."

"So are you going to tell me why you called so early?" she asked.

"Yes. We have not located Sergey Goncharov."

She didn't answer, so he continued.

"License plate readers and credit card records indicate that about two days ago he left Philly, and it looks like – headed west. We know he got as far as Ohio and was taking cash out along the way. And then it stopped."

Maddy did not respond. Liz made a quizzical gesture, with her hands, indicating she wasn't sure who Sergey Goncharov was. Maddy shook her head at Liz and frowned, as if to say "not now."

"Rabbit? Listen, I also talked with the police there, in Bloomington, just to brief them. If they see him, they can stop him for questions. But in the meantime, it would be important for you to stay in public places – and I've asked Professor Carlyle to put you up, starting tonight."

"Ugh, Wolf, that is so fucking awkward."

"No," he replied, "it isn't."

Liz pointed repeatedly to the floor in a somewhat frantic gesture, as if to say *you can stay here*. Maddy shook her head firmly at Liz.

"No, Rabbit, it's not awkward – and it doesn't matter if it is awkward. It's just until we sort it out. I asked him about whether there was somewhere you could stay, and he offered. He told me he has a place outside of town, on fifteen acres, with a security system on the house, and – "

"Yeah, Wolf," said Maddy, annoyed. "I've been there plenty of times for departmental functions." She thought about Professor Carlyle's homestead, a modern take on a cabin, about eight miles from campus out in the woods and fields, dotted with hills and a creek that ran through. She remembered the cattle grate at the base of his drive near the road, meant to keep the cows from the neighbor's place from coming up onto his land where they would eat the grass in the places he kept as fields to attract pheasants. The convent had had a cattle grate just like it.

"Well, Rabbit, Carlyle said he has the space, and he has two hunting dogs himself, so he won't mind Hunter. It's just for a couple of days at the most, I think. Hunter will like being with other dogs and having the space to run. You can run with them."

"Okay," she said. "I gotta go, Wolf. Liz is bugging me."

She hung up the phone without further ado. The emotion she was feeling surprised her. It was mild anger at Wolf.

Somehow, in her tired state, smelling vaguely of Phoenix Dumpling and being sent by Wolf to bunk with her awkward and elderly dissertation director, her mind was calculating that this was all Wolf's fault. If he had let her go and shoot The Jerk when she intended to, just after his letter had arrived, then she wouldn't have had to fully take up the problem of Wilhelm, to make up for Katie. And if Wolf hadn't made Maddy care about what he thought of her, then she wouldn't have held back so long before telling the police what she knew about Wilhelm. Yes, this all certainly seemed to be Wolf's fault.

Liz could see her friend was in a knot.

"You want coffee, Mad, or too early?"

"Long day ahead," sighed Maddy. "So yes, please."

She followed Liz from the little front room to the kitchen.

Liz filled the hot pot with water and turned it on as Maddy sat down at the table.

"You want to talk about it now?" Liz asked.

"No," said Maddy. "Later. Much later. I have to go soon."

Liz set up the pot and turned it on.

"Okay. So how was Professor Butterfly?" Liz asked.

"Meh," answered Maddy. "I'll try him again in a few days or something. It wasn't terrible."

Liz pulled the French press down from the shelf above the sink and set it on the counter next to the cannister of coffee.

"Can I ask you something, Lizard?'

Liz nodded and scooped several spoons of grounds into the bottom of the pot.

"What do you think sex is for?" Maddy asked.

"I'm not sure what you're asking, Mad. Do you mean me, personally?"

Maddy didn't answer, so Liz continued.

"Sex for me is for pleasure. But do you mean in terms of contemporary human life in a civilized society – in terms of the ways sex is used to create alliances and bonds? Or do you mean in terms of evolution – like why do we reproduce sexually instead of asexually? Or do you mean politically – what it's used for by different groups?"

Maddy still didn't answer for a moment. Then she said, without a hint of sarcasm, "That was a very helpful answer. I'll be glad to mull that."

The hot pot was starting to make the noise of water being brought to a boil.

"But Liz, when you have sex with Margie, what is it for – is it just pleasure?"

"I guess I do it *primarily* because it feels good to me," Liz answered, somewhat pensively. "But I also want it to feel good for her, so she'll stay with me." She scrunched up her face and thought a little more. "I guess I also just want her to feel good, even if it doesn't make her feel bonded to me. It just makes me so happy when she feels good, I don't even care who causes it. But I love when it can be me."

Maddy found herself a little taken aback. This, she thought, was perhaps the least cynical thing she had ever heard Liz say. Maddy thought Liz must have been thinking something similar, as she had her head tilted quite far sideways, like she had surprised herself with what she had just said.

"Are you *in love* with Margie?" Maddy asked.

"I think maybe so, Mad Girl, although I'm not sure what love is, exactly."

The hot pot switch flipped to off, and Liz poured the water into the French press.

"I think about Margie *a lot*," said Liz, "and I worry about her sometimes. But then I think about *you* a lot, and you know I worry about you. And while I suppose I love you, I don't love you romantically. It's definitely not the same."

"You feel a specific sexual desire for her?"

"Definitely."

"Is that the difference between true friendship and romantic love?"

"Sheesh, I don't know, Mad," said Liz, stirring the coffee a little with a bamboo spoon Maddy knew she kept for this purpose. "I think of these things in terms of hormones and behavior. I think about us as big rats. I don't know how to talk about it the way you do in the humanities."

"You don't feel any sexual desire for me, right?"

"Correct," answered Liz. "No offense, but the thought of fucking you is – well, it is disgusting. It's not your body, or even your orientation. But the idea of having sex with you is – well, it is truly repulsive to me."

They were quiet again for a while. Maddy thought Liz was probably having the same thought – how good it was to have a friend you could say this to without worrying it would cause hurt feelings.

Liz gave the pot another stir and then plunged the top of the pot down. She pulled down two mugs and took the milk out of the refrigerator to pour a little in each mug. Just then Maddy stood up and gave Liz a sudden embrace.

"What the fuck, Mad? You're going to make me spill the milk."

"It just makes me so happy to hear that you're repulsed by the idea of having sex with me, Liz," Maddy answered, wiping a tear out of her left eye with her fingertips.

"Why?"

"I'm sure the idea must repulse you because it hits the incest taboo – the feeling of disgust we naturally feel at the thought of sex with a sibling. I think this is proof you've come to think of me as a sister. And I think that's how I think of you now."

Maddy started to wipe tears away faster and faster.

"And now I have to go, and I have to stay away from you, so I don't get you killed."

"What the fuck are you talking about?" Liz asked, but Maddy did not answer. "Well, at least give me that thermos to wash out and fill with coffee."

Liz hastily washed out Wolf's thermos while Maddy put her coat on and started to gather up her things. She hooked Hunter's leash to his collar and put on her backpack. Liz poured in coffee and milk and handed it to Maddy, and then gave Maddy a hug. Maddy hung onto her a little longer than Liz expected. Then she went out the front door, gave Hunter time to pee on the lawn, and started trudging her way, with suitcase and backpack and thermos and dog, toward the offices of her department.

-29-

The university's main library was quiet save for the steady hum of the ventilation system and the occasional dinging of the elevator bells. Here on the tenth floor, within the building's thick and windowless walls, the sounds from the street could not reach. The only audible variation came from the handful of other grad students and faculty here quietly retrieving books and turning pages. When Maddy listened carefully, the subtle sounds of scholars working quietly reminded her of the night sounds of the mice at work in the convent.

In the random study carrel she had chosen to use for today, Maddy tried again to read from the book she had pulled on the history of late-nineteenth-century American medical education. She was trying to make sure she understood what other historians had found about the use of cadavers in this particular era.

"This seems like a good day for *secondary* sources," Professor Carlyle had told her in his departmental office a few hours earlier, as she had let out another long sigh. "I know that much of your primary sources are with the police, so you don't have them. So, Maddy, just spend today with the secondary."

When she did not answer, he made himself clearer:

"I would advise staying away from the tertiary for today."

She understood his implication. Until she got back her photocopies of the primary sources she had collected from the nineteenth century, she should focus on the secondary – contemporary historians' straightforward accounts of the past. She should stay away from the tertiary – the historiographical – because these were the more theoretical texts that would engage the greater philosophical questions of the field: how we think of evidence; how we know the truth.

Today was not a day to engage epistemological theory. Today, epistemology was no theoretical problem in her life.

As he gave this advice, Carlyle had reached out to her a box of tissues, assuming any woman who needed advice to adhere to the secondary would also require a tool for composing herself. He seemed to do this almost ritualistically with women under stress – hand them a box of tissues – as if it were a prophylactic.

She had taken one so that he would take the box back.

"Yes, go to the library," he had said, carefully setting the box back in its place on his famously well-organized desk, "and work only there today. Maybe just have lunch at the cafeteria there."

"It's no good," Maddy had replied.

She had realized as soon as she had said it that he probably thought she had meant the idea was no good. But she had meant the food at the library cafeteria.

As if he had hoped he could at least get one animal in the room to listen to him, Carlyle had called Hunter to him to come sit next to him. Then he had rewarded the animal with a firm series of pats that Hunter seemed to see as some kind of sweet treat.

"Good boy," Carlyle had said in a soft voice. "Maddy, you and Hunter go to the library and just stay there the whole day with some good secondary sources. If you do that, I believe that everything will feel relatively normal. And we'll know roughly where to find you if we need to. And around four o'clock, after my afternoon seminar ends, you can come back here and we can pack your things and my things into my car and go to my home and introduce the dogs, yours and mine. I have some cold cuts there, things to make sandwiches. Mustard and things."

She wondered if he had some newfound respect for her, for having a dog? Not that he didn't generally respect her. But Carlyle was serious about dogs, particularly working dogs.

"You know, Maddy, I'll tell you a little secret: Going to the library is what I do when I'm dealing with something stressful like what you are dealing with. With Philadelphia. With what is happening with your work in Philadelphia."

He had almost made it sound as if the police had seized her work because she had done something suspicious. Her eyes had started to tear-up at that, and she cut it off by blowing her nose loudly into the tissue.

She had felt ridiculous at the thought of crying to him. It would be neither professional nor the sort of thing with which he wanted to deal – a weepy female. But she was labile from the lack of rest. Almost loopy.

"I could see if Professor Mastromonaco would give you lunch today?" Professor Carlyle had said, pulling the box from his desktop to reach it over to her again.

"No, thank you!" she had answered, a bit too loudly, taking another tissue. "I mean, I don't want to have to talk about my research trip today, Professor Carlyle."

She had run into Giovanni in the department hallway shortly before, and he had looked so startled.

"I didn't know you were back, Maddy!" Giovanni had exclaimed, making it sound, she thought, as if she were a chronic case of shingles. "You look quite exhausted!"

Maddy had noticed he was grasping his travel coffee mug between his palms as if his wrists were handcuffed together.

"I am sorry – I should ask, Maddy, when did you get back?" Then before she could say anything, he had added, "My God, you look unwell."

"Last night," she had told him. "I got back last night. And yes, I could use a bath and a place to take a long rest," she had continued, realizing too late it sounded like she was asking him to provide those things. "I had a complicated trip research-wise, a lot more complicated than I had expected, and I'm looking forward to getting back to my *own* space, my *own* apartment."

"But Professor Carlyle said you and your – your service dog, is that what he said? – that you would be staying with him for a few days."

She had not corrected him. She wondered what exactly Professor Carlyle understood to be going on from Wolf, and what Carlyle was telling people.

Whatever. Now, sitting at this carrel on the tenth floor of the library in the stacks where the Dewey decimal system put the volumes related to her research interests, she was trying mostly to stay awake until near four o'clock. The coffee she had had with the dreadful library lunch was wearing off, and Hunter was asleep on her feet. It felt almost as if his doziness were being transmitted to her.

She reached under her laptop and pulled out from there the letter Carlyle had given her about the dog – a letter he had suggested that morning that she have at the ready at the library in case someone questioned her taking Hunter into academic buildings. He had printed it out on departmental letterhead, signed it quite officially, and given it to Maddy in an envelope to carry with her. She read it again.

To whom it may concern: Madeline Shanks is a doctoral candidate in our department in good standing. The white German shepherd that she has with her is necessary to keep with her for the purposes of research work. Questions may be directed to me as her dissertation director.

He bothered to mention the breed? Like she might slip in a substitute dog and try to get away with something?

This letter was even weirder than the letter he had given her when she went to Europe, when the two of them realized she might be carrying home nineteenth-century images that could look concerning to border control officers – images of naked children with various inborn conditions. Then, Carlyle had given her a letter explaining that her research required her to have medical images that might seem strange to a modern eye.

That, she thought to herself, was going to be the main problem with the Wilhelm issue – getting people to understand the strange idea of a present-day doctor killing patients for research material so that he could have unlimited access to a whole body – unlimited in time and space. What an anachronistic scene. Was she even right, or had she simply read onto this what she knew of the history of specimen acquisition and the ethical lines that had been crossed over and over again in the last few hundred years? What if the police found nothing further to support her hypothesis? What if they didn't understand what to look for? What if they deferred to his social status and power, deferred to their reluctance to drag the name of a good local hospital and university through the mud? What if they concluded that she was probably just hysterical and that Wolf was too attracted to her to think straight?

What if Wolf was?

And what if they decided she was right and it made it all the way to trial and the jury was a bunch of stupid people, the Philadelphia equivalent of a collection of her dullest Hoosier undergrads, and the jury acquitted after Maddy was publicly known to have accused Wilhelm?

She was getting so tired of these same thoughts looping around again and again. What should she hope – that the search warrants showed up nothing and they dropped the whole thing? Even then, Wilhelm would try to ruin her and would have influence enough to make her life a lot harder.

What should she hope for? The Catholics had it so easy – simply praying for God's will. Sometimes even believing it would make a difference.

She closed and rubbed her eyes with her hands, and heard a voice next to her say, "I need you to take my history."

She instantly thought it must be one of her friends from the department come over to say hello with an odd little joke. *Take a history* – the phrase used in medicine to refer to obtaining and recording a patient's oral account of his or her own history.

"And do what with it?" she asked, opening her eyes and turning to look at the man standing next to her, this thin man looking down at her. It was not anyone she knew – he was no grad student. He was middle-aged and looked, she thought, a bit homeless. Had a homeless man wandered up here? To what end?

"I need you to take my history, Miss Shanks," he said, "and give it to the police. So they know what to look for."

Now his slight Slavic accent was evident. But she didn't need it by that moment to understand who he was. No, she didn't need the accent, not with a good look at his frame and his face, not with his reference to medicine and to the police. This was Sergey.

She jumped up suddenly and took off down the aisle of books. He began running after her, calling, "Wait – please wait! There are things I have to tell you about!"

Her dash had startled awake Hunter. He had scrambled to his feet and was now running toward her to catch up. She reached the end of the shelves of books and turned the corner to run towards the elevators and stairwell, but Sergey ran in a direction that cut off her path.

"Wait!" he cried out again. "I need to talk to you, Miss Shanks! Shirley told me – wait!"

Hunter was trying to run ahead of her just enough to look at her face, to ascertain the purpose of this tearing about. Was this a game or something very bad?

She ran toward the center of the floor where pairs of carrels side-by-side interrupted the tall metal bookcases. Feeling Sergey behind her, she quickly calculated she could approach the carrels as gymnastic devices – weirdly-shaped horses. She ran toward the first back-to-back set, jumping up fast to the desk of the first and using her hands to provide balance and lift to get over the bookcases that formed the backs of the carrels. This put the carrels between her and Sergey. He could not easily mount them as she had. She leapt over one more back-to-back set of carrels to get another aisle of books away from him.

Hunter, like Sergey, wasn't sure what to do about the carrels that Maddy treated as if they were mere puddles. The man and the dog both took off down the row of stacks to try to catch up with her in the next row, or the next.

At this point, the handful of other patrons who had also been up on this floor had all stood up, alarmed.

One asked loudly, "What the hell is going on?"

Sergey and Hunter kept after Maddy as she jumped over the carrels and tried again to loop around to the bank of elevators and stairwell. But Sergey again cut her off.

"Please, wait!" he yelled to her. "I want to tell you what I did – what he did – "

Maddy was rapidly scanning her mental map of this floor for another way out and down. There was no external fire escape, she knew – just the interior stairwells. And then it came to her: the book elevator. The dumbwaiter the clerks used to return books from other floors back up to this floor, the dumbwaiter they used to send books down for interlibrary loan requests.

She could almost certainly fit herself into it if she curled up completely.

She took off in that direction, now with Hunter galloping toward her, Sergey not far behind. As she approached the book lift, she could see the door to it was closed. It had not occurred to her it would not be on this floor. But of course, what were the odds it would be?

While running past it, she pushed the button twice fast to call the lift to this floor. She took off down a long aisle again, stopping again in the middle section to leap again over the carrels. This time she did so less elegantly, knocking over someone's neatly compiled collection of books. Now Hunter was barking, as if to scold her for the mess. She could occasionally hear the sound of his nails tapping and scratching on the hard floor surface as he tried to catch up with her.

From down the aisle, she could see the door to the book lift open. She took off as fast as she could toward it. Arriving at the wall where it was located, she pulled as much of herself as she could into the tiny open car, shoved her knees up into her chest, and bent her head over her knees. She reached out to push the button on the wall just outside the car to send it back down to the first floor.

The door closed and darkness descended on her. She could feel the device starting to go down and could feel the air around her mist up from her hot panting. The sound of Hunter's distressed barking was fading.

Only then did it occur to her how stupid she had been not to just give Hunter the orders she had at her disposal to protect her. What the fuck was wrong with her, that she was just now remembering what Wolf had taught her about using Hunter as a self-defense mechanism! The dog must think her absolutely batshit – he must have been wondering if this was some weird chase game. He must have been waiting the whole time for some command. Why hadn't she practiced with Wolf and Hunter rather than just verbally going over the commands with Wolf?

The elevator stopped and the door slowly opened to reveal the clerk's area of the first floor. Maddy pushed herself out of the elevator, spilling onto the floor. A young woman clerk manning the desk turned and looked at her, thoroughly confused.

"That's not for people," she said to Maddy, who was down on the floor crawling toward the corner of the clerk's area nearest the elevators and stair-well. She figured if she plastered herself up against this counter that formed a barrier between the clerk's area and the public space, then, when Sergey came down, he would not see her.

"Tell him I ran out the front door," she said to the young woman in a loud whisper.

"What?"

"When a tall older man appears – he's wearing a blue jacket and he has graying hair – when he comes down the elevator or the stairs, point at the front door and tell him 'She ran out that way.' For God's sake, please just do that!"

Just then she could feel the woman push her legs up next to Maddy. The clerk was clearly concealing her as best she could. The fabric of her chinos brushed up against Maddy's face.

"She ran out that way!" the woman said, and Maddy could feel the motion of her pelvic turn and the bodily jerk created by her thrusting her hand forward.

"Okay, he's gone," she said to Maddy a moment later, backing away from her and looking down at her. "He ran out the front door."

Just then, someone else appeared at the desk, another woman. She said to the clerk, rather breathlessly, "Something weird is going on, up on the tenth floor – there's a dog up there, running all around."

Maddy stood up, startling the woman.

"It's my dog," she said. "I'll go get him."

She bent over for a moment to try to get the blood back into her head.

-30-

One of the good things about Professor Carlyle, Maddy realized at this moment, was that he didn't have a need for small talk. He didn't seem to care that he and Maddy were both silent on the way to his home. Her suitcase and backpack were tucked into in the trunk of his Subaru, with Hunter sitting up straight in the backseat, occasionally leaning his head forward to give the back of Maddy's or Carlyle's head a soft poke and a sniff.

She was glad the dog couldn't talk. If he could, he would probably tell Carlyle about the madness of him and Maddy and Sergey running all over the tenth floor of library not long before, of Maddy suddenly disappearing into a hole in the wall, of Maddy reappearing on the tenth floor a few minutes later to call him over to her as if nothing had happened – though she was obviously, in fact, as rattled as him. If he had human language, Hunter would tell Carlyle how something had caused Maddy then to throw all her things so quickly in her backpack and hasten herself and Hunter back to the department with her acting unusually impatient as he stopped to relieve himself just outside the library. He might tell how, as he peed, Maddy kept looking up at the big limestone-covered tower of the library and then scanning the area all around her.

It was especially good, Maddy thought, that Hunter couldn't dial a phone and speak English. He would tell Wolf all that, and Wolf would ask why the hell she hadn't given Hunter the commands to protect her, to attack Sergey, if necessary.

She had called Wolf not long after she and the dog had returned to the department because the main secretary had told her John Wolf had called three times during the day, trying to reach her. Maddy had taken the liberty of letting herself into Carlyle's office and dialing Wolf from there. But before she might tell him anything about Sergey, Wolf told her that there had been "a communication error" about someone calling NYPD. No one had called to ask them to secure Schlesinger 1888. And no one had called to ask them to check on Jimmy.

Now, Wolf had said – as if this were sufficient – *now* they were on it.

"Jesus fucking Christ!" Maddy had exclaimed, realizing too late she should have shut Carlyle's office door.

Before hearing of this screw-up, she had thought about telling Wolf about Sergey. On the fast walk over to the departmental office from the library, across the cement campus paths that passed through the basin of the creek-like Jordan River, though the tall oaks and maples, she had been trying to figure out what to do about Sergey if he showed up again. *When* he showed up again.

Sergey had clearly wanted to tell her something, and it seemed he was not going to be thwarted. The more she had thought about it, the less it seemed he had been there to harm her. He had said he wanted Maddy to take his history and give it to the police? Why would he say that if his goal had been to do her harm? He had invoked Shirley's name – Shirley must have told Sergey that Maddy was going back to Indiana? Why would Shirley do that if Shirley thought he would harm Maddy? And why had he stayed on the tenth floor and repeatedly begged Maddy to stop and listen to him, even after the other people on the floor had become aware of his presence through the commotion?

Why hadn't he taken Maddy's laptop when he had the chance, when she had disappeared into the book elevator? Why, when he had descended from the tenth floor, had he tried to catch up with Maddy in what would un-doubtedly be an even more public place rather than trying to flee the scene? If Sergey had known that she was back in Indiana – which he obviously knew – then surely he knew also that the police were involved. It could not be that he thought or hoped she had the power to call off the police – that he could convince her to stop the police. In fact, he had mentioned the police – saying he wanted her to give his history to them. What history did he want her to take and give the police?

All she could think of was Shirley's remarks about doctors wanting historians for their legacies.

So, she did not tell Wolf. What good were the police anyway? They had failed with the communication between New York and Philly. They had let eight years pass with The Jerk.

She reached her hand back now between the Subaru's front seats and gave Hunter a few firm scratches behind his ear. She wondered if Professor Carlyle would be okay with Hunter sleeping inside, in the same room as her. She knew his dogs slept outside together, in a pen with a well-built doghouse. She was trying to figure out how to get up the nerve to ask Carlyle to let her keep Hunter in her room. Maybe she could call Wolf and ask him to ask Carlyle?

But now she was just annoyed with herself for feeling like she had to ask a man to ask another man to let her do something that she ought to be able to just do. How the fuck had she gotten herself in this position – a position so reminiscent of the first days after the accident, where she had to rely on well-meaning men to rely on other well-meaning men to protect her from The Jerk. If girls and nuns were simply issued guns, and men were not, the whole world would be so much simpler.

Fucking patriarchy.

Just past where the strip malls of oil-change and fast-food joints petered out, Professor Carlyle turned off the main road to the country road that would take them through the lightly forested hills to the area where he lived. Here, not far from town, Maddy knew from prior trips out to his place, the road would start to run a half-mile between manmade structures, and barns and trailers would come at about the same rate as houses and garages. She was looking forward to taking a shower in Carlyle's guest bathroom, to washing off the lingering odor of Colin. She was tired of wearing what she had worn on the train. She was especially looking forward to trying to sleep.

She let out a heavy sigh and was then glad that Carlyle either didn't hear it or opted to say nothing about it. It was hard not to think herself incredibly stupid for not having told Wolf about Sergey. But what was he going to do about it? Wrap her in useless and frustrating safeguards at most.

Despite there being no other vehicle anywhere on the road, Carlyle flipped on the car's blinker to turn into his half-mile-long driveway. As the tires bumped over the cattle grate, Maddy asked him why he had a security system for the house. He replied that after someone had broken in and stolen his television set, his hunting rifle, and some bottles of good scotch, he realized that he didn't want to worry when one of his graduate students was house- and dog-sitting for him while he was away.

As they got out of the car and Carlyle let his dogs out of the pen, the dogs all behaved as solid working dogs do: Carlyle's pair and Hunter treated each other warily for about sixty seconds, and then shifted into acting as if they were all old chums. Standing near the car at the top of the drive by the house, Carlyle reminded Maddy that the yellow Labrador retriever was named Daisy, and the chocolate lab, Pago.

Undoubtedly Carlyle's verbal and physical cues to them had helped the dogs understand they were supposed to get along. Finished greeting Hunter, Daisy and Pago ran a few happy circles around Maddy. As Carlyle opened the trunk to retrieve Maddy's suitcase, the three dogs came over to see what he was doing.

"Gah!" Carlyle said in a friendly tone, pointing away from the house. The dogs trotted away together down the driveway.

"Detective Wolf said you might go running with the dogs while you are here," Carlyle said as he let Maddy into the house, carrying her suitcase. "I don't quite understand this business of intentional exercise myself, beyond a hearty hike, but you are welcome to run the dog trail – it goes all around the property, as I think you know."

"Thank you," she said, following him to the guest room.

And here it was – the warm rustic-modern-cabin version of the convent, of Wolf's house, of it all.

Here she went again, into another monastic guest room.

She tried so hard to focus on what was so lovely about this room – the bed neatly made with a colorful handmade quilt, extra heavy wool blankets folded and stacked on the wooden chest. The Persian rug. The desk all set up for working, with a ceramic mug full of pens and pencils, and a proper desk lamp.

But Jesus. It all just felt like one more round of tenuous housing.

This had to stop.

This had to stop.

This had to stop.

"Time for dinner," Carlyle said, slapping his hands together and startling her out of her mental fugue.

Maddy had forgotten she was back in the land where people thought five o'clock was the right time for the last evening meal.

Following him back to the kitchen, she watched as he pulled out the makings for sandwiches. Then, as he made them each a roast beef sandwich with lettuce, tomato, mayo, and mustard, he asked her something she didn't expect: he asked her to tell him how she had done the research on Wilhelm in Philadelphia and what exactly she had found.

Maddy realized that Carlyle had asked it in the voice he would use in a grad seminar when asking a student to recount what she had found in her course-related research project. His request was straightforward and Socratic, with not a hint of worry that she was too fragile to talk about it. It felt to her just like a scholar asking another scholar about her work.

And so, as he sliced the tomatoes with a sharp serrated knife on his wooden cutting board and used a butter knife to apply the mayo to the factory-produced whole-grain bread, she answered in kind – young scholar to old scholar, realizing she didn't have to do any of the explaining of historical method she had felt the need to do with the police.

She told him about the feeling of anachronism she had had in Wilhelm's lab; her timelining of the specimen acquisition as evident in his published papers; her obtaining his grant reports via the Freedom of Information Act. She explained what she found when she compared the grant reports to the published records to what she knew from various members of the little people organization. She described the disjuncture between some of the death certificates and his own accounts of the deaths of people who became his specimens. And she told Professor Carlyle especially about Schlesinger 1888 – although she did not tell him that she had purposefully marred it with an inky fingerprint, because, she thought, there were limits to what mischief he could tolerate, and a scholar marring a text was beyond those limits.

He asked little as she presented the work, eating his sandwich while standing with her at the kitchen counter, nodding a lot, and making small noises of appreciation at her perseverance and her findings.

She realized what a relief it was to not have to try to speak of this in one or two sentences – "something happened in Philadelphia, and I discovered what I think was a series of homicides" or some such. What a relief it was to lay out the research properly! It was like the difference between trying to write one of those awful, tortured 50-word abstracts for a conference paper and getting to give the whole paper itself. And nothing in her method was so different from what historians do, really, that he would think it bizarre, the way some of the police seemed to think it.

"Well, well," he said, when she had finished the mainline of the story. He gestured to her sandwich to suggest she eat. "You've not done what I would have done, Maddy, but what you've done seems to me very interesting and very important."

She took a bite of the sandwich feeling so much happier than she had just an hour before. Sure, he should have toasted the bread, and this sandwich was badly wanting the company of a well-aged dill pickle. But all in all, this was what she had needed: reasonably good, slightly fatty food, and a senior colleague who understood her.

Carlyle pulled down from the top of the refrigerator a bag of potato chips, opened them, and spilled some out into a bowl he put between them.

"I guess you have been stuck doing what amounts to some oral history work, Maddy, with this?"

She nodded as she ate a few chips.

"And we haven't given you any training in that – you know, we don't expect our Ph.D.'s to do much oral history work."

"It's okay," she said. "I'm good at interviewing people to get information out of them, so I was able to get a lot of what I needed."

"But perhaps this is something we should add to the program, in case – "

And then they both laughed at the idea that any other graduate student would ever find herself or himself in this position again.

"Can I ask you something historiographical, Professor Carlyle?"

He had pulled out two glasses now and was pouring them each some root beer from a plastic soda bottle pulled from the fridge. It was as if it did not occur to him to serve a meal with all its parts together.

"Of course you can ask me something historiographical," he replied.

"When I was with the police, one of them said something about obtaining justice for the dead. And the curator Ms. Anseed and I – well, we just looked at each other, because – well, it made me realize that I find it odd to talk about justice for the dead. The dead are dead."

Carlyle drank a bit of the root beer pensively, and then ate another chip.

"I'm not sure how this is a historiographical issue, Maddy? Are you asking about history and justice?"

"Professor Carlyle, do you believe in God and an afterlife?"

"No, Maddy."

"So, you're an atheist, like me."

"Well," he answered, "I would have to say 'agnostic' – we don't know what we don't know. But I seriously doubt there is a God or an afterlife, and I don't bother spending time considering otherwise."

"Then *you* get," Maddy said so earnestly that her own tone surprised herself a little, "that the reason we pursue justice in the case of suspected homicide – the reason we try to figure out the history of what happened – is for the *living*. Not for the dead, but to protect the living. But also – because also we have to *know*. We just have to *know*."

"I think that is right," he said. "I am not sure everyone values the knowing, but I can understand your desire. The desire to just know."

For a while, they both said nothing more. The sounds in the room included only the loud ticking of the clock on the fireplace mantle in the attached sitting room and the crunching of the potato chips.

"Maddy, you must really want to know Wilhelm's motivation," said Carlyle finally. "I mean, you understandably assume he wanted the bodies for his research, his grants. But you must wish you could look into his head and his heart and see what is there."

"Yes! When I think on that, it always reminds me of a lecture you gave us once, in the first-year course on historiography, Professor, when we were reading that awful biography of Newton that suggested his sexual repression somehow explained his scientific genius. You talked about how we could speculate about motivation in history, but in fact, we could never know."

"Never?" Carlyle asked. "Did I say 'never'? Maybe not never. But even if a subject tells us his motivation, records it very specifically in his journal, say, how can we know he understands his own mind well enough to know? How can you know what motivated you to pursue this line of inquiry, Maddy, about Wilhelm?"

She thought about it – how complex her motivation had been. Her professional annoyance of the stuffy M.D.'s attitude toward the young women Ph.D. in history; the dream that set her off from the strange feeling that something wasn't right; the curiosity about what FOIA might tell her that other sources might not; the need to not deal with The Jerk and her guilt over Katie; the desire to engage and impress Wolf.

She would never have thought that a conversation with old Professor Carlyle could make her feel so – so thrilled – *so very thrilled* by it all, by the whole intellectual constellation of What Happened in Philadelphia. She remembered now the thought that she had had, on the blanket with Giovanni not so very far from here, among the southern Indiana cedars, on the bluff above the stream.

Isaac Newton might have used The Calculus to figure out the entire area under the curve, but sometimes in life the best thing to do is to just live in one section under the curve of a whole life, live in one perfect narrow section of the area under your life's whole curve, for just a few hours.

And here was one perfect hour with Professor Carlyle. One perfect hour that reminded her the reason why she had *not* gone to medical school or to law school where the career path would have been so much easier but had instead pursued the questions of how we know the past and what we do with it, given a world that lacks a St. Peter to sort it all out later, the credit and the blame.

"I need to feed the dogs and run them a bit," Carlyle said, looking out the kitchen window to the drive where the dogs were lying about together. "Did you want to come?"

"I need to call my friend Liz, so she doesn't worry," Maddy answered, and he nodded and pointed to the phone.

Carlyle grabbed a Tupperware bowl and headed out the front door. Maddy could see the three dogs all stand up quickly at the sight of him, expressing the way dogs do that combination of obedience and delight at the site of a worthy human master. She watched while he fed the dogs from a big metal bin of dog food, using the plastic bowl as a dish for the visiting Hunter. Then they all took off along the dog trail, Pago staying close to Carlyle's side, Daisy and Hunter running ahead a little. She felt happy to have given poor over-traveled Hunter this time with his own.

It was just as Maddy was dialing Liz that she could see a car coming up the drive. Just as Liz answered, Maddy realized she was going to have to go tell this person that Carlyle was momentarily off running the dogs and would not be back for a little while.

"How are you?" asked Liz, hearing Maddy's voice.

"Okay," Maddy replied.

But then she thought, no. She was not okay. For the person getting out of the car was Sergey.

The speed at which her brain made the next decision surprised her. Perhaps it should not have. The "pro" column had already been all stacked up, like a bin of seed filled to the brim, ready to be dispensed from the bottom. It had already occurred to her, since he disappeared out the library's front door, that Sergey could tell her so much: his own part in it, the methods, perhaps even more about the motivation than she understood.

If he gave her his history and she gave it to the police, the case might be so much less circumstantial. If she stayed calm and talked to Sergey, the living might be made significantly safer. And most of all, she might know things she so badly wanted to know.

The only "con" was her physical self. It wasn't as if she didn't value that – her physical self. But just at this moment, this atheist, this materialist – she felt as if she were more than that.

It was something like the decision to risk bad sex occasionally, she thought to herself. In the search for knowing something more, something better, something different. It was like that, right?

"Maddy?" said Liz.

"I have to go, Liz, sorry." Then she added, in a quieter voice, "Liz, no matter what happens, please know I love you. So, so much."

"Maddy?" said Liz, a little alarmed. "Are you about to do something very stupid?"

"I don't think so," Maddy answered. "I think I am about to do something quite reasonable."

She hung up the phone.

-31-

"Could you bring me a glass of water?" Sergey asked, as soon as Maddy had stepped outside the front door.

She went back inside and brought him out a glass of water. She handed it to him but noticed he did not drink it.

"Can we sit somewhere to talk?" he asked.

"You're not going to come at me again, like in Philadelphia that night?"

"It was just meant to scare you off," he said. "If you had looked, you would have seen the knife was completely dull. It was a stupid thing, that, but Dr. Wilhelm thought it would make you go away – that you would not go to the meeting in Washington, and you would leave Philadelphia and you would go back to the nineteenth century. We didn't know you were living with a policeman."

She was scanning his face, trying to understand why she felt as if he were an honest man, knowing what she knew. But what did she know?

"Please, can we sit somewhere so I can tell you some things?"

She motioned to a bench up the hill above the house, a couple hundred feet up a winding path, set in a clearing among the trees, past the store of Carlyle's stacked firewood. Sergey walked up toward the bench, and she followed. They sat down and he held the glass of water between his hands, still not drinking any.

"I think there is not a lot of time," he said.

She was struck by how exhausted he looked. His eyes were encircled in gray skin, and his body gave off a light shake. She wanted to tell him to come inside and rest, but she thought he must be right – that there would not be a lot of time.

"Shirley told you I was coming back to Indiana – she told you we had gone to the police?"

Sergey nodded.

"Why didn't you just tell Shirley what you want the police to know?"

"Then they will think she was a part of it," he answered. "She didn't know she was a part of it, until now. She didn't understand how he used her to get the donation forms and a couple of times to deliver medications to patients who – "

He did not finish the thought.

"But you were part of it?"

"Yes," he said. "Not at first on purpose. Even for him, for Dr. Wilhelm, it was not at first on purpose."

Maddy asked him what he meant.

"The first patient – I don't even know the name. Dr. Wilhelm told me that it was just the case that the patient was suffering horribly from sickle cell, and the young man begged Dr. Wilhelm to give him enough morphine to just end it. Dr. Wilhelm was interested in the case because the man's growth had been so stunted by a very terrible version of the disease, and Dr. Wilhelm did what the patient wanted. He pushed the morphine to end the pain. And then he had the body, to study."

"What was the first one for you?"

"Not that different – a man with dysplastic dwarfism, he had a bone cancer and we thought the dwarfism and the cancer might be linked in a way that could tell us something about the mechanism of bone growth and this particular type of carcinoma – it could be important – but the man wanted to go to Europe to see his family there for the last time, and it was into stage-four – terminal. And he was in pain – bone cancer can be so painful."

"Wilhelm didn't want the body going away and not coming back."

Sergey nodded.

"He had me sit with the man and do the morphine push, so that he would not be in the room when it happened – the idea was we could delay the medical response if I acted like I had to supposedly go look for Dr. Wilhelm when the breathing stopped."

Maddy winced a little.

"Shirley did not tell you, perhaps," said Sergey, "that I was dependent upon Dr. Wilhelm for my green card. And if I lost my green card, I would be sent back to Russia."

"And why was your green card worth this?" Maddy asked bitterly.

"Because in Russia, I fell in love with the wrong man's woman."

She didn't reply.

"Perhaps you would not kill a man near death to save your own life," he said, dipping his finger into the water and putting the wet fingertip into his mouth. "But add to the calculation the possibility that in obtaining the man's body, you might come to understand something very meaningful for humanity, about osteosarcoma?"

Maddy was trying to think about what she would want to know so badly that she would hasten a person's death. She might hasten it if they were pointlessly suffering?

"The next one," said Sergey, cutting off her thoughts, "the next one, that was different – another cancer, lymphoma. We knew it was a very interesting body that Tom Maupisand had. Asymmetrical growth, with evidence of a bilateral genetic mosaicism – Tom had two different color eyes, I remember."

"And the method?"

"Overdose of the chemotherapy. Not hard to make that look accidental."

Maddy wondered if she was right in detecting in his voice some remorse.

"Why are you telling me these things?" she asked. "Why didn't you just go to the police and confess, if you are confessing to me?"

"You are a historian – I think there is a chance you will understand, I didn't set out to do this. It started and then, well, then he could use what I had done so far to make me do more. If you write the history, maybe you record how I didn't set out to do this. Maybe you capture the subtleties and not tell a simple story about good and evil, where I am evil."

She did not reply.

"And also, I am telling you because, if I go and tell the police myself, then I will spend the rest of my life in jail. Perhaps much of it in Russia if they deport me. If I tell you, you tell them, and they know. But I die without imprisonment."

She looked at his face and looked down at the glass of water. There must be a reason he was not drinking it yet. She could now guess the reason.

"What substance?" she asked. "I would like to know what I am facing in – in the next – the next period of time."

"Cyanide," he answered. "Not reversible. Not very pleasant, but it won't take too long."

"It causes the central nervous system to collapse, correct?"

She was trying to remember what she had read in a nineteenth-century treatise on poisoning.

"Dizziness, confusion," he said, "the heart gives up eventually, after not too long. You can go while it takes effect. You don't need to see."

"But in prison," she said, thinking back to the convent and wishing she might drag him there mentally, "while you are in prison, you can always *read*."

"To what end?" he asked. "And it is not even as if they will let you read what you want. Either Dr. Wilhelm will try to pin it all on me, in which case I will go to jail forever, or we will both be found guilty, in which case I will go to jail forever. The math is not difficult, Miss Shanks."

The two of them heard one of the dogs bark. The sound was a long way off, but it seemed as if it were a sign they might be coming back in this direction, the direction of the house.

"There is not a lot of time, I think," he said. "Listen carefully?"

"Let me go get paper and pen?"

"You'll remember enough."

He went on to tell Maddy a list he had obviously made in his head: which bodies should be tested for which substances; which prescriptions Dr. Wilhelm had written for Sergey to make it look as if Sergey were the patient, to obtain drugs they needed to effect various deaths; at which gym Sergey had a locker in which the police could find a large stash of useful records, including notes from Dr. Wilhelm to him, including requests to pull various papers on the toxicology of the substances they were considering using at any given time.

Sergey stopped suddenly then, and Maddy followed his gaze down the hill. Carlyle had reappeared with the dogs, and he was standing behind the car looking at the license plate. He would see the car registered in Pennsylvania.

"Maddy!" Carlyle yelled, standing up suddenly and looking all about.

The dogs visibly startled at his piercing cry, Hunter in particular.

Carlyle's eyes settled on the two of them sitting on the bench.

"Call Wolf," Maddy yelled down to him, "and tell him Sergey is here and that I am finding out important things. I will be down later."

"Who?" Carlyle yelled back. And Maddy realized that somehow, in telling Carlyle the history over the sandwiches, Sergey had not even seemed worth mentioning.

"Sergey!" said Maddy. "I will explain later!"

Carlyle hastened into the house, the dogs unsure what to do. Hunter jogged up the hill to come to Maddy, moving a little slowly as he approached. He clearly recognized Sergey from the library earlier in the day. Maddy slapped her thigh to let him know it was okay to approach.

"Who is Sergey?" Sergey said, letting out a short laugh. "I am nobody – nobody in his papers, nobody in his grants. But now I will be so important in his stories about it all! Because he will try to say it was all just me."

He petted Hunter like a man who loved dogs, and Maddy wondered if the feeling of a dog might convince him not to end his life. But as if he could sense Sergey's lethargy, Hunter soon turned and trotted back down the hill toward Daisy and Pago.

"Listen," Sergey said, "the dogs remind me – there is at least one body in the lab that is misidentified. There might be more."

"What do you mean?" asked Maddy.

"One woman – her family wanted her body back not too long after the death. The family was okay with a little bit of research after the death, but only for a few days. So Dr. Wilhelm said he'd return her body cremated, soon. He told them it would have to be cremated because of the kinds of tests he was running, that it wasn't safe to send the body without cremation. But what he did was give the family ashes of some dogs he had euthanized. So, the name in the lab, the name associated with the specimen, it is fake."

Maddy was taken aback by this. She then wondered to herself why this felt particularly shocking after all she had already heard.

"There may be more of those," said Sergey. "He didn't tell me where everything came from, or where it went. DNA analysis on the bodies should show who they all are."

At this moment, Sergey and Maddy realized that Carlyle had reemerged from the house and was now slowly approaching them, his hunting rifle drawn up to his shoulder and pointed toward Sergey. He was about seventy feet away by Maddy's calculation.

"Jesus, Professor Carlyle, no!" she yelled, leaping up and putting her body in front of Sergey's. "I'm taking a history!"

"Detective Wolf told me who this is, Maddy," Carlyle yelled to her. "Move aside."

"Jesus Christ, Professor, Wolf doesn't understand all of what's going on!"

Sergey had put the glass of water down next to the bench and was now also standing, holding on to Maddy's shoulders, staying positioned behind her, ducking his head down. She started to wonder whether he was suicidal, or if there was just more he absolutely needed to tell her.

"Go away!" Maddy said, flipping her hand up and down as if this would shoo away an old man with a long gun. To her surprise, Carlyle lowered the weapon.

"What would you have me do?" Carlyle asked.

"Go in the house and wait," she said.

Carlyle backed down the hill, called Hunter to him, bent down, and quietly gave Hunter a command. Hunter sat and cocked his head. Carlyle gave it again, and Hunter began to creep up the hill, his head and tail lowered.

Maddy figured out that Carlyle must have given Hunter an order, something like to attack Sergey.

"Hunter!" she yelled sharply. "Come!"

She pointed at the ground in front of her and the dog trotted up to her and looked at her, his head cocked again. He let out a small whine.

"Let's go back to the bench," Maddy said to Sergey. "If we put the dog in your lap, he won't shoot you. He would not dare to hurt the dog."

They settled on the bench, and Maddy ordered Hunter to come up and lie across Sergey. The dog and the man both looked uncomfortable positioned like this, but Maddy held out hope the heat of a vibrant animal against him might somehow bring back in Sergey a will to live.

He began to pet the dog, and Hunter seemed to calm down.

"Tell me where Schlesinger 1888 came from?" Maddy asked.

"Well, it came from Dr. Wilhelm," said Sergey. "When someone in the little people group started saying that it seemed like a lot of people were dying after joining his clinic – by then, it wasn't just the people with cancer dying – he tried to claim the reason was heart complications of the growth conditions. He cited a paper he claimed existed – Schlesinger 1888. And then when someone in our area of research wanted to see it, he had to produce it."

"So where did it come from?"

"Dusseldorf," answered Sergey. "There was a printer there, an old printer, he had access to blank paper from the period, he knew what it would look like. Dr. Wilhelm told him that he wanted this pamphlet recreated, a replica, because it had been written by my grandfather and lost to history, and he wanted to give it to me as a gift."

"Do you think the printer believed him?" asked Maddy.

"I think when you pay someone like that enough, they are happy to believe you," answered Sergey. He shifted to adjust Hunter's weight on his lap and gave the dog another series of pats on the head.

"Would the printer tell the police that Dr. Wilhelm came and ordered it?"

"I expect so," said Sergey. "You know why he did it as a pamphlet?"

"To explain its absence in all the historical indices," answered Maddy, and Sergey nodded. "And then he faked the destruction in the fire, to move it to New York, to get it into the library indices and make it look like there had been at least two copies extant all along."

Sergey nodded and was about to say more when Carlyle emerged from the house and walked partly up the hill, warily, still holding his hunting rifle.

"Maddy, I have summoned the police!" he yelled.

Sergey and Maddy looked at each other.

"You could take off into the woods," she said, as he pushed the dog off to her. He reached into his pocket and pulled something out. He leaned over and retrieved the glass of water.

"I don't think I could get very far," said Sergey. "And Dr. Wilhelm will try to pin it all onto me. But I think that will not be possible now, with what you know."

"You were not in Washington when Nick died, were you? They could prove that was just Dr. Wilhelm, on his own."

"No," said Sergey, "I was not in Washington. They will be able to prove I was in St. Louis, at a meeting. And the same with Jimmy."

Maddy felt her heart go up into her throat.

"What do you mean, with Jimmy?"

"I wasn't in New York. That was just Dr. Wilhelm."

Sergey could see by Maddy's expression that she had not known.

"But why – why would he kill Jimmy? His body was so boring – just achondroplasia."

"I expect to prove something to you," answered Sergey. "I believe he has the body now."

When Maddy did not answer, he went on: "That one wasn't going to be hard, he told me. Alcohol poisoning. Dr. Wilhelm told me his plan was to go to Jimmy and tell him that you had been working for Dr. Wilhelm – that you had gone to New York to find out what Jimmy knew specifically so you could report back to Dr. Wilhelm. He knew it wouldn't be hard to get

Jimmy drunk with that suggestion, that he had been had by you. And from there, well, it would not be difficult to enact alcohol poisoning that would appear self-inflicted."

The way he stated all of this so matter-of-factly, now she had no sympathy for him. Or was it that she wanted all the guilt of this death transferred from her to him?

The sound of sirens cohered, the light of the police cars came spinning up the long drive, through the dusky air.

Sergey brought his hand to his mouth, took the capsule, bit down, raised the glass, and drank the water. Maddy pushed Hunter off her and stood up to turn and watch. It was not long before Carlyle was standing next to her, and it was not long before Sergey's face flushed and his limbs started to flail with a seizure. He fell down off the bench, hitting his head on the edge, and vomited. Her first instinct was to turn him over, to clear the vomit out of his airway. And then she realized there was no point. She crossed her arms across her body and thought she might feel better if she could pray. If only one of the sisters were here, she would be obliged to pray with them. If only Wolf were here –

"What is going on?" Carlyle asked with horror in his voice, the dogs all now at his side, all in evident distress. "Dear God, dear God."

"Cyanide," said Maddy quietly, mentally noting that Carlyle had joined her in this involuntary slide into the desire for a deity.

"Dear God, dear God," he said again, as Sergey made noises Maddy had never heard come from a human, noises she hoped she would be able soon to forget.

She looked now at Professor Carlyle's face, seeing a twisted visage of terror, a portrait worthy of Hieronymus Bosch. And she realized it was true: It was not the dying or the dead about whom she had to be concerned. She would hold in her conscience forever not the deaths of her parents, of her sister, of Nick, of Jimmy, or of Sergey. She would hold in her conscience the life of dear old Professor Carlyle, perhaps irreparably wounded – wounded by bearing witness to the consequences of her own selfish and insatiable need to know.

-32-

In the fading blue light of the mid-November dusk, the flock of black birds swirled around and around and around the old school's chimney, looking like static on a television screen. Hundreds of seemingly identical swifts, circling hundreds of times, getting ready for the moment when the shift in movement would begin – when one by one, then two by two, these birds would drop down into the chimney and settle in, to bunk together until the morning.

The way the flock held off on descending into the rectangular brick column for the night – circling and circling – always reminded Maddy of a group of squealing young children dashing out to the end of a frighteningly high diving board, looking over the edge, and then backing away, over and over until finally one jumped, then the next, then the next.

She was sitting next to Wolf in the outdoor fabric fold-up chairs lent for the evening by the undergrads who lived in the flat next door to hers. She had told them she wanted to show her friend visiting from Philadelphia the sight of the funneling chimney swifts at the Harmony School at sunset. She was surprised that the young men had no idea what she was talking about. But perhaps she should not have been; no wonder so often when she came to watch this natural delight, she was the only one around. Few in

Bloomington seemed to have noticed this remarkable daily dance of nature, the one that marked the start of night, when the sun would be gone to make its daily visit to the other side of the earth.

The evening was the chilliest it had been this fall, and Maddy was wearing her winter coat. She was glad Wolf had thought to bring a real coat for himself when he hastened his way by car from Philadelphia the morning after Sergey's death. For his part, Hunter seemed unfazed by the low temperature as he walked around the parking lot, sniffing out smells, tasting weeds, and coming back to where they were sitting every now and then. They had brought Wolf's thermos, filled with the hot tomato soup he had just made at her little apartment. From his coat, Wolf pulled out two grilled cheese sandwiches wrapped in tin foil and handed her one.

"I feel a little funny," she said, "that I have comfort food and good company and maybe Professor Carlyle has neither?"

"He seemed to be okay today, Rabbit," answered Wolf. "I talked with him when we took the dogs out together. He told me the story of the death three times. I reassured him he did everything right. I think he believes me now."

"I asked the EMTs to do me the favor of not declaring the death until they were off his property, so that in the records, Sergey will not have died on Carlyle's property. I thought that might make it a little easier on his psyche."

"Good thought," Wolf answered, raising his eyebrows, opening the thermos, and pouring some soup into the cup. He sipped it to see if it was good, made a noise of satisfaction, and handed it to her.

It had been two days since the death, two days since the searches of Dr. Wilhelm's lab and house. With the information Maddy had obtained from Sergey, the police had already been able to find more evidence that was going to help. Today, they had located the printer in Dusseldorf.

Wolf had explained to her, soon after he arrived, that what Sergey had told her about the deaths, about the motivations – none of that would be admissible in court. A woman claiming she remembered what a man on the verge of suicide said, that would count legally as mere hearsay.

But much of the physical evidence Sergey had left behind in the gym locker or had otherwise told her about – that physical evidence would be admissible.

Wolf told Maddy that he was rather glad the prosecutors would be using evidence not tied to Maddy because it made it unlikely she would be called to testify very much, if at all. And that meant she could just focus on her own life, her intended profession, and move on.

The two of them watched the birds in silence for a while. Maddy was wondering how long Wolf might stay. His excuse for coming here had been to deliver her back her dissertation materials. Now that he had done that, Wolf didn't have much reason to stay. But he was making no noises yet about leaving. Presumably he would stay tonight.

She hoped so. She was looking forward to another night like the last – sleeping in her own bed on his arm, waking to the feeling of order in the universe. Although...she was also looking forward to when he would be gone and her life would return to something like normal – when she could always call him by phone but could also have her own space back to herself. When she could do what she felt and not worry about him knowing.

"Thank you for meeting with my dissertation committee today," she said, handing him back the empty thermos cup.

"It was good to put names to faces," he answered, "and I think it helped Professor Carlyle feel like he didn't have to explain it all to them. I liked hearing from Professor Parnelle about how she had always been impressed by your ability to go down paths other scholars wouldn't be able to see."

Wolf poured more soup into the cup.

"She's always been very supportive," Maddy said. "I can always count on her to tell me that I can manage whatever I have to manage. Like you."

"And Professor Mastromonaco. He's the one who gave you the dresses."

She thought it interesting that Wolf didn't intone it as a question. She was wondering how he had figured that out.

"What was it, Rabbit, that Shirley Anseed said in the car about why brides in China wear red?"

"Because there it is the color of good luck, good fortune – happiness. White is worn here because it is the color of virginity – of naiveté."

"Right," said Wolf. "So, I think you should wear that red dress he gave you to your dissertation defense. To signal that you are very happy and very fortunate indeed."

He smiled a devilish smile, and Maddy started laughing.

She had noticed at the meeting the way Giovanni was looking from her to Wolf. Giovanni had not looked happy, especially when Wolf briefly put his arm around Maddy after the meeting was over and they had all stood up and Professor Parnelle told Wolf what a good thing it had turned out to be that Maddy accidentally ended up in a police detective's home, given where her research had taken her.

"Rabbit," he told her now, "you should invite me back out to

Bloomington for that – for your dissertation defense."

"I will, Wolf. And hopefully you will manage to come again without Father Tad, like this time."

She took the cup of soup from him and drank some more. Again, in silence, they watched the birds. Some were now starting to drop into the chimney, but only one every twenty seconds or so. There was still a good five or ten minutes, she knew, from the moment when there would be the sudden big funneling of dozens of birds per minute dropping down.

"I have to say, Rabbit, it is difficult for me to imagine how a feeling of pure happiness can constitute sinfulness."

"What do you mean?" she asked, wondering what he was talking about.

"I think that Father Tad feels I should confess the happiness you make me feel – confess it as a sin. But, Rabbit, it makes much more sense to me to think of sin in terms of acts – not feelings."

"Neither acts nor feelings are sufficient for sin," she replied. "You need both – the bad act and the conscious motivation. We don't blame people for accidentally killing their children."

"Not usually," he said pensively. "Anyway, remember the observation you made to me about Catholic confession – that you go to a stranger rather than the person you've wounded?"

She nodded.

"I think," he said, "I will go to a stranger for my next confession."

Seeing Hunter was wandering around carrying something, Wolf called him over. He checked Hunter's mouth and saw it was just a stick and let the dog trot away with an affectionate light slap on the rump.

"He's acting like a retriever now. He's losing all his training around you," said Wolf.

"Everybody does," said Maddy.

She was not meaning to make a joke, but Wolf let out a laugh. He paused and then laughed again.

"*Everybody*, Rabbit. What do you think of the food?"

"Oh, Wolf," she said, turning toward him, "when I left Philadelphia – it's hard to believe that was just a few days ago – but when I left Philadelphia, I think I didn't thank you for putting me up all that time. And feeding me. And all."

"You're welcome," he said. "I'm glad you came. I am glad it was not Matthew at my door after all."

She settled back into her chair, soaking up the violet-blue of the sky. It was now the color of the fabric the local Amish used for the men's shirts – a sort of deep and ethereal indigo.

"It's funny, Wolf, but I don't even feel like Wilhelm was the most significant thing that happened in those two months in Philadelphia."

"The Jerk's letter and all?" he asked. "That?"

"No. All the things you made me think about."

She zipped up her coat a little more.

"Sometimes I think I will be thinking about some of our conversations for the rest of my life."

"I think the same thing," he said, leaning back in his chair, tipping it back a little.

A car drove by on the street near the school's parking lot momentarily brightening the space with its headlights. Soon, the darkening of the evening descended again.

"It is almost that time of night," she said, "when it feels like everything will be known."

But not in the sexual sense, she thought to herself. She thought it not with a feeling of disappointment, but one of fascination.

"Do you *really* think, Rabbit, that everything in the world is material – that there is nothing more than the physics of the world, that all we feel is merely chemical?"

She thought about his question for a moment. One of the wonderful things about conversations with Wolf, she thought, was that she never had to think about what he *wanted* to hear. He wasn't needy that way, and he wasn't interested in pat answers.

She ate a little of the sandwich and noticed how he had managed once again to find the right kind of cheese for the tomatoes life had happened to give him that day.

"I mean, do you *really* think, Rabbit, that everything in the world is merely material – that there is nothing more to us than our flesh?"

The flow of the birds was starting to create lines of descent into the chimney.

"I don't think I told you, Wolf, that Dr. Wilhelm had painted on the ceiling of his home library a reference to an old medieval idea, about the human person being the microcosm to the macrocosm of the universe," she said. "It captured this idea that everything in the person had a corresponding element in the universe."

"Why are you telling me this now, Rabbit?"

"Because I think what Philadelphia taught me is the enormity of the universe contained within the individual human. How there is so much that can be within one – how there can be almost anything?"

He waited for her to go on and, after a moment, she did.

"Do I think everything is material? I do not believe there is any 'me' that is not part of my anatomy," she said. "I may have permeable boundaries that let in light and odor and even fluid. I *do* have such permeable boundaries. But I am still a self-contained material object."

Again, he did not reply. She pointed her finger to the chimney to make sure he was watching there.

"Here is what I think now, since Philadelphia, Wolf: That within this anatomy, within this sac of cells and fluid that is me, *within that* can be experienced the entire universe, if my life is lived correctly."

"That certainly sounds like a *spiritual* sensation, Rabbit," he answered with a tone of interest rather than criticism.

She noticed now how, as the birds dropped rapidly, so did the light, so did the temperature of the air. Night was descent; day ascent. Life on earth was a bird?

"It's so funny, Wolf," she said, "that everything that to *you* feels exquisitely spiritual feels to *me* exquisitely primal. Everything that to you feels *transcendent* feels to me – *transcendently phylogenetic*."

"Meaning?"

"The enormity I feel, when I feel the enormity, it represents the culmination of our species' journey through time and space. What feels to you like it goes all the way up to heaven feels to me like it goes all the way back in time! That's it!"

"History," he said.

"Biologic history," she answered. "And don't take this the wrong way – sometimes when you ask me something and you confuse me, I think the truth is that you and I think all the same things, we have the same worldview, we just stick them in different frames."

"I think you may be right, Rabbit. Mine may require a priest. But we are both interested in doing the right thing – we are both interested in trying to understand the right thing."

She pointed again at the chimney. He put the thermos on the ground, inched his chair closer to hers, and took her hand in his. The heat of his palm met the cold of hers. She focused on the sensation for a moment and obtained exactly the feeling she was looking for in her chest – the feeling of a boat's anchor touching the sea floor.

"Do you think justice will be brought to Dr. Wilhelm and The Jerk?" she asked.

"You know I will do what I can," he said.

"I hate having to rely on the fucking patriarchy to get it right," she sighed, and he did not laugh, for he knew she was not joking.

"Do you not have faith in me, Rabbit?"

"Oh, Wolf," she said, squeezing his hand but keeping her gaze focused on the birds. They were now falling into the chimney faster and faster, like water running down a slide. She wondered if the swifts felt in that chimney the way she had felt in his house all those times late at night, on a work break, when he made her something to eat, and put on some music, and gave her something to drink. "Oh, Wolf, I have such *enormous* faith in you."

He rubbed the back of her hand with his thumb.

"Wolf, I have so much *faith for you* that I don't honestly care how much trouble I have been to you. The faith I feel for you removes what guilt I have for all the trouble I have been."

He must have understood, she thought, her prepositional choice.

"Rabbit!" he replied in such a fashion that he caused Hunter to come rushing to his knee. "Rabbit, you have been *no trouble at all.* You have never for a moment been of trouble to me."

She was glad it was dark now. He could not see the tears on her cheeks.

"Rabbit, just as you have felt faith for me," he said, "it has been my great good fortune to have had you be the subject of so much of my charity. I feel in me a desire to be in a charitable state with you forever more, and for that, I feel so very grateful to you."

She closed her eyes, imagined for just a moment what his face must feel like, and then opened her eyes again.

And the birds spun down and in, and the stars came out.

The End.

Maddy Shanks will return
in *Book Two: The Difficult Subject*

THE
DIFFICULT
SUBJECT

Book Two of
the MADDY SHANKS *Mystery Series*

-1-

Madelaine Shanks arrived Minneapolis with the singular goal of becoming a complete nobody again. The nondescript commercial district abutting the University of Minnesota's east-bank campus where her office would be felt like the perfect setting for her plan. A big-chain drug store; a Vietnamese lunch place; a coffee shop; an all-purpose commuter shop selling umbrellas, messenger bags, notebooks, and the kinds of birthday cards you grab at the last minute. Perfect. Aside from the fact that the sidewalks along Washington Avenue were Midwestern-tidy and seemingly devoid of homeless people, in the late summer warmth of 2004, this scene felt like it could easily be almost anywhere in North America. Which meant Maddy could just be some academic nobody again, and not who she had lately become.

Looking up, she felt that the architecture of the university's medical complex would only help. With an utter lack of aesthetic imagination, it combined the most soulless, institutional styles of the last century, each new building section having been pasted to the last like chunky warts and benign tumors grown upon a hard concrete face. The tallest bit, Moos Tower, looked to Maddy as if it had been designed by an unimaginative undergraduate taking a mechanical drawing class; she pictured an angsty fellow who had understood his grade to depend on how many right angles he could work in. The ill-shaped structure loomed above the complex, covered in a drab pebble facing that seemed to grab ahold the soot of passing delivery trucks. At the ground level, a steady stream of people entered and exited the various doorways carrying backpacks, briefcases, and lunch sacks, looking like they had been handpicked by a stock-image photographer to represent Any Man and Any Woman going and coming to work, earnestly, wearily, thoughtlessly.

She tightened the cinch of her straw sunhat under her chin a little more to keep it from blowing off in the updrafts caught between the buildings.

Yes. She could do this. She could be just another young, underpaid instructor with a Ph.D. — just another short-term humanities hire with little job security and no fashion sense, working in a grinding state-university machine.

Of course, this plan would require avoiding reporters. And upon arrival, Maddy had been disappointed to discover her office would not be in a secured section of the complex. This left the possibility that a journalist could show up at her fifth-floor closet of an office and catch her off-guard.

But the solution to that was simple: avoid her assigned office and work instead in the nearby History of Medicine library. Since her unit's administrator had stuck her in the only empty office he could secure quickly — an eight-by-ten-foot closet of a room in a wing mostly occupied by neurology researchers — odds were good no one would notice if she did not frequent her official location. Productivity was what mattered, not sticking to one's assigned office. The neurologists weren't going to think twice if a visiting assistant professor in the history of medicine didn't show up very much. In fact, it would just match their stereotype of the lazy humanities prof.

The chief librarian of the history of medicine collection — a maternal, gregarious, corn-fed Minnesotan who sported a strawberry-blonde coif and a dip of meaty cleavage — told Maddy she'd be perfectly happy to give Maddy regular space to work in the small library's main reading room. The space wasn't big, but it was at least five times the size of Maddy's office, and the windows looked out across a series of flat commercial roofs right down to the thick, sliding serpent that was the Mississippi River. The furnishings felt humane: antique wooden tables; simple leather chairs; low, incandescent lighting. Not fancy, but not spartan.

"But of course you can work here, Professor Shanks! It's always a joy to have a real historian of anatomy in the house!" the librarian had cried out in answer to Maddy's request.

Unasked, the librarian also offered to provide space in the break room for Maddy to meet with her students if they came for her help and another patron wanted quiet in the library's central space. There was a linoleum-topped lunch table in the break room with a few chairs alongside a kitchenette.

Maddy had instinctively lied when she sought this kind of accommodation from the librarian, never mentioning the problem of reporters. She just said she found her tiny assigned office more than a little depressing, with a window facing a brick wall and tossed-off furnishings that looked like army-surplus, all of it too far from old books.

Well, that wasn't a complete lie.

"You prefer the company of the dead," the librarian had said to her with a wink.

"I like old books," Maddy had answered. "I guess I'm a typical historian that way."

"The dead are so much easier to deal with than the living," the librarian replied with a sing-song voice and a broad smile, as if Maddy had never answered.

"Eighteenth-century books smell so good, don't you think?" Maddy observed in return, picking up a circa-1750 midwifery manual from one of the display shelves and giving it a sniff as if it were a wildflower plucked in a field on an afternoon walk. That unique aromatic blend of dried book-mold and aged leather binding always made her feel calmer, more in her natural place. She breathed it in again and thought to herself that some chemist in some sparkling clean New Jersey corporate laboratory should concoct a perfume that matched this scent. "Thesis," it could be called, marketed in tiny bottles that looked like those of late-nineteenth-century opioid tinctures, with a tea-stained paper label. She would sprinkle it in her evening bath.

"Old books smell better than pickled bodies, I'm sure!" the librarian exclaimed. "But you would know better than I?"

Maddy forced a lip-closed smile, paused, and asked if the collection here included an original Vesalius De Humani Corporis Fabrica? (The best way to distract a history of medicine librarian, Maddy had long-since learned, was to ask to see her first-edition Vesalius.)

The librarian suddenly fluffed like a chicken disturbed by a farmer come to collect her eggs.

"I'll get the key to the vault!" she cried out. "You'll want to see our Harvey, too."

. . .

All this work of holding off people's curiosity – it was already exhausting, and it had only been a couple of days here so far. Maddy had imagined before arriving that she might manage to have a clean slate here. When she had called to tell her best friend Liz that the Minnesota job offer had come through, Maddy had even burst into tears in relief at the idea of a fresh start.

She had met Liz, a behavioral rat researcher, through a cross-departmental grad course on gender and science at Indiana University, where they had both been earning Ph.D.'s. On the call, Liz just waited until Maddy composed herself. Maddy knew well that Liz didn't much care for crying women, unless they were specifically crying on her shoulder – in which case, she found them irresistible.

"Freedom?" Liz had asked, when Maddy had stopped sniffling.

"Freedom," Maddy answered, blowing her nose. "I can move on, get out of Indiana, get back to work. Get on with the rest of my life."

"The trial will be going on."

"But that won't matter. That won't matter," Maddy said firmly again, as if trying to discipline the unruly dog that was the anxiety in her gut. "I'll get a couple of articles out, get an academic book contract in the works. The teaching load is light—two and two—and it'll position me well. It's just a two-year—so being on the market again no later than next year will be hard. But it's something."

"It is something," Liz agreed.

Liz thought about what it was going to be like without Maddy to share a six-mile run or a pitcher of cheap beer in the dull of Bloomington weekday evenings. Then she realized she should be sounding happier for Maddy.

"Seriously, congratulations! It's something! Something is what we all hope for. Something is what we aspire to when we go for a Ph.D. Something is what everyone wants to put on her c.v.!"

Liz paused, wondering if Maddy was annoyed with her joking.

"Would you like a couple of little young fellas to take with you to Minneapolis? They're not as good company as me, but they also eat a lot less than me."

"I can't, really," Maddy said, although she liked the idea of a pair of rats from Liz's line to hang out with during the lonely moments. Without the lab's principal investigator noticing, Liz had managed to breed one subgroup to be particularly smart and welcoming of human companionship. Liz had taught Maddy the visceral pleasure of a small, furry, sleeping creature on her belly, tucked under her shirt, when everything else felt like a shit-show. Liz wasn't supposed to take rats out of the lab, but she told Maddy that it wasn't as if anyone noticed or cared. The lab's research was behavioral, not of the biohazard sort.

"Why can't you, really?" Liz asked in a tone that suggested Maddy might be acting a bit snobbish regarding Liz's species preferences. "You know they'll keep each other company if you're busy. And you'll have some mammals to come home to. Warm, short-term mammals who like how you smell and who will be happy when you drop crumbs all over. That's the best kind of mammal to come home to, and you know it."

"The associate dean who offered me the job also offered to put me up in a small house he owns, and I can't bring rats to someone else's house."

"Oh?" asked Liz, her voice rising.

"Oh, come on, Liz," Maddy answered. "It's not like that. It's an empty house. Well, I mean it has furniture. Probably grownup furniture, not grad-school furniture. More something! I just have to pay the utilities. It'll save me a fortune, especially compared to what a whole nice house would cost to rent. And I'll be living alone. You can come visit. You can drive and bring my palm tree since I won't be able to ship it or fly it there with me."

"It's not a setup?" Liz asked.

Maddy didn't answer.

"He installs you in a tenuous position and in his house at the same time, Maddy?"

Liz's voice had that low timbre it took on when she felt that combination of annoyance and vigilance about her friends.

"He knew I'm coming on short notice to take over for Alex Shugar. So, he offered me what had been her house since it's sitting unused anyway. He says it's a nice small house in a quiet spot in the Lake Minnetonka area, twenty-five or thirty minutes west from school. If there's no traffic. If there's traffic, more."

"That's kind of far. You're going to waste a lot of work time getting there and back. And is that how you say her name? SHUG-er?"

"Yeah, apparently they used to say, 'Shugar, rhymes with slugger,'" Maddy answered. "I guess that made it easy to remember. Alex Shugar was a bit of a slugger by all accounts. Anyway, he has her house because he inherited it. She was his wife. Well, his ex-wife."

"Oh," answered Liz. "Oh. And he hired her replacement....Hang on. How are you going to get from there to the university? Is he giving you a ride every day?" Liz asked.

"He's lending me her car," Maddy answered, sounding annoyed with Liz. She was in fact annoyed with herself. She hadn't thought about this all as a possible arranged entanglement. Why hadn't she? Desperation in terms of jobs? No other offer had come through. Of course, she had barely applied for positions, being afraid of being offered interviews by search committees only interested in meeting a fifteen-minute celebrity and having been assured by her dissertation director that she could stay in Indiana one more year – that the college would find a way to make it work if she needed one more year given everything that had happened. The dean didn't seem to mind the good publicity.

"Well," Liz said, "with all the money you're saving, what with being lent a house and a car of the ex-wife you're replacing, you can afford to install a couple of fresh deadbolts, to ward off any drunken late-night visits that might occur when this associate dean forgets where he lives now."

"Stop, Liz," Maddy pleaded. "Stop. Honestly, he a dorky academic, not a player. He's remarried. For fuck's sake, Liz, he's a sociologist. And it'll be great. Because you can come visit."

"There is a bar there in Minneapolis that I like," Liz answered. "Had a good time there during a genetics conference a couple of years ago."

"I was actually thinking you'd be visiting with me," Maddy replied, a little exasperated.

"Don't worry, Chicken Little. You can always bring another friend if we go out. You make friends easily enough."

To be continued ...

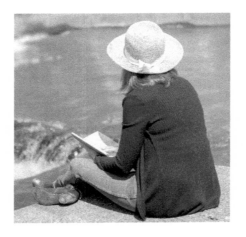

Molly Macallen is the author of the Maddy Shanks mystery series. Beginning with *The Index Case,* the series follows the life of Maddy Shanks, a young historian of anatomy, as she tries to figure out the truth behind a succession of suspicious deaths – while also dealing with the challenges posed by her own complex past and present.

Visit mollymacallen.com to learn more about the series.

Write to the author at molly@michigoose.com.

Lightning Source UK Ltd.
Milton Keynes UK
UKHW010112100223
416722UK00012B/871/J